The EVOLUTIONARY PLATE

FROM TASTE TO TRANSFORMATION

By

Yolanda Trevino

First Edition

Lightbody Publishing

www.lightbodypublishing.com

Published by Lightbody Publishing, LLC
PO Box 151, Lafayette, CA 94549
www.lightbodypublishing.com

First Edition: August 6, 2024

Hardback ISBN: 978-1-7371595-6-8

Dedication

To everyone embarking on a journey of transformation, seeking balance and well-being in their lives. This book is for you.
And to all who believe in the power of holistic wellness to heal and transform, may this guide serve as a beacon of hope and a source of lasting change.

In health and wellness,

Yolanda Trevino

Acknowledgments

Creating this book has been a journey filled with dedication and collaboration. I am particularly grateful to Safia Nijam, whose exceptional skills and hard work have transformed this manuscript into a beautifully formatted book. At a critical moment when my project needed immediate assistance, Safi stepped in and took on the challenge with unwavering dedication. His creative formatting and tireless effort, even working through the night, were instrumental in bringing this book to its final form. Thank you, Safi, for going above and beyond.

CONTENTS

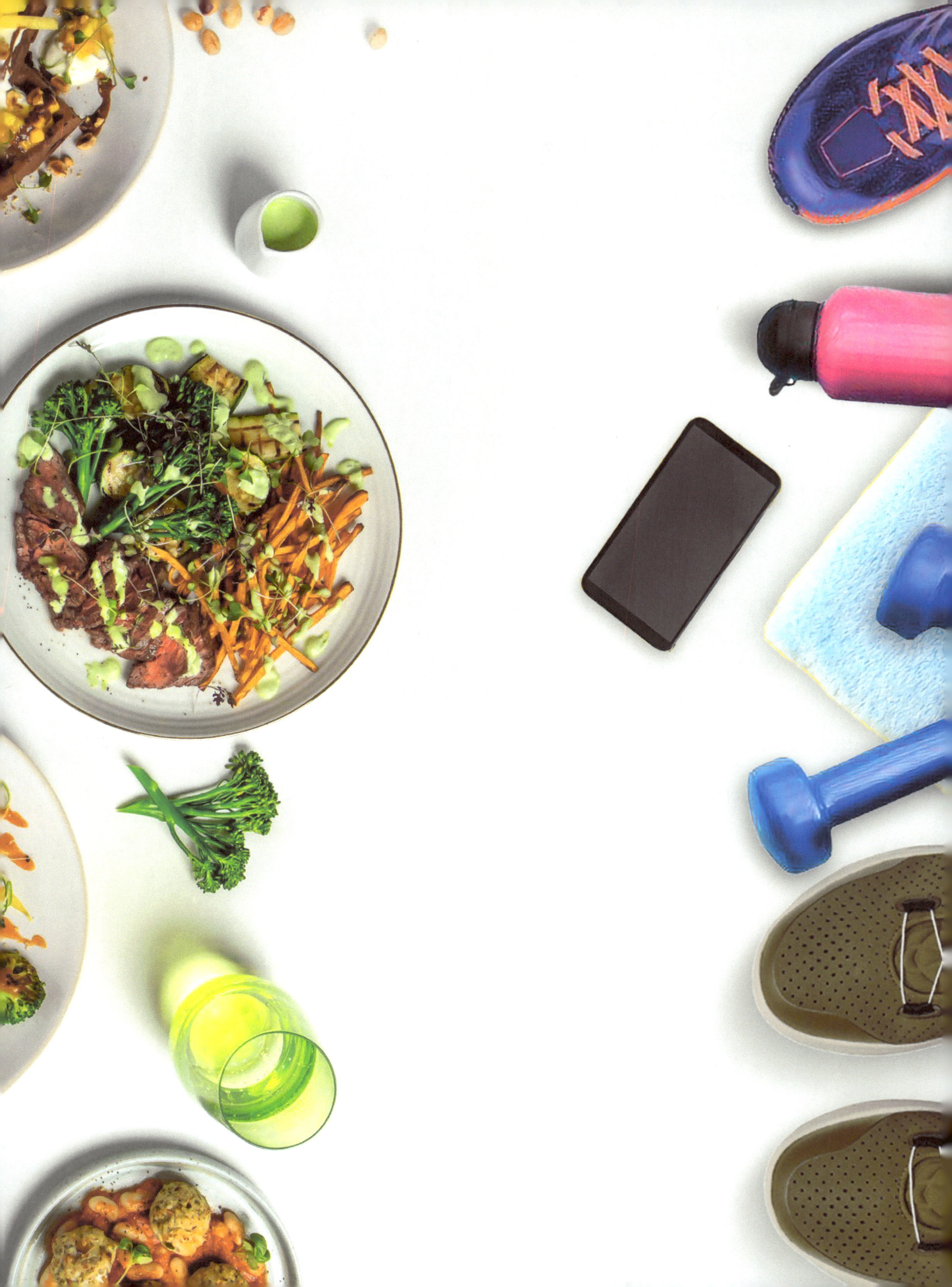

SECTION 1

INTRODUCTION

WELCOME Message

Dear Reader,

Welcome to "The Evolutionary Plate: From Taste to Transformation." I'm Yolanda Trevino, the founder of Evolutionary Body System, and I am thrilled to share this transformative journey with you. This guide is not just about recipes; it's about embracing a holistic approach to wellness that nourishes your body, mind, and spirit.

Throughout my life, I have faced many challenges, from significant weight loss to overcoming personal traumas. These experiences have taught me the importance of a balanced lifestyle that integrates nutrition, mindfulness, and physical activity.

Originally launched as a simple ebook with a meal plan and a modest collection of recipes on my website in 2023, this book has evolved into a comprehensive wellness guide packed with holistic health information. The entire book has undergone significant changes, including a new cover and a wealth of additional content such as over 50 recipes, special recipe collections, a comprehensive 4-week meal plan, personalized fitness plans, mindful eating practices, information on detoxification methods, insights into herbal supplements, a 21-day health goal smoothie challenge, a 4-week wellness transformation plan, and more. These enhancements provide valuable resources for maintaining health and wellness through all seasons.

This book is a culmination of my journey, offering practical insights and guidance to help you achieve your wellness goals. Thank you for joining me on this path to holistic health. Together, we will explore the practices and principles that lead to a vibrant and fulfilling life.

With warmth and gratitude,

Yolanda Trevino

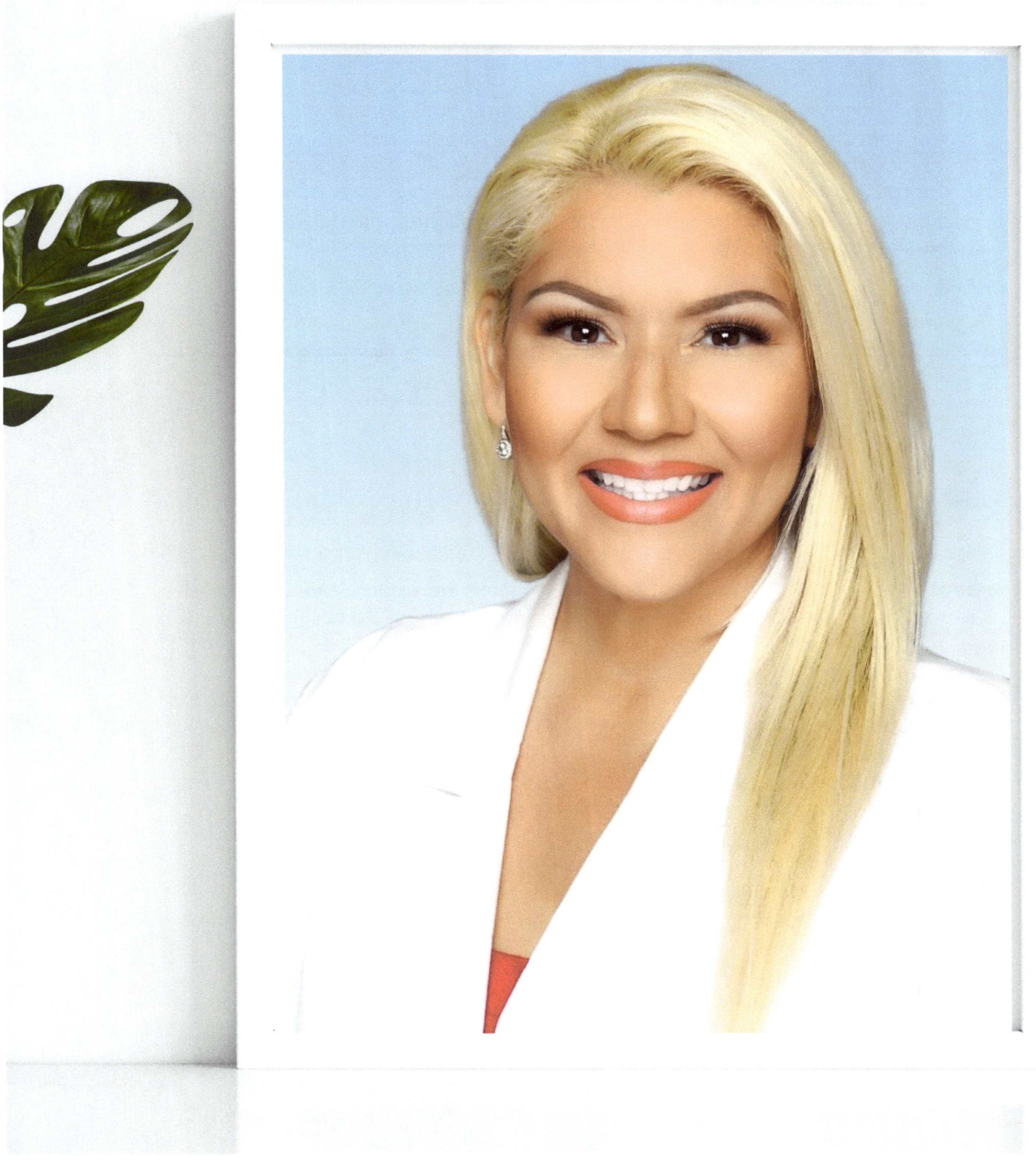

PURPOSE The Book

"The Evolutionary Plate: From Taste to Transformation" is designed to be your comprehensive guide to holistic wellness. This book simplifies your journey to balanced and sustainable health by providing you with practical advice on nutrition, mindful eating, personalized fitness plans, and holistic health practices. Whether you're looking to transform your life or simply incorporate healthier habits, this guide provides the resources you need.

BENEFITS OF The Book

Holistic Health Guidance
Learn about the importance of holistic wellness and explore comprehensive practices that integrate body, mind, and spirit for improved well-being.

Nourishing Recipes
Discover over 50 delicious and nutritious recipes inspired by Mediterranean and global cuisines.

Special Recipe Collections
Explore unique collections such as meat marinades, salad dressings, seasoning blends, smoothies, and wellness shots to enhance your culinary repertoire.

Comprehensive Meal Plans
Follow a 4-week meal plan complete with grocery lists to make healthy eating simple and stress-free.

Mindful Eating Practices
Gain insights into how to eat mindfully, enhancing your relationship with food.

Personalized Fitness and Nutrition Plans
Complement your nutrition journey with customized meals and dynamic workout plans tailored to your body type and wellness goals.

Sustainable Lifestyle
Embrace the 80/20 rule for balanced eating, allowing for indulgence while prioritizing nutritious choices.

Detoxification
Discover natural methods to effectively support your body's detox processes and improve your overall well-being.

Herbs and Supplements
Understand the benefits of common herbs and supplements, and how they can support your overall health.

Seasonal Wellness Tips
Get tips on how to maintain wellness throughout different seasons.

Self-Care Practices
Learn essential self-care practices like meditation, journaling, and gratitude to support your mental and emotional
well-being.

Interactive Elements
Discover video links to guided meditations, and quizzes to deepen your understanding and practice of holistic health.

Tracking and Progress
Utilize tools to track your workouts, meals, and overall progress towards your wellness goals.

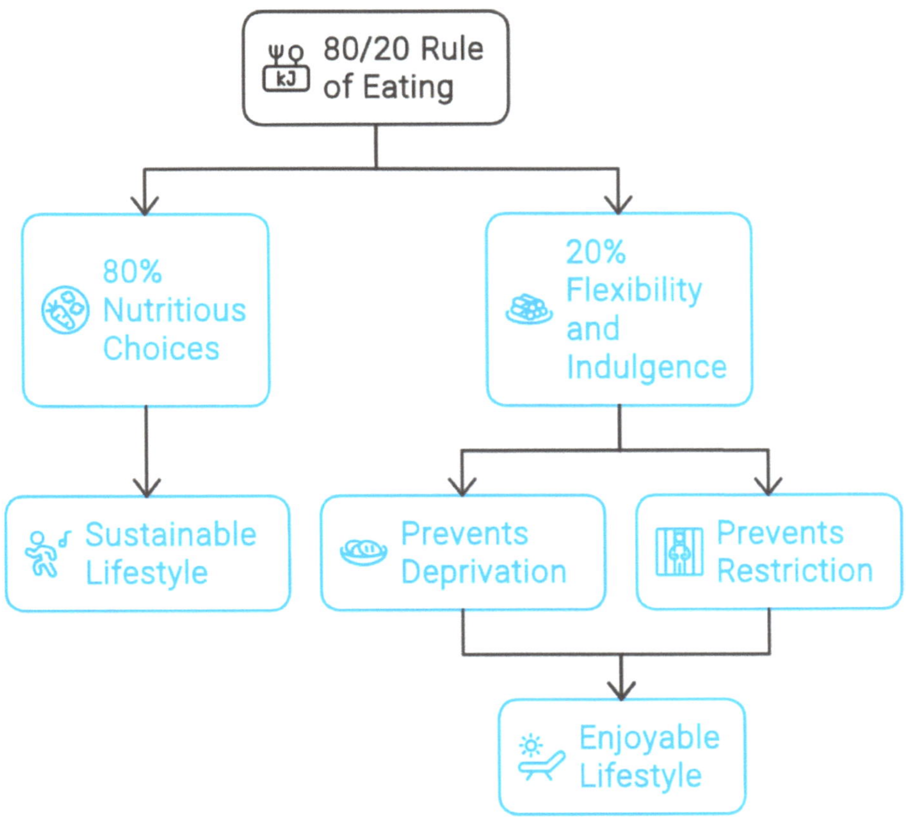

BRIEF SUMMARY OF Yolanda's Holistic Healing Journey

My journey to wellness began not just with a desire to lose weight, but with a need to reclaim my health and life. After years of struggling with my weight and facing various personal challenges, I decided to take a holistic approach to my health. This meant addressing not only my physical needs but also my mental and emotional well-being.

I started by transforming my diet, focusing on whole, nutritious foods that energized and healed my body. The recipes in this book are a reflection of this transformation, offering the flavors and nutrients that supported my journey. But nutrition was just one part of the equation. I incorporated mindful eating practices, personalized fitness routines, and holistic wellness strategies that helped me regain my vitality and balance.

Through these dedicated practices, my healing journey profoundly reshaped every part of my life. I didn't just recover – I thrived. It was a process of reclaiming my health, building relationships, and rediscovering my true self. Self-reflection and personal growth transformed challenges into opportunities and adversity into resilience. Today, I live a life filled with vitality, authenticity, and a deep belief in the power of personal healing.

This transformation was pivotal in rebuilding my life, resulting in losing 77 pounds. Through dedication and a holistic approach, I discovered the power of integrating body, mind, and spirit. I founded Evolutionary Body System to share these principles with others, offering comprehensive programs and tools designed to help individuals achieve their wellness goals and embrace a balanced, healthy lifestyle.

This book is a testament to the power of holistic healing. As you explore these pages, I hope you find the inspiration and tools you need to transform your health and your life.

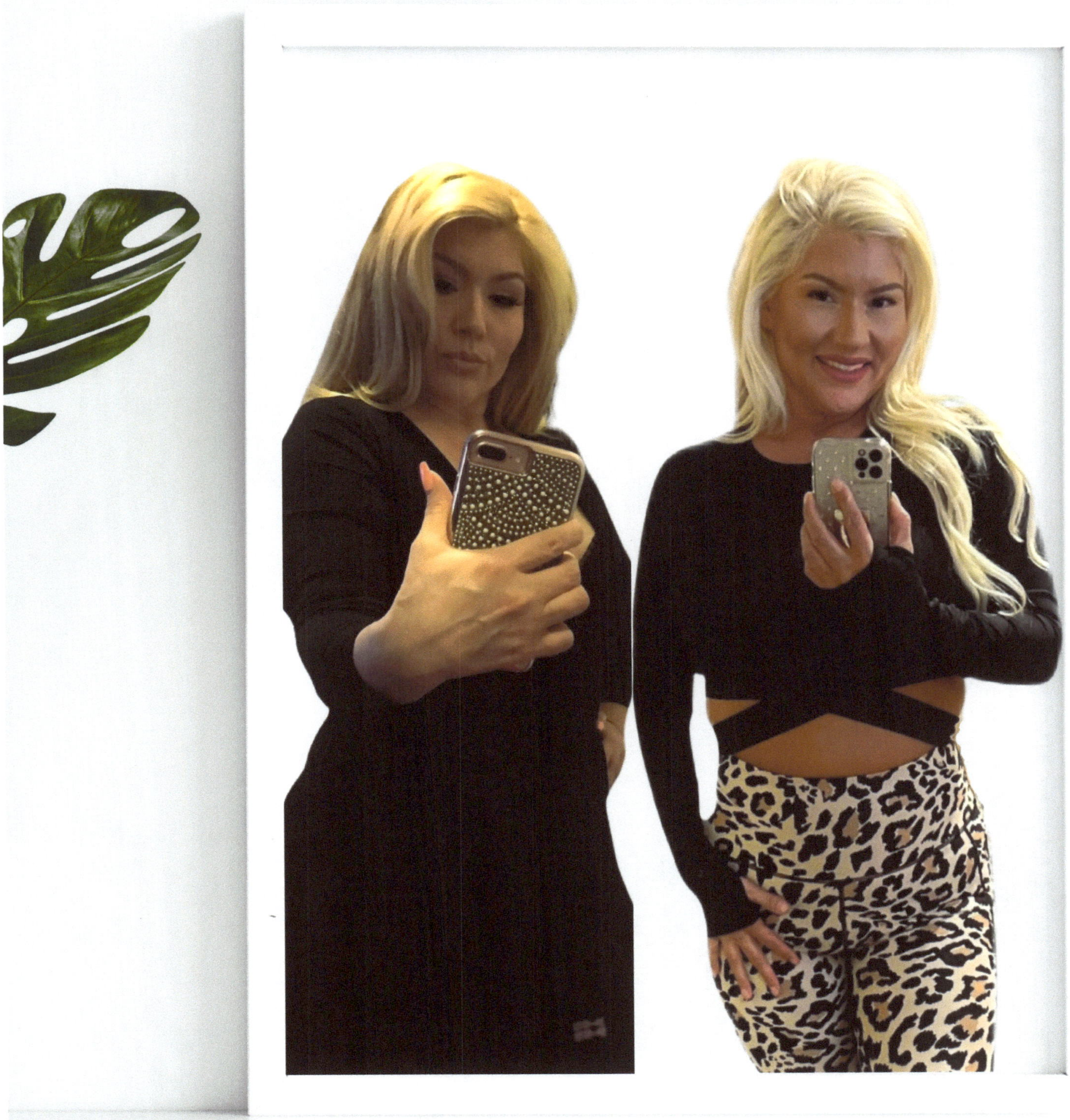

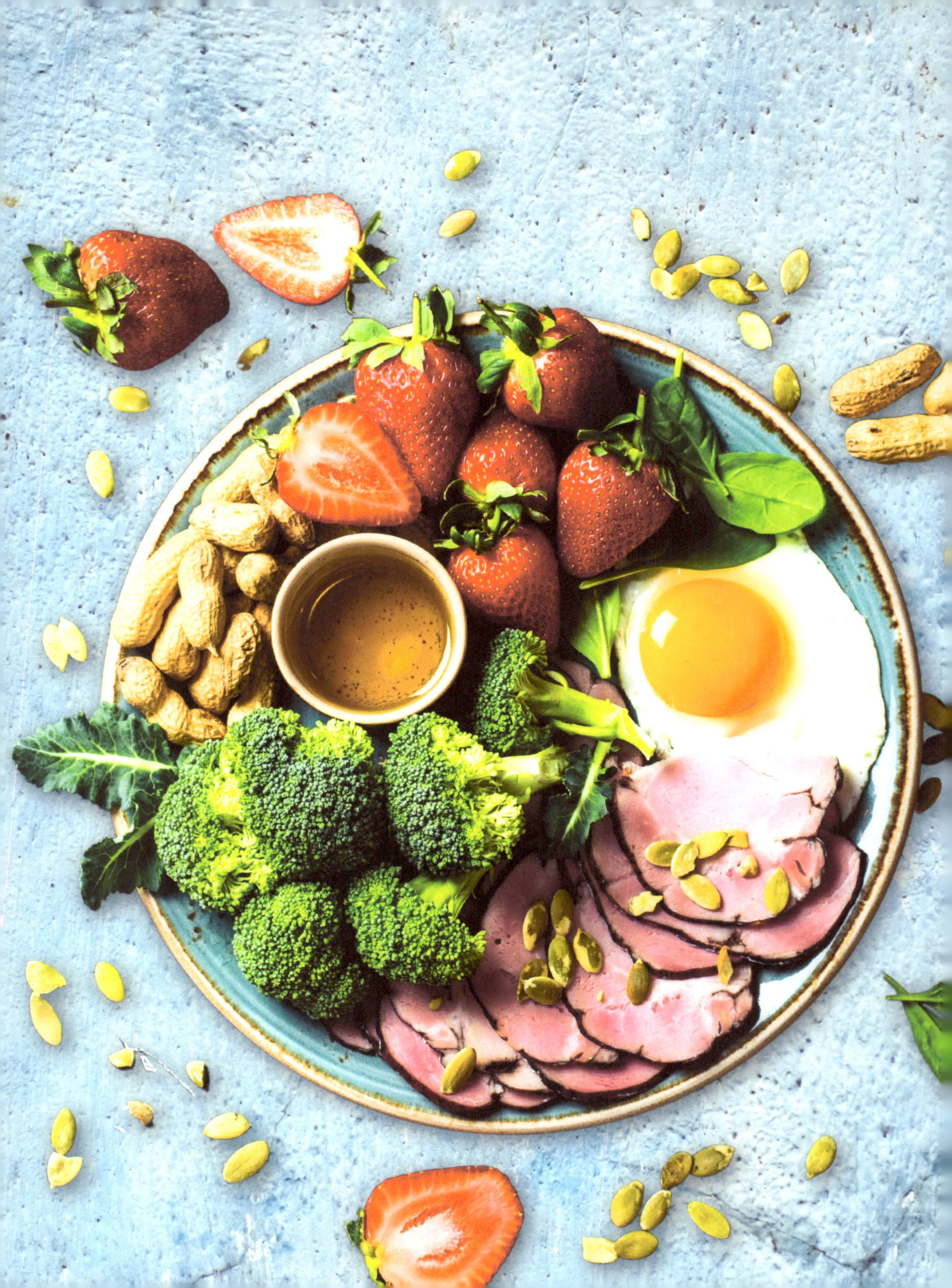

SECTION 2

THE EVOLUTIONARY Plate Philosophy

EXPLANATION OF HOLISTIC nutrition and wellness

Holistic nutrition is an approach to health that considers the whole person—body, mind, and spirit. It emphasizes the importance of eating whole, unprocessed foods that are rich in nutrients, while also recognizing the impact of lifestyle choices, mental well-being, and emotional health on overall wellness. This philosophy is about more than just what you eat; it's about how you live and the choices you make to nurture your entire being.

In "The Evolutionary Plate," we focus on:

Whole Foods: Emphasizing fresh, nutrient-dense foods such as fruits, vegetables, whole grains, lean proteins, and healthy fats.

Balanced Meals: Creating meals that provide a balance of macronutrients—carbohydrates, proteins, and fats—to support your body's needs.

Mindful Eating: Practicing mindfulness in your eating habits to enhance your relationship with food and recognize the signals your body sends you about hunger and fullness.

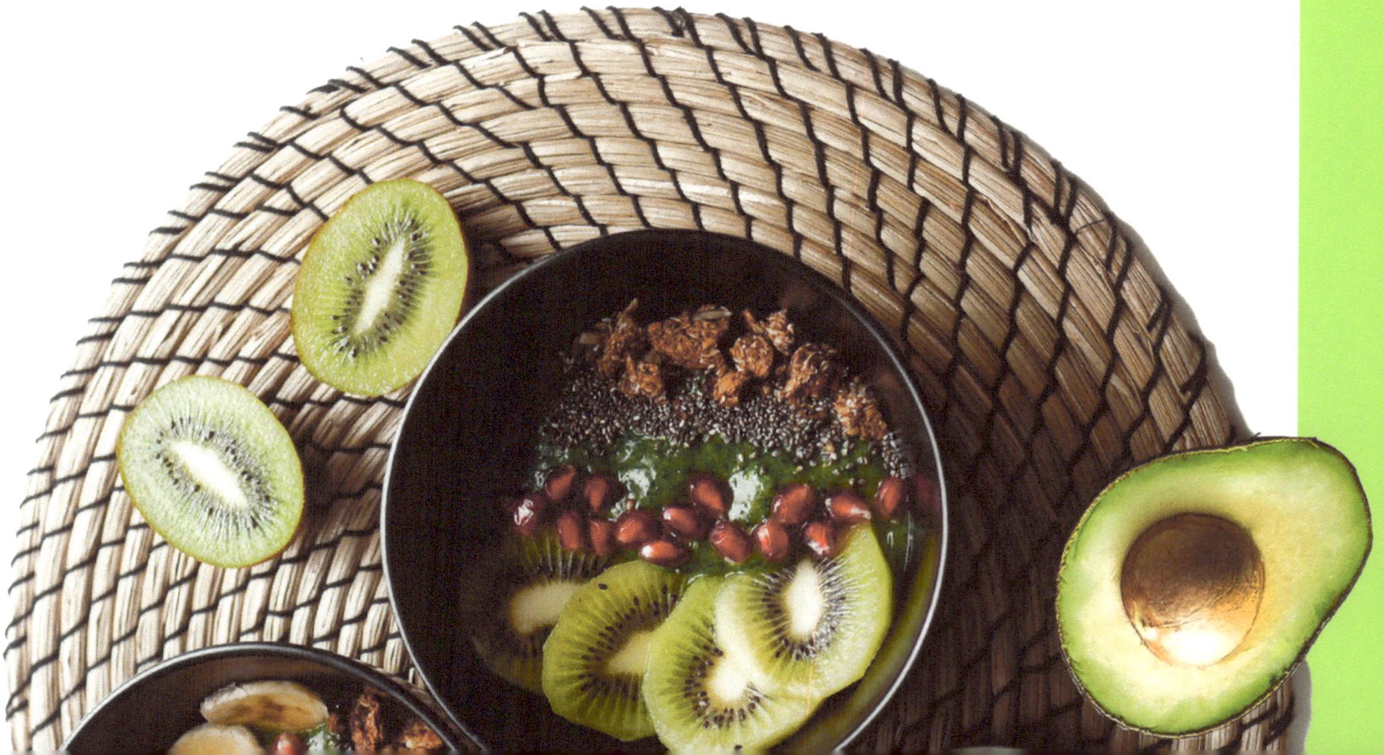

IMPORTANCE OF BALANCED Meals and the 80/20 Rule

Balanced meals are key for maintaining energy levels, supporting bodily functions, and promoting overall health. A well-balanced meal includes:

- *Proteins:* Essential for building and repairing tissues, and supporting immune function.
- *Carbohydrates:* The body's primary source of energy, especially important for brain function and physical activity.
- *Fats:* Necessary for absorbing vitamins, protecting organs, and maintaining cell membranes.
- *Fruits and Vegetables:* Provide essential vitamins, minerals, and fiber, which are vital for overall health and disease prevention.
- *Water:* Essential for hydration, digestion, and overall bodily functions.

The 80/20 rule is a practical approach to balanced eating, where 80% of your food choices are nutritious and beneficial to your health, and 20% allow for flexibility and indulgence. This rule helps maintain a sustainable and enjoyable lifestyle without feeling deprived or restricted.

A TASTE OF MEDITERRANEAN and Global Flavors

The Mediterranean diet is renowned for its numerous health benefits, including reduced risks of heart disease, diabetes, and certain cancers. It emphasizes:

- *Fresh Vegetables and Fruits:* These provide essential vitamins, minerals, and antioxidants that protect against various diseases and promote overall health.
- *Whole Grains:* Such as quinoa, barley, and brown rice, which are rich in fiber and nutrients, helping to maintain steady blood sugar levels and improve digestive health.

- *Healthy Fats:* Found in olive oil, nuts, and seeds, these fats support heart health by reducing bad cholesterol levels and provide anti-inflammatory benefits.
- *Lean Proteins:* Including fish, poultry, beans, and legumes, these sources of protein offer essential amino acids and nutrients necessary for muscle repair and growth.

HEALTH BENEFITS OF THE Mediterranean Diet

- **Improved Heart Health:** The Mediterranean diet is celebrated for its heart-protective effects. Healthy fats from olive oil, nuts, and fish help reduce bad cholesterol (LDL) levels while increasing good cholesterol (HDL). This combination lowers the risk of heart disease and stroke.
- **Better Weight Management:** The diet's emphasis on whole foods, lean proteins, and high fiber content helps promote satiety and prevent overeating. This focus aids in maintaining a healthy weight and supports long-term weight management.
- **Reduced Risk of Chronic Diseases:** Regular consumption of antioxidants from fruits and vegetables lowers the risk of developing certain cancers and diabetes. The diet's anti-inflammatory properties also help prevent chronic diseases.
- **Improved Insulin Sensitivity:** Whole grains, legumes, and fiber-rich foods in the Mediterranean diet help stabilize blood sugar levels and improve insulin sensitivity, which is essential for preventing and managing type 2 diabetes.
- **Reduced Inflammation:** Anti-inflammatory foods like olive oil, nuts, and fatty fish help reduce inflammation in the body, which is linked to various chronic conditions, including arthritis and cardiovascular disease.
- **Lower Cortisol Levels:** Nutrient-dense foods and a balanced diet can help regulate cortisol levels, reducing stress and improving overall well-being.

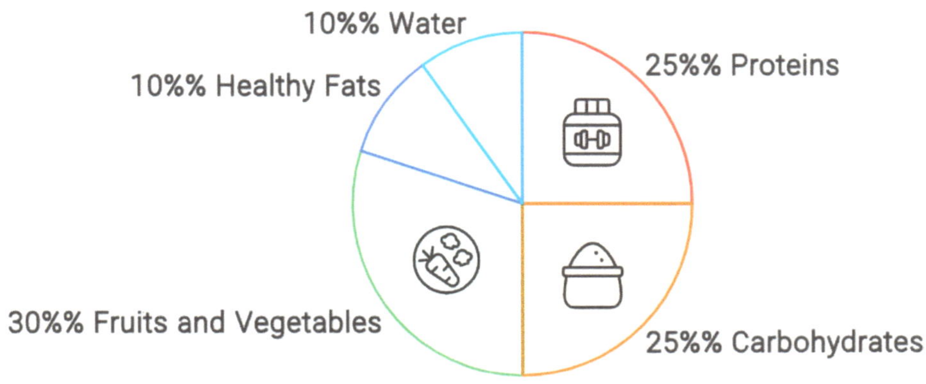

Key Components of a Balanced Meal

GLOBAL FLAVORS FOR a Diverse Palate

In addition to Mediterranean flavors, "The Evolutionary Plate" incorporates diverse global cuisines to add variety and excitement to your meals. Exploring different culinary traditions not only broadens your palate but also introduces you to a wide range of nutrients and health benefits. By embracing a variety of global flavors, you can enjoy delicious meals while reaping the health benefits of a diverse and balanced diet.

"Wellness Insights: *Did You Know?*"

- ***Did you know...*** that the colors of fruits and vegetables are linked to specific health benefits? For example, red foods like tomatoes support heart health, while green vegetables like spinach boost bone health.
- ***Did you know...*** that adding lemon juice to your water can aid digestion and help detoxify your liver?

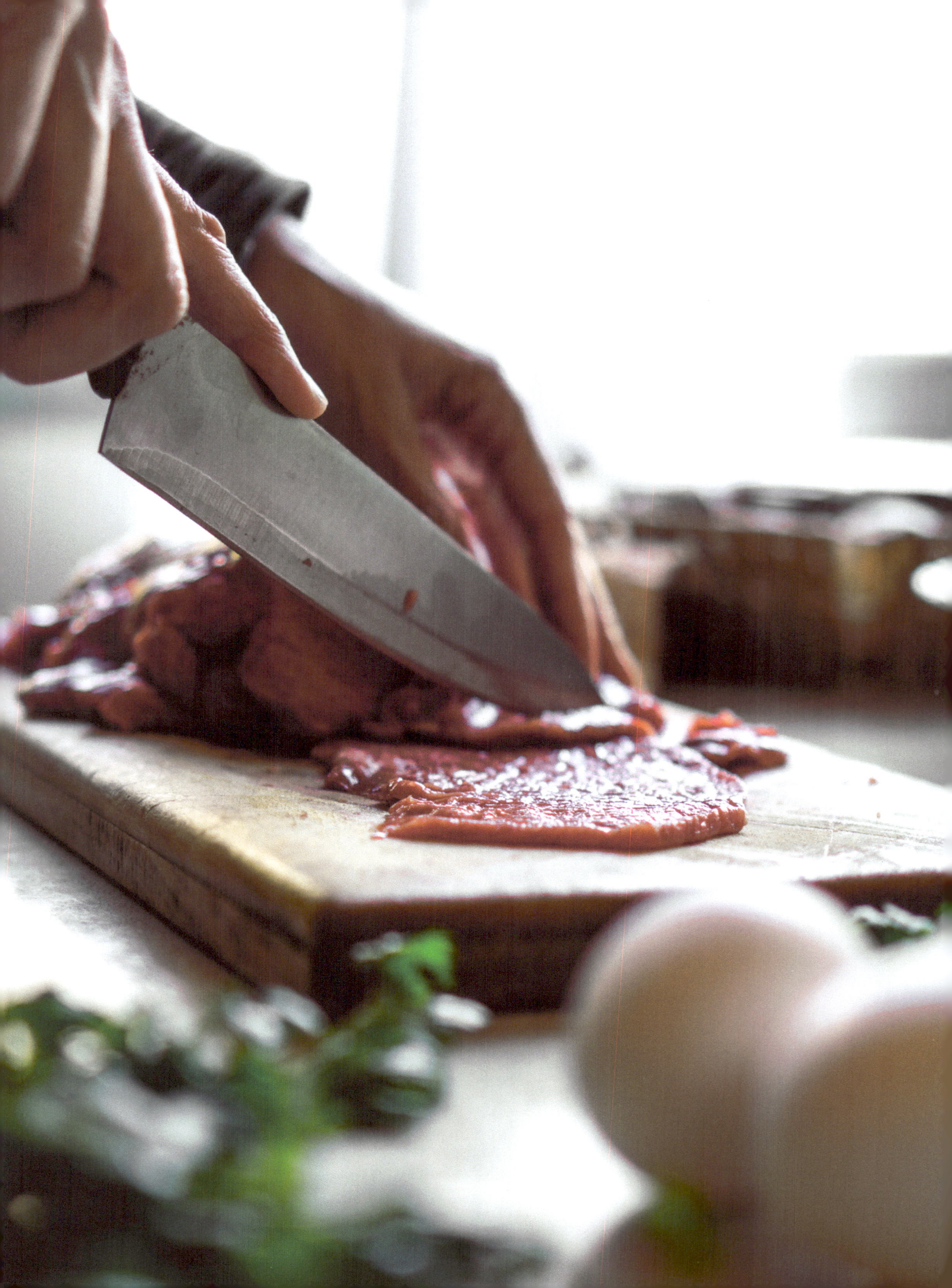

EVOLUTIONARY

SECTION 3

MEAL PLANNING and Preparation

FOUNDATIONS FOR Success

Welcome to the Meal Planning and Preparation section of "The Evolutionary Plate: From Taste to Transformation." This section will guide you through a comprehensive 4-week meal plan that emphasizes nutritious and delicious meals, tailored to support your holistic wellness journey.

HOW IT Works:

Foundation for Nutrition

The 4-week meal plan offers a variety of recipes and meals designed to ensure you receive a wide range of vitamins, minerals, and macronutrients. All recipes in this guide are under 500 calories per serving, ensuring they are both nutritious and suitable for a healthy lifestyle. It is structured to help you transition smoothly into healthier eating habits by eliminating guesswork and making it easier to stick to a nutritious diet. This plan serves as a foundational blueprint that anyone can follow to maintain a healthy diet and establishes the groundwork for a more tailored approach provided in the customized meal plans later in this book.

Convenience and Efficiency

Most of the recipes in this book are designed for 2 servings and are quick and easy, taking 30 minutes or less to prepare. This approach allows for convenience in having leftovers for the next day, easily expanding to accommodate a larger number of people, or making meal prep straightforward and efficient.

Enhancing Variety and Nutrition

You can swap any of the grains in the recipes with alternatives like quinoa, barley, or cauliflower rice. These substitutions offer a variety of flavors and nutritional benefits, such as added fiber, vitamins, and minerals. Similarly, you can substitute any meats, including beef, pork, poultry, or seafood, with your preferred options. Don't shy away from trying new ingredients and flavors; cooking is an act of self-love and self-care, helping you prioritize your wellness and set an example for others to do the same.

Einkorn: The Superior Grain

In this book, you'll notice that I've chosen Einkorn as the primary flour. Einkorn is an ancient grain that has remained largely unchanged for thousands of years. Unlike modern wheat, which has been heavily modified, Einkorn retains its original genetic structure. It contains more protein, essential fatty acids, phosphorus, potassium, and vitamins B6 and B12. The simpler gluten structure in Einkorn can be easier for those with gluten sensitivities to digest. By choosing Einkorn, you're opting for a grain that supports your health without sacrificing taste or texture.

Choosing high-quality, unprocessed grains like Einkorn provides essential nutrients and energy without the negative effects associated with heavily processed carbs. However, those with conditions like celiac disease or other gluten-related disorders should still avoid all forms of gluten. For most people, incorporating Einkorn into your diet supports a sustainable and balanced lifestyle, allowing you to enjoy bread and other baked goods in a healthier way.

The 80/20 Rule

Integrating the 80/20 rule into your eating habits can make maintaining a healthy diet more manageable and enjoyable. The idea is simple: eat nutritious, whole foods 80% of the time, and allow yourself to enjoy less nutritious treats the other 20% of the time. This balanced approach helps you stay on track without feeling deprived, making it easier to stick with healthy eating long-term.

This approach supports natural weight loss by allowing for flexibility and reducing the psychological stress associated with strict dieting. When combined with organic, non-GMO foods, the 80/20 rule ensures that most of your diet consists of nutrient-dense, high-quality foods. This leads to better digestion, more energy, and improved overall health. Organic foods, free from harmful chemicals and additives, further enhance the benefits of this balanced approach, helping to reduce inflammation and support a healthy metabolism.
By focusing on whole, unprocessed foods for the majority of your meals, you provide your body with the essential nutrients it needs to function optimally. The occasional indulgence, making up the remaining 20%, allows you to enjoy your favorite treats without guilt, promoting a sustainable and enjoyable way of eating. This not only promotes a healthier relationship with food but also encourages long-term adherence to a balanced diet, ultimately leading to sustained weight management and overall wellness.

Adjusting the Meal Plan for Your Body Type

Each individual has unique nutritional needs, and adjusting your meal plan to suit your body type can help you achieve optimal health and wellness. While the 80/20 rule provides a balanced approach to eating, tailoring your meals further can enhance your results. Here are a few tips on how to adjust the meal plan for different body types:

1. *Ectomorphs (Lean and Long)*
   - Focus on increasing healthy carbohydrates and proteins to support muscle growth and energy levels.
   - Include nutrient-dense foods like sweet potatoes, quinoa, and legumes.
   - Eat more frequently throughout the day to maintain energy levels.

2. *Mesomorphs (Muscular and Well-Built)*
   - Balance your intake of carbohydrates, proteins, and fats to maintain muscle mass and overall health.
   - Include lean proteins like chicken, fish, and tofu, and complex carbs like brown rice and whole grains.
   - Monitor portion sizes to avoid overeating.

3. *Endomorphs (Higher Body Fat)*
    - Focus on reducing carbohydrate intake and increasing protein and healthy fats to support weight loss and muscle maintenance.
    - Incorporate plenty of vegetables, lean proteins, and healthy fats like avocados and nuts.
    - Avoid processed foods and sugars to help manage weight.

You can learn more about identifying your body type and specific dietary recommendations in the later sections of this book.

Importance of Organic and Non-GMO Foods

Purchasing organic produce, pasture-raised meats, grass-fed products, non-GMO foods, and wild-caught fish is important for your health. Many foods today appear healthy but contain hidden health risks due to chemicals like glyphosate. Glyphosate, a common herbicide, has been linked to various health disorders, including cancer, hormonal disruptions, and digestive issues. Choosing organic options helps avoid these harmful chemicals.

Wild-caught fish are another important aspect of healthy eating. Farmed fish often contain higher levels of contaminants, antibiotics, and lower levels of beneficial nutrients like omega-3 fatty acids. Wild-caught fish, such as salmon, cod, and tuna, provide superior nutritional benefits and are free from harmful additives.

Organic foods offer superior taste and nutrient density. Berries are sweeter, fruits are naturally flavorful, and greens have distinctive tastes. Herbs and spices are more potent in flavor when they are organic. Over time, you will notice and feel the difference, as real nutrients improve your energy, balance hormones, and clear brain fog, allowing you to live a more vibrant and engaged life.

In the long run, opting for premium, healthy foods such as organic produce, other minimally processed organic items, pasture-raised, grass-fed, and wild-caught protein options is financially beneficial. While the initial cost may be higher, these foods provide superior nutrients and keep you more satiated, reducing the need for excessive food consumption. This leads to better overall health, fewer medical expenses, and an enhanced sense of well-being.

Hydration and Water Quality

Staying hydrated every day is essential for maintaining overall health and well-being, especially when following a structured meal plan. Clean water is important, so I recommend using a high-quality water filtration system to remove contaminants like heavy metals, parasites, bacteria, viruses, and harmful chemicals. Personally, I use the Berkey system because of its long-lasting filters and countertop convenience. This system has worked best for me, and while I have no affiliations with any brands throughout this book, I share these recommendations based on my own positive experiences.

Cooking as Self-Care

Cooking is not just about making meals; it nurtures your body and soul. By prioritizing your health through nutritious food and mindful eating, you create a foundation for overall wellness. Each recipe in this book has been carefully selected to provide a variety of nutritious and delicious meals. If you have specific dietary needs or health conditions, please consult with a healthcare professional to determine which recipes best fit your requirements. Many recipes focus on whole foods and balanced nutrition, but some may be higher in certain nutrients or ingredients. Please select recipes accordingly and consider portion sizes to maintain a balanced diet that suits your individual needs.

Meal Prep

Meal prepping involves preparing meals in advance to save time and ensure healthy eating throughout the week while streamlining your cooking process. The grocery lists may sometimes include larger quantities of certain items. These extra ingredients are intended to be saved for use in the following week's dishes or can be used for meal prep, helping you to reduce waste and make the most of your groceries.

For example, when baking bread as part of the meal plan, allow the loaf to cool completely before slicing it. Once sliced, you can freeze the pieces for later use. When you're ready to enjoy the bread, simply defrost the slices by toasting or warming them up. Proper meal prep not only saves time but also ensures you have healthy meals ready throughout the week. To learn more about effective meal prepping strategies and tips, refer to the upcoming section dedicated to Meal Prepping.

Benefits of Sea Salt

I've also suggested using sea salt in the recipes. Sea salt offers several benefits over regular table salt, including trace minerals like magnesium, calcium, and potassium, which act as electrolytes and help maintain proper fluid balance. Sea salt comes in different grinds, allowing you to choose the texture that best suits your needs or even grind your own if necessary. If you prefer, you can use Celtic sea salt for a higher concentration of these minerals and a slightly briny taste. Additionally, pink Himalayan salt, which contains similar trace minerals, can also be a good alternative. You can even add a pinch of either sea salt or Himalayan salt to your water to improve hydration by replenishing electrolytes.

Understanding Macronutrients and Micronutrients

Before diving into the meal plan, it's essential to understand the roles of macronutrients and micronutrients in your diet. Macronutrients, including carbohydrates, proteins, and fats, provide the energy and building blocks your body needs for various functions. Micronutrients, such as vitamins and minerals, are integral for supporting bodily functions, from immune health to bone strength. By incorporating a balance of these nutrients into your meals, you can ensure optimal health and well-being.

Macronutrients are the powerhouse nutrients that our bodies need in large amounts to function optimally. They include carbohydrates, proteins, and fats. These nutrients are fundamental to providing the energy we need for daily activities, supporting growth and repair, and maintaining overall health. Each macronutrient plays a unique and vital role in maintaining health, contributing to various bodily functions. By understanding the role of each macronutrient, we can make informed choices that contribute to a balanced and nutritious diet.

HOW MACRONUTRIENTS IMPACT HEALTH:

Carbohydrates

- Function: Provide energy, especially for the brain and muscles during exercise.
- Health Impact: Essential for energy but consuming too many simple carbs (like sugars) can lead to weight gain and blood sugar spikes. Complex carbs (like whole grains) are better for sustained energy and digestive health.

Proteins

- Function: Build and repair tissues, make enzymes and hormones, and support immune function.
- Health Impact: Essential for muscle repair and growth, and overall body maintenance. High-protein diets can aid in weight management by promoting satiety.

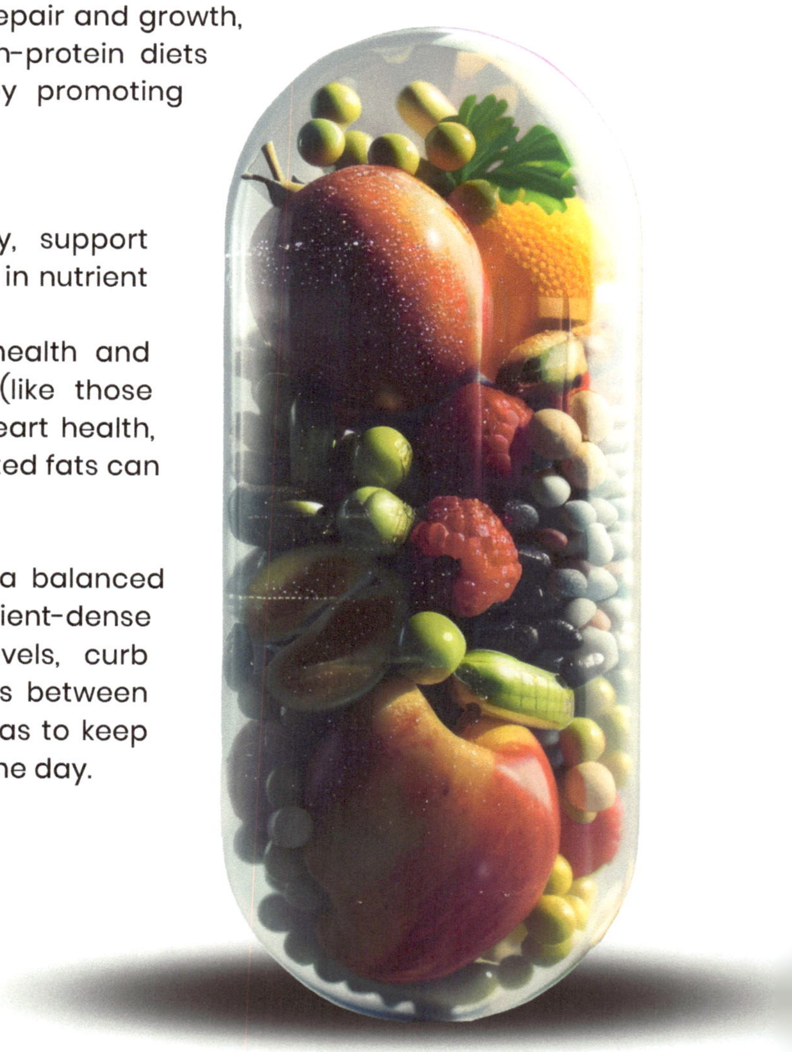

Fats

- Function: Provide long-term energy, support cell growth, protect organs, and help in nutrient absorption.
- Health Impact: Essential for brain health and hormone production. Healthy fats (like those from avocados and nuts) support heart health, while trans fats and excessive saturated fats can increase the risk of heart disease.

Snacking can be an important part of a balanced diet when done mindfully. Choosing nutrient-dense snacks can help maintain energy levels, curb cravings, and provide essential nutrients between meals. Here are some healthy snack ideas to keep you satisfied and nourished throughout the day.

HEALTHY Snacks

Fruits and Vegetables:
- Apple slices with peanut butter
- Carrot sticks with hummus
- Greek yogurt with fresh berries

Nuts and Seeds:
- A handful of almonds, walnuts, or sunflower seeds
- Trail mix with dried fruits and nuts

Whole Grains:
- Whole grain crackers with cheese
- Air-popped popcorn

Protein-Rich Snacks:
- Hard-boiled eggs
- Edamame
- Cottage cheese with pineapple

Smoothies:
- Blended fruits and vegetables with a scoop of protein powder or Greek yogurt

HIGH-PROTEIN Foods

Animal Sources:
- Chicken breast
- Turkey
- Lean cuts of beef or pork
- Fish (salmon, tuna, cod)
- Eggs
- Greek yogurt
- Cottage cheese

Plant Sources:
- Lentils
- Chickpeas
- Black beans
- Quinoa
- Tofu
- Tempeh
- Edamame
- Nuts and nut butters
- Seeds (chia, hemp, flax)

Incorporating these foods and snacks into your diet can help you maintain a balanced intake of macronutrients, supporting overall health and well-being.

MICRONUTRIENTS:

Micronutrients, although required in much smaller quantities than macronutrients, are no less critical to our health. These essential vitamins and minerals support a wide range of physiological functions, from immune support and bone health to energy production and cellular repair. Even though they don't provide energy like macronutrients, their role in maintaining overall health and preventing disease is indispensable. Learning about the different types of micronutrients and their benefits can help us ensure we're getting a well-rounded and nutrient-rich diet.

Types of Micronutrients Vitamins Fat-Soluble Vitamins: Stored in the body's fatty tissue and liver.

- Vitamin A: Important for vision, immune function, and skin health.
- Vitamin D: Essential for bone health and calcium absorption.
- Vitamin E: Acts as an antioxidant, protecting cells from damage.
- Vitamin K: Important for blood clotting and bone health.

Water-Soluble Vitamins: Not stored in the body and need to be consumed regularly.

- Vitamin C: Important for immune function, skin health, and antioxidant protection.
- B Vitamins: Include B1 (thiamine), B2 (riboflavin), B3 (niacin), B5 (pantothenic acid), B6 (pyridoxine), B7 (biotin), B9 (folate), and B12 (cobalamin). They are necessary for energy production, brain function, and cell metabolism.

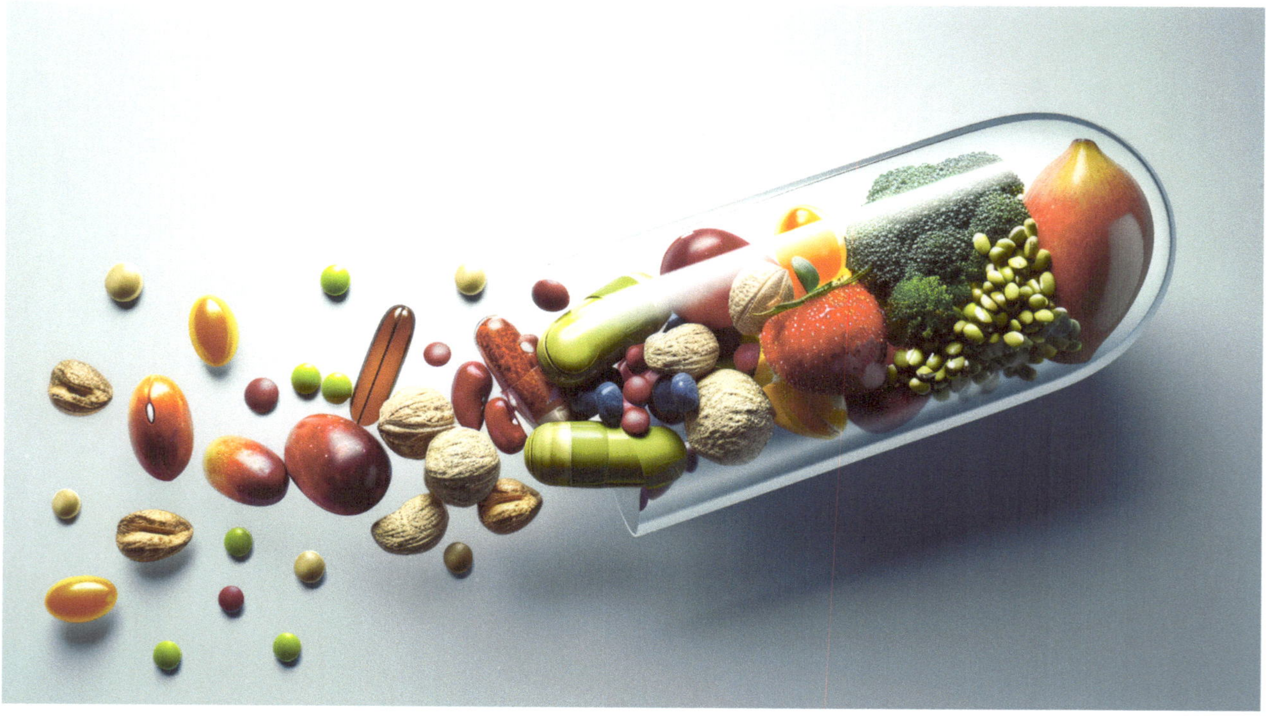

Minerals Macrominerals: Required in larger amounts.

- Calcium: Essential for bone health, muscle function, and nerve signaling.
- Phosphorus: Important for bone and teeth formation and energy metabolism.
- Magnesium: Involved in muscle and nerve function, blood sugar control, and bone health.

- Sodium: Important for fluid balance, nerve function, and muscle contraction.
- Potassium: Helps regulate fluid balance, muscle contractions, and nerve signals.
- Chloride: Maintains fluid balance and is part of stomach acid.

Trace Minerals: Required in smaller amounts.

- Iron: Essential for oxygen transport in the blood.
- Zinc: Important for immune function, wound healing, and DNA synthesis.
- Iodine: Necessary for thyroid hormone production.
- Selenium: Acts as an antioxidant and supports thyroid function.
- Copper, Manganese, Fluoride, Chromium, Molybdenum: Involved in various biochemical processes.

Meal Plan Instructions

After understanding the importance of macronutrients and micronutrients, it's time to put that knowledge into practice with your 4-week meal plan. Each week, you can alternate between the two options for breakfast, lunch, and dinner. For more variety, mix and match any of the breakfast options across the entire 4-week plan. This flexibility allows you to enjoy a wider range of meals while maintaining a balanced diet. Follow this meal plan for 5 days a week, and for the other 2 days, decide on whatever you'd like to eat, either from the recipes in the book or your own meal choices. The grocery lists provided cover the meal plan, but feel free to make other meal choices as well.

Final Thoughts

Incorporating this meal plan and the provided tips into your routine will help you take significant steps toward a healthier and more balanced lifestyle. Remember, cooking and eating well is an act of self-care that has far-reaching benefits for your overall well-being. Enjoy the process, try new things, and feel the positive changes in your life.

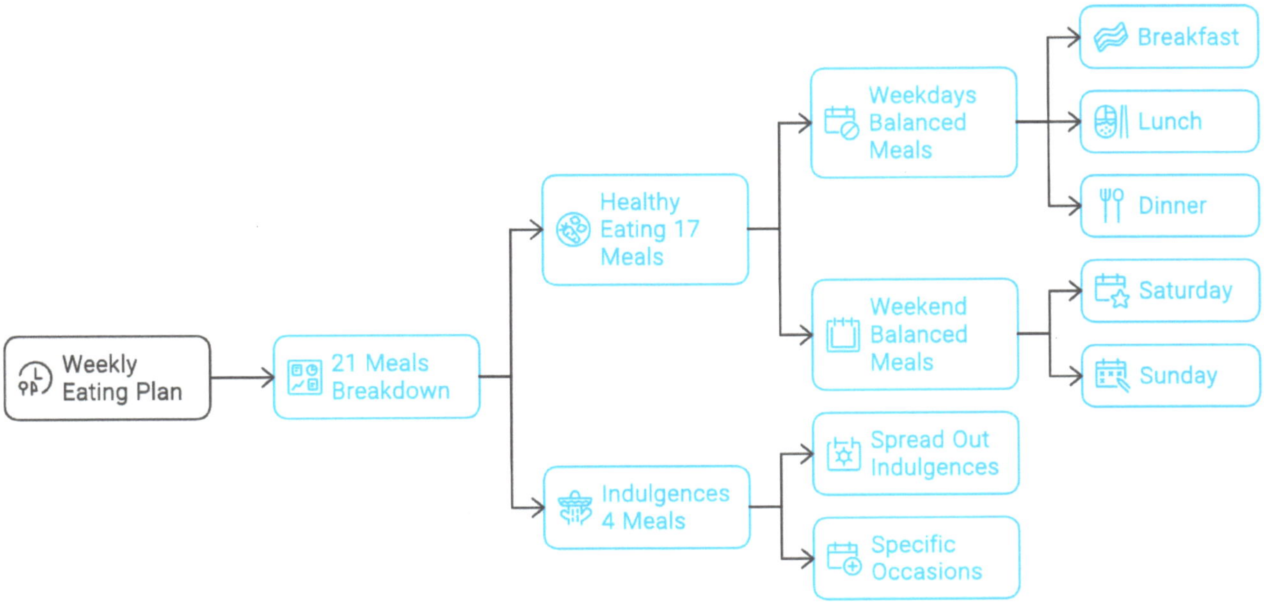

COMPREHENSIVE 4-WEEK Meal Plan

WEEK 1:

Breakfast:

- Blueberry Bliss Protein Smoothie
- Spinach and Veggie Egg Bites

Lunch:

- Mediterranean Orzo Pasta Salad
- Chipotle Chicken Salad Bowl

Dinner:

- Pan-Seared Salmon with Lemon Dill Sauce and Sautéed Asparagus
- Sweet and Spicy Crispy Pork Stir Fry with Rice Noodles

Snacks/Desserts:

- Homemade Organic Granola
- Dark Chocolate Cacao Cookies

WEEK 2:

Breakfast:

- High-Protein Sweet Banana Nut Overnight Oats
- Avocado Toast with Jammy Eggs

Lunch:

- Savory Lettuce Wraps with Peanut Sauce
- Quinoa Bowl with Roasted Eggplant and Hummus

Dinner:

- Shrimp Tacos with Creamy Citrus Sauce
- Baked Cod in Luscious Tomato Sauce

Snacks/Desserts:

- Strawberry Chia Yogurt Parfait
- Creamy Chocolate Protein Mousse with Cacao Powder

WEEK 3:

Breakfast:

- Bagels & Lox Protein Deluxe
- Peanut Butter & Jelly Toast

Lunch:

- Savory Chicken & Spinach Tortilla Wrap
- Greek Chicken Souvlaki Wraps with Tzatziki Sauce

Dinner:

- Mediterranean Salmon with Quinoa & Green Pea Purée
- Sensational Shakshuka

Snacks/Desserts:

- Granola Breakfast Bowl
- Blueberry Cobbler

WEEK 4:

Breakfast:

- Protein Packed Belgian Waffle
- Breakfast Tacos with Chorizo, Eggs, and Salsa

Lunch:

- Falafel Bowl with Zesty Tahini Dressing
- Hearty Cinnamon Spiced Sweet Potato Hash

Dinner:

- Grilled Salmon with Quinoa, Mango Salsa & Wilted Veggie Bed
- Golden Seafood and Chicken Paella

Snacks/Desserts:

- Raspberry Chia Yogurt Cups
- Protein-Rich Dreamy Hot Chocolate

"Wellness Insights: *Did You Know?*"

» ***Did you know...*** that using herbs like basil, oregano, and thyme in your cooking can provide antioxidant properties while enhancing the flavor of your dishes?

» ***Did you know...*** that creating a weekly meal plan can help you save money, reduce food waste and learn the habit of making more balanced and nutritious food choices?

GROCERY LISTS FOR EACH WEEK OF COMPREHENSIVE 4-Week Meal Plan

WEEK 1 GROCERY LIST

Protein:

- Eggs (1 dozen)
- Chicken breasts (2 boneless, skinless)
- Salmon fillets (2 fillets)
- Pork loin strips or pork belly (1 pound)
- Vanilla ice cream flavor protein powder (1 container)
- Feta cheese (1 package)

Produce:

- Wild Blueberries (1 package fresh or frozen)
- Spinach (1 bunch)
- Grape or cherry tomatoes (1 pint)
- Red bell peppers (2)
- Spring onions (green onions, 1 bunch)
- Yellow bell pepper (1)
- Romaine lettuce (1 head)
- Tomato (1)
- Fresh cilantro (1 bunch)
- Fresh limes (2)
- Fresh dill (1 bunch)
- Asparagus (1 bunch)
- Orange bell pepper (1)
- Garlic Bulb (1)
- White onion (1)
- Red chili peppers (2)
- Green chili peppers (2)
- Fresh basil (1 bunch, optional)

Dairy:

- Greek yogurt (8 oz.)
- Butter, Grass-fed (1 package)

Pantry Staples:

- Black beans (1 can)
- Corn kernels (1 can or equivalent fresh/frozen)
- Unsweetened applesauce (1 jar)
- Grapeseed oil (1 bottle)
- Unsweetened nut milk (1 carton)
- Einkorn flour (1 package)
- Orzo pasta (1 package, organic Montebello brand)
- White or brown rice (1 bag)
- Rice noodles (1 package)
- Rolled oats, Organic Non-GMO (1 container)
- Nuts, Organic (almonds, cashews, or walnuts, or a mix of all, 12 oz.)
- Seeds, Organic (pumpkin or sunflower seeds, 4 oz.)
- Baking soda (1 box)
- Brown sugar (1 box)
- Coconut oil (1 jar)
- Vanilla extract (1 bottle)
- Olive oil (1 bottle)
- Vegetable oil (1 bottle)
- Soy sauce (1 bottle)
- Oyster sauce (1 bottle)
- Honey (1 jar)
- Rice wine vinegar (1 bottle)
- Sesame oil (1 bottle)

Pantry Staples:

- Black beans (1 can)
- Corn kernels (1 can or equivalent fresh/frozen)
- Unsweetened applesauce (1 jar)
- Grapeseed oil (1 bottle)
- Unsweetened

Herbs, Spices, and Condiments:

- Sea Salt, Fine Ground - Substitute for regular salt; provides added minerals and health benefits (1 container)
- Black pepper (1 container)
- Chipotle chili powder (1 container)
- Ground cumin (1 container)
- Smoked paprika (1 container)

- Cayenne chili powder (1 container)
- Dried oregano (1 container)
- Ground cinnamon (1 container)
- Cacao powder (1 container)

WEEK 2 GROCERY LIST

Protein:

- Eggs (1 dozen)
- Ground chicken (1/2 pound, or substitute with pork, beef, turkey, or tofu)
- Shrimp (24 large, peeled and deveined)
- Cod fillets (2)

Produce:

- Bananas (2)
- Avocado (2)
- Pea shoots (1 package)
- Butter lettuce (1 head)
- Carrots (2)
- Button mushrooms (1 package)
- Fresh ginger (1 piece)
- Eggplant (1 small)
- Grape or Rainbow Cherry tomatoes (1 pint)
- Baby spinach leaves (1 bag)
- Red cabbage (1 head): Use leftovers if meal prepping; otherwise, save for next week.
- Limes (4)
- Onion, small (1)
- Fresh basil leaves (1 bunch)
- Lemon (1)
- Strawberries, fresh or frozen (32 oz)

Dairy:

- Cottage cheese (8 oz.)
- Greek yogurt (16 oz.)
- Unsweetened almond milk, Malk brand (1 carton, sold in refrigerator aisle)

Pantry Staples:

- Maple syrup, Grade A (1 jar)
- Organic cane sugar (1 bag)
- Baking powder (1 container)
- Natural organic peanut butter (1 jar)

- Tahini (1 jar)
- Tri-color quinoa (1 package)
- Chia seeds (1 bag)
- Canned chickpeas (2 cans, 15 ounces each)
- Apple cider vinegar (1 bottle)
- Mission Carb Balance Taco Size Soft Flour Tortillas (or use Almond Flour, Cassava Flour or White Corn) (1 package)
- Chicken stock (1 carton)

Herbs, Spices, and Condiments:

- Mayonnaise, avocado (1 small jar)
- Low-sodium soy sauce or tamari (1 bottle)
- Red pepper flakes (1 container)
- Dried basil (1 container)

Miscellaneous:

- Dark chocolate bar, small (for shavings, optional)

WEEK 3 GROCERY LIST

Protein:

- Boneless, skinless chicken breast (1)
- Smoked salmon (4 slices)
- Eggs (1 dozen)
- Salmon fillets (2, about 12 ounces total)
- Ground beef (1 pound)
- Ground lamb (1 pound)

Produce:

- Avocado (3)
- Spinach (2 bunches)
- Tomato (3)
- Garlic (2 bulbs)
- Fresh dill (1 bunch)
- Fresh mint (1 bunch)
- Fresh parsley (1 bunch)
- Fresh cilantro (1 bunch)
- Red onion (1)
- Lemon (4)
- Lime (1)
- Radishes (1 bunch)

- Red bell pepper (2)
- Green peas (1 cup fresh or frozen)
- Red cabbage (1 head)
- Spring mix lettuce greens (5 oz.)
- Romaine lettuce (1 head)
- Cucumber (2)
- Carrot (1)
- Asparagus (1 bunch)

Dairy

- Greek yogurt (1 quart)
- Cream cheese, whipped (1 container)
- Whipped cream (1 can, optional)

Pantry Staples

- Dijon mustard (1 bottle)
- Rice vinegar (1 bottle)
- Crushed tomatoes (14 oz. can)
- Black beans (1 can)
- Chickpeas (1 can)
- Spinach Tortillas (1 package)
- Naan bread, Stonefire Organic (1 package)
- Almond milk (1 carton)
-

Miscellaneous:

- Wooden skewers
- Pea shoots microgreens

Week 4 Grocery List:

Protein:

- Salmon fillets (4, about 6 ounces each)
- Mexican chorizo (4 oz, casing removed)
- Fresh falafel patties (8)
- Chicken breasts (2, boneless, skinless)
- Shrimp (1/2 lb., large, peeled and deveined)
- Squid (1/4 lb., cleaned and sliced)
- Mussels (1 lb., fresh, cleaned and debearded)

Produce:

- Avocado (3)
- Spinach (10 oz.)
- Tomato (4)
- Fresh dill (for optional garnish)
- Fresh mint (for optional garnish)
- Fresh parsley (for optional garnish)
- Red onion (1)
- Lemon (4)
- Red bell pepper (1)
- Green bell pepper (1)
- White onion (1)
- Jalapeño (1, medium)
- Cilantro (1 bunch)
- Lime (1)
- Mango (1 ripe)
- Heirloom grape tomatoes (1 pint)
- Spring mix greens (16 oz container)
- Sweet potatoes (2 medium)
- Broccolini (1 bunch)
- Zucchini, Green (1 medium)
- Asparagus (1 bunch)

Dairy:

- Greek yogurt (8 oz.)
- Feta cheese (1 container)

Pantry Staples:

- White corn tortillas (or use Almond Flour, Cassava Flour or Mission Carb Balance Taco Size Soft Flour)
- Arborio rice (16 oz. bag)
- Native Forest Organic Coconut Milk (no guar, BPA Free) – 1 can
- Ground turmeric (1 container)
- Chicken or vegetable broth, Kettle & Fire Organic Bone Broth (32 oz., low-sodium)

Miscellaneous:

- Peppermint extract (optional)

MEAL PREPPING TIPS and Strategies

Meal Prepping Tips:

1. Plan Ahead: Take some time each weekend to plan your meals for the week. This will help you stay organized and reduce stress during busy weekdays.

2. Batch Cooking: Prepare large quantities of staples like grains, proteins, and vegetables that can be used in various recipes throughout the week.

3. Portion Control: Use containers to portion out meals and snacks. This helps with portion control and ensures you have ready-to-eat options available. Consider using glassware for storing your portions, as it is more durable, eco-friendly, and free from harmful chemicals that can leach into your food from plastic containers.

4. Portion Sizing: A good rule of thumb for protein portions is to use the size of your palm for a serving. For example, one palm-sized portion of chicken, fish, or tofu is a suitable serving size for most adults. For carbohydrates like rice or pasta, a cupped hand is a good measure, while fats like butter or oil can be measured using the size of your thumb.

5. Freezer-Friendly Meals: Prepare and freeze meals that can be quickly reheated, such as soups, stews, and casseroles. To do this, cook your meals as usual and let them cool completely. Portion them into airtight, freezer-safe containers or freezer bags, label them with the contents and date, and lay them flat in the freezer. When ready to eat, thaw the meal in the refrigerator overnight and reheat thoroughly before serving.

6. Labeling: Label your containers with the date and contents to keep track of what needs to be eaten first.

Strategies for Success:

- **Stay Flexible:** It's okay to switch up meals based on what you have available or what you're in the mood for. The key is to have a variety of options ready.

- **Use Versatile Ingredients:** Choose ingredients that can be used in multiple dishes to keep meals interesting without overcomplicating your shopping list.

- **Healthy Snacking:** Keep healthy snacks, like cut-up veggies, fruits, and nuts, readily available to prevent unhealthy choices.

- **Stay Hydrated:** Drink plenty of water throughout the day. Herbal teas and infused water can add variety to your hydration routine.
- **Listen to Your Body:** Pay attention to your body's hunger and fullness cues. Eating mindfully can help you enjoy your meals more and prevent overeating.

MEDITERRANEAN Eating Essentials

Embracing the Mediterranean lifestyle is more than just following a meal plan—it's about prioritizing fresh, wholesome, and nutrient-rich foods. This list is designed to guide you through the essential groceries you'll need long-term to incorporate into your daily routine, categorized for your convenience. From vibrant vegetables and fruits to hearty whole grains, lean proteins, and healthy fats, you'll find everything you need to enjoy the delicious and healthful benefits of the Mediterranean way of eating.

Balanced Meal Cycle

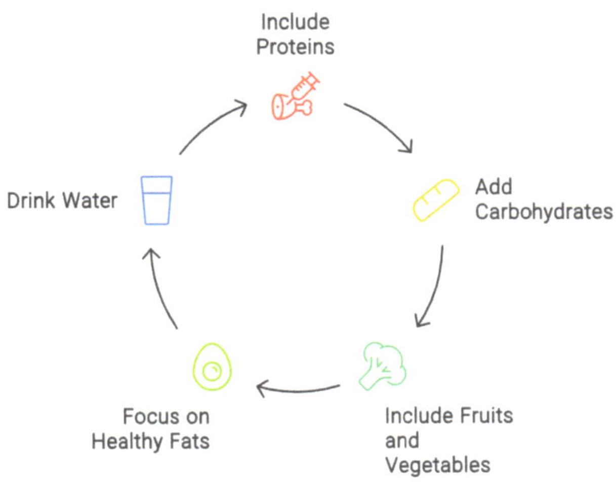

Whenever possible, choose organic produce, pasture-raised and cage-free poultry, grass-fed meats, and wild-caught fish to ensure the highest quality and nutritional value. Happy cooking and enjoy the journey to a healthier you!

The following table provides a comprehensive list of Mediterranean food staples categorized for your convenience. Use this as a handy reference for your grocery shopping and meal preparation.

Vegetables, Fruits, Legumes, Nuts, and Seeds:

Vegetables	Fruits	Legumes, Nuts, and Seeds
Tomatoes	Apples	Chickpeas
Cucumbers	Oranges	Lentils
Bell peppers	Bananas	Black beans
Zucchini	Grapes	Kidney beans
Eggplant	Berries (strawberries, blueberries, raspberries)	Cannellini beans
Spinach	Figs	Almonds
Kale	Dates	Walnuts
Broccoli	Lemons	Pistachios
Artichokes	Melons	Pine nuts
Onions	Peaches	Chia seeds
Garlic	Plums	Flaxseeds
Carrots		Pumpkin seeds
		Sunflower seeds
		Sesame seeds

Whole Grains, Fish and Seafood, Dairy, Healthy Fats, Herbs and Spices, Beverages:

Whole Grains	Fish and Seafood	Dairy	Healthy Fats	Herbs and Spices	Beverages
Whole wheat bread	Salmon	Greek yogurt	Extra virgin olive oil	Basil	Herbal teas
Whole grain pasta	Sardines	Feta cheese	Avocados	Oregano	Water
Brown rice	Tuna	Ricotta cheese	Olives	Thyme	Red wine (in moderation)
Quinoa	Mackerel	Parmesan cheese		Rosemary	
Barley	Trout			Parsley	
Oats	Shrimp			Mint	
Farro	Mussels			Dill	
Bulgur	Clams			Cinnamon	
				Cumin	

CALORIC CONTENT OF Common Foods

Many people are unaware of the caloric content of the foods they consume. This comprehensive list provides the caloric values of common items, including many staples of the Mediterranean way of eating. While the goal is to move beyond strict calorie counting, understanding the calories in your food can support a balanced and healthy lifestyle.

Knowing the caloric content helps manage daily intake, ensuring you consume the right amount of energy for daily activities and overall health. This awareness is beneficial when planning meals, balancing higher-calorie foods with those lower in calories but rich in nutrients.

> **Let food be thy medicine and medicine be thy food.**
> *— Hippocrates*

The Mediterranean diet emphasizes whole grains, fruits, vegetables, lean proteins, and healthy fats. Recognizing the caloric values of these foods can transform your eating habits, making it easier to create balanced meals that support your health.

Categorized caloric information for fruits, vegetables, grains, proteins, and more helps you see how different foods contribute to your daily intake. Whole, unprocessed foods ensure your diet is rich in essential nutrients while managing caloric intake effectively. Processed foods often contain hidden sugars and fats, increasing calorie consumption without substantial nutritional benefits. Choosing natural, whole foods offers better nutrition and controlled calorie intake.

Use this guide to make more informed choices and enjoy a diverse and wholesome approach to nutrition.

Vegetables, Fruits, Legumes, Nuts, and Seeds:

Vegetables	Calories	Fruits	Calories	Legumes, Nuts, and Seeds	Calories
Tomatoes (1 medium, 123g)	22	Apples (1 medium, 182g)	95	Chickpeas (1 cup, 164g)	269
Cucumbers (1 medium, 301g)	45	Oranges (1 medium, 131g)	62	Lentils (1 cup, 198g)	230
Bell peppers (1 medium, 119g)	24	Bananas (1 medium, 118g)	105	Black beans (1 cup, 172g)	227
Zucchini (1 medium, 196g)	33	Grapes (1 cup, 151g)	104	Kidney beans (1 cup, 256g)	215
Eggplant (1 medium, 458g)	115	Strawberries (1 cup, 152g)	49	Cannellini beans (1 cup, 177g)	225
Spinach (1 cup, 30g)	7	Blueberries (1 cup, 148g)	84	Almonds (1 ounce, 28g)	164
Kale (1 cup, 67g)	33	Raspberries (1 cup, 123g)	64	Walnuts (1 ounce, 28g)	185
Broccoli (1 cup, 91g)	31	Figs (1 medium, 50g)	37	Pistachios (1 ounce, 28g)	159
Artichokes (1 medium, 128g)	60	Dates (1 date, 24g)	66	Pine nuts (1 ounce, 28g)	191
Onions (1 medium, 110g)	44	Lemons (1 medium, 58g)	17	Chia seeds (1 ounce, 28g)	138
Garlic (1 clove, 3g)	4	Melons (1 cup, 160g)	60	Flaxseeds (1 ounce, 28g)	151
Carrots (1 medium, 61g)	25	Peaches (1 medium, 150g)	59	Pumpkin seeds (1 ounce, 28g)	151
		Plums (1 medium, 66g)	30	Sunflower seeds (1 ounce, 28g)	165
				Sesame seeds (1 ounce, 28g)	160

Whole Grains, Fish and Seafood, Dairy, Healthy Fats:

Whole Grains	Calories	Fish and Seafood	Calories	Dairy	Calories	Healthy Fats	Calories
Whole wheat bread (1 slice, 28g)	69	Salmon (3 ounces, 85g)	177	Greek yogurt (1 cup, 245g)	149	Avocados (1 medium, 150g)	234
Whole grain pasta (1 cup, 140g)	174	Sardines (3.75 ounces, 106g)	191	Feta cheese (1 ounce, 28g)	75	Avocado oil (1 tablespoon, 14g)	124
Brown rice (1 cup, 195g)	216	Tuna (3 ounces, 85g)	99	Ricotta cheese (1 cup, 246g)	428	Extra virgin olive oil (1 tbsp, 13.5g)	119
Quinoa (1 cup, 185g)	222	Mackerel (3 ounces, 85g)	223	Parmesan cheese (1 ounce, 28g)	122	Grapeseed oil (1 tablespoon, 14g)	120
Barley (1 cup, 157g)	193	Trout (3 ounces, 85g)	143			Olives (1 cup, 134g)	155
Oats (1 cup, 81g)	154	Shrimp (3 ounces, 85g)	84				
Farro (1 cup, 173g)	200	Mussels (3 ounces, 85g)	73				
Bulgur (1 cup, 182g)	151	Clams (3 ounces, 85g)	126				

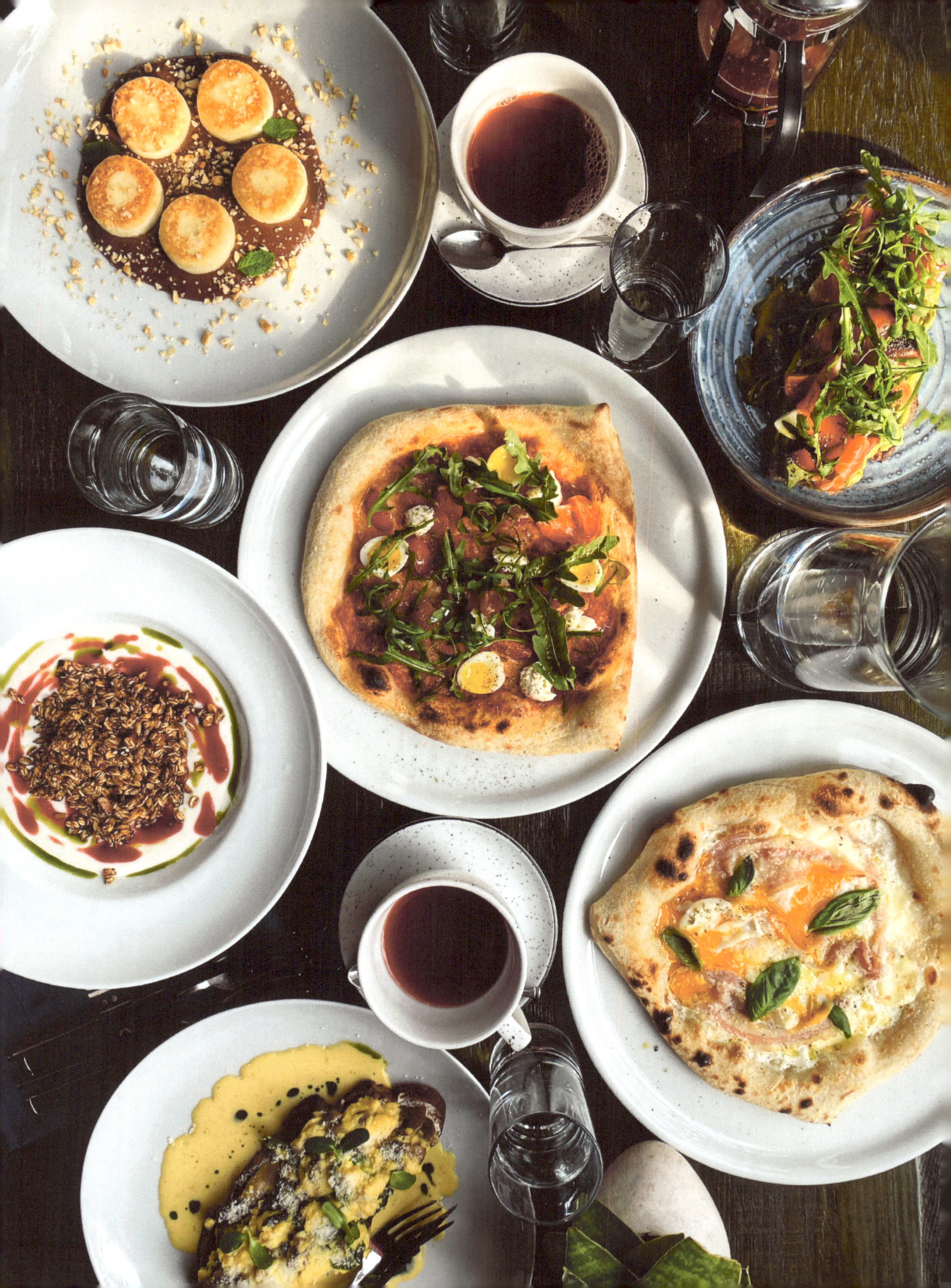

SECTION 4

RECIPES

Poultry

- Buffalo Chicken Flatbread Pizza

Vegetarian

- Cranberry Kale Salad with Quinoa and Butternut Squash
- Creamy Broccoli Mac 'n' Cheese
- Vegetable Zucchini and Pumpkin Stew

AMERICAN CREATIONS

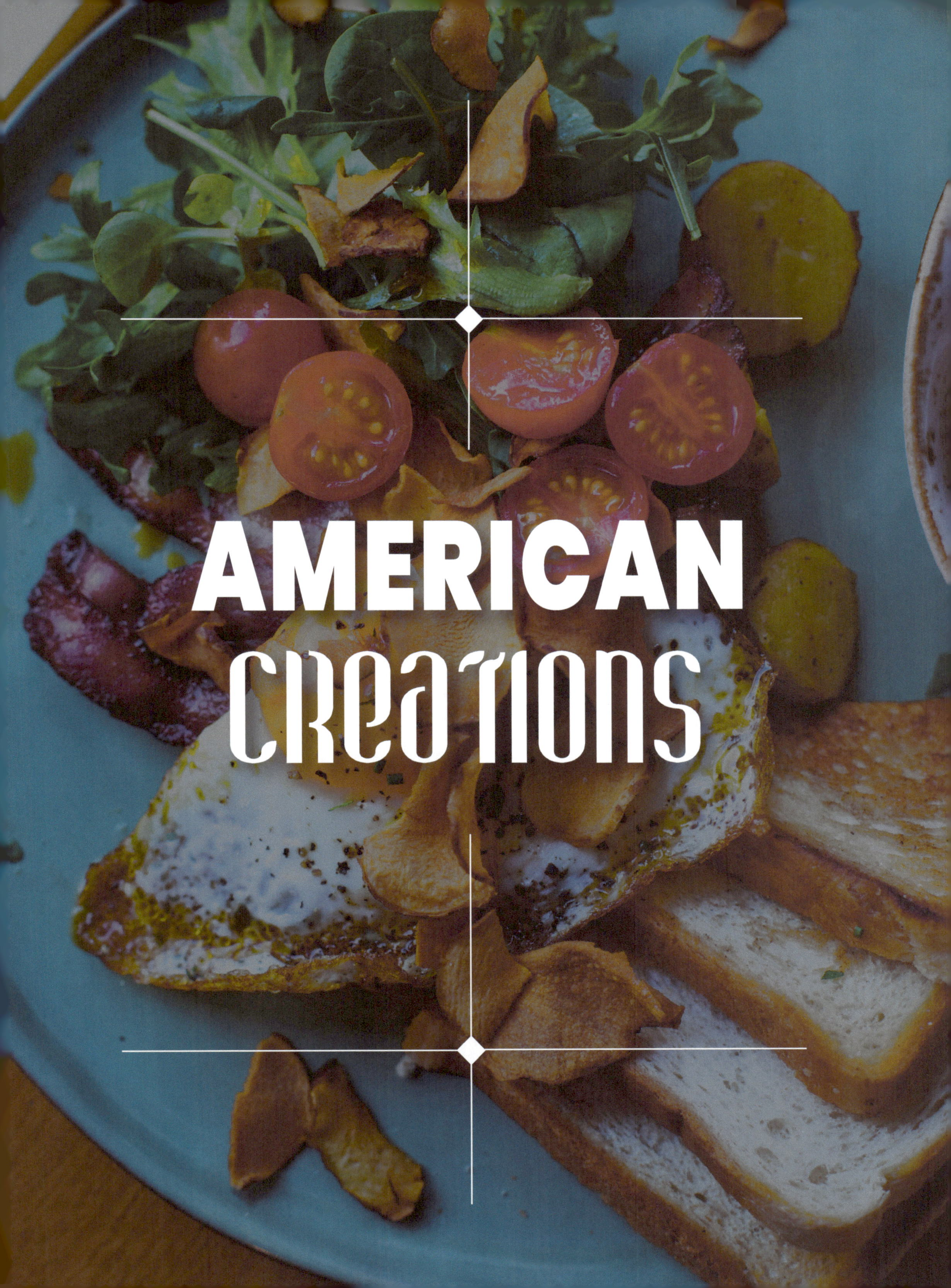

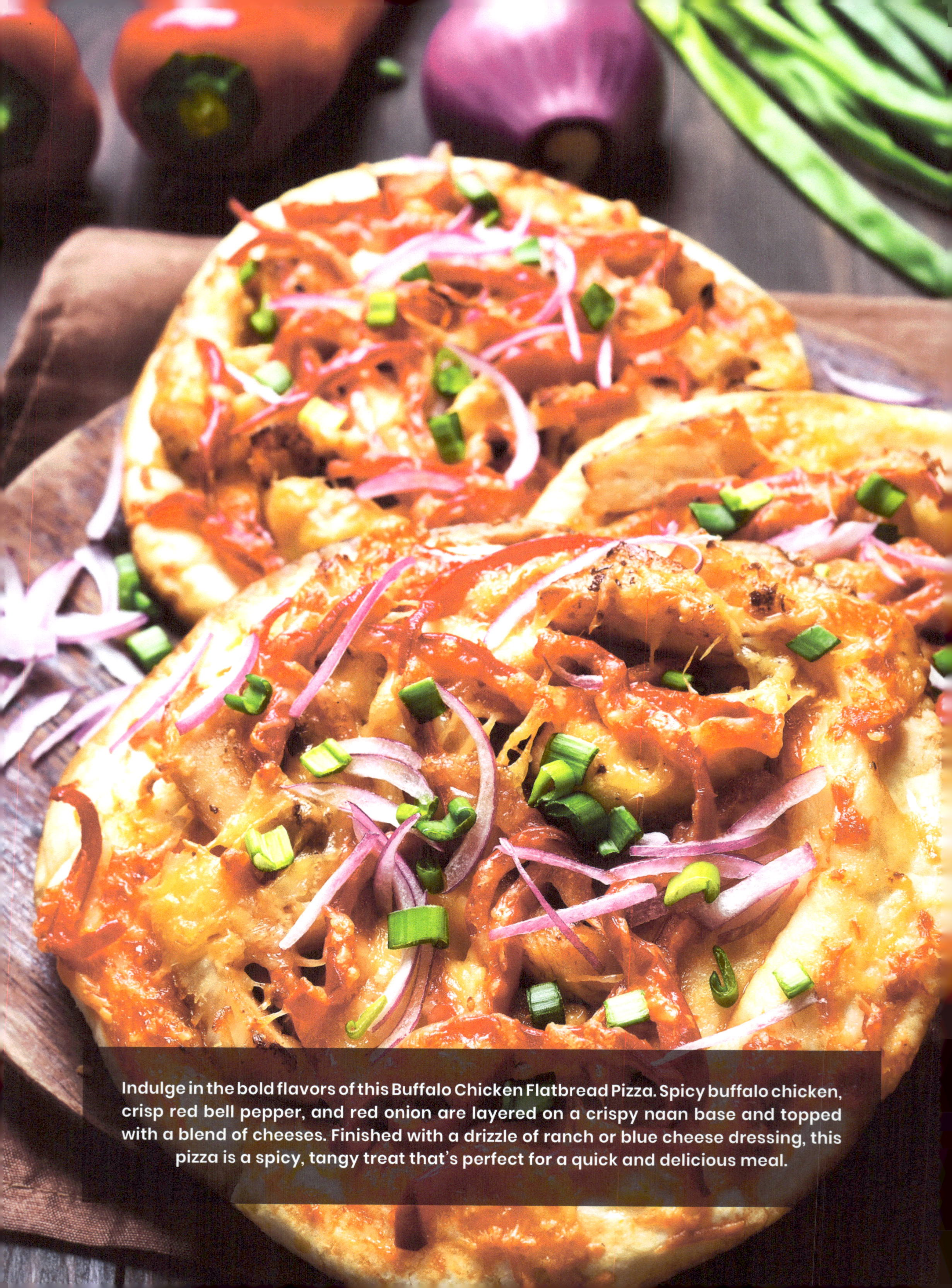

Indulge in the bold flavors of this Buffalo Chicken Flatbread Pizza. Spicy buffalo chicken, crisp red bell pepper, and red onion are layered on a crispy naan base and topped with a blend of cheeses. Finished with a drizzle of ranch or blue cheese dressing, this pizza is a spicy, tangy treat that's perfect for a quick and delicious meal.

POULTRY

BUFFALO CHICKEN FLATBREAD PIZZA

2 servings	21g P | 28g C 21g F	385 per serving	Prep Time: 10 minutes	Cooking Time: 10 minutes	Total Time: 20 minutes

INGREDIENTS

- 2 pieces of Stonefire Organic Original Naan
- 1 cup cooked chicken cut into small pieces
- 1/2 cup finely sliced red bell pepper
- 1/4 cup finely sliced red onion
- 2-3 green scallions, thinly sliced
- 1/4 cup shredded white cheese blend (mozzarella, provolone, or your choice)
- 1 tablespoon grated Parmesan cheese
- Ranch or blue cheese dressing for drizzling (optional)

DIRECTIONS

1. Preheat the Oven: Preheat your oven to 400°F (200°C).
2. Place the naan bread on a baking sheet or pizza stone.
3. In a separate bowl, combine the cooked chicken pieces with the Buffalo wing sauce until well coated, set to the side.
4. Distribute the shredded white cheese blend evenly over each naan bread.
5. Place the buffalo chicken pieces onto the naan bread.
6. Place the finely sliced red bell pepper and red onion over the chicken.
7. Sprinkle the grated Parmesan cheese over the top.
8. Place the baking sheet or pizza stone in the preheated oven and bake for about 10-15 minutes, or until the cheese is bubbly, and the edges of the naan bread are golden brown.
9. Garnish with fresh green scallions.
10. If desired, drizzle ranch or blue cheese dressing over the cooked pizza.

VEGETARIAN

CRANBERRY KALE SALAD with QUINOA and BUTTERNUT SQUASH

2 servings	12g P | 45g C 14g F	380 per serving	Prep Time: 20 minutes	Cooking Time: 25 minutes	Total Time: 45 minutes

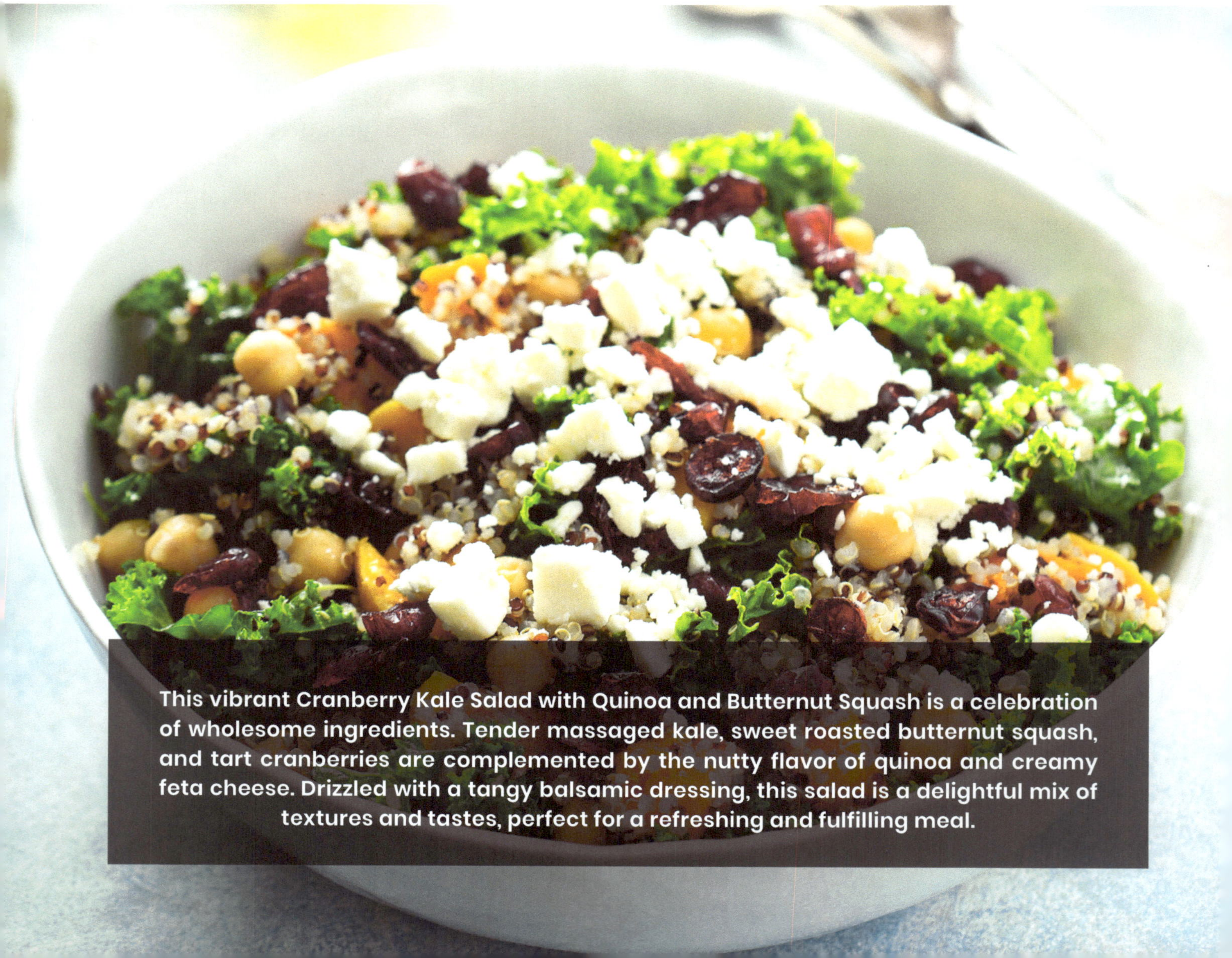

This vibrant Cranberry Kale Salad with Quinoa and Butternut Squash is a celebration of wholesome ingredients. Tender massaged kale, sweet roasted butternut squash, and tart cranberries are complemented by the nutty flavor of quinoa and creamy feta cheese. Drizzled with a tangy balsamic dressing, this salad is a delightful mix of textures and tastes, perfect for a refreshing and fulfilling meal.

INGREDIENTS

For the Salad:

- 1 cup multigrain quinoa, cooked and cooled
- 2 cups kale, stems removed and leaves massaged
- 1 cup roasted butternut squash
- 1/2 cup chickpeas, cooked and drained
- 1/4 cup dried cranberries
- 1/4 cup crumbled feta cheese
- Salt and black pepper to taste
- 2 tablespoons extra-virgin olive oil

For the Dressing:

- 2 tablespoons balsamic vinegar
- 1 tablespoon honey
- 1 teaspoon Dijon mustard
- 1 clove garlic, minced
- 1/4 teaspoon salt (or to taste)
- 1/4 teaspoon black pepper (or to taste)

DIRECTIONS

For Roasting the Butternut Squash:

1. Preheat your oven to 400°F (200°C).
2. Peel the butternut squash, remove the seeds, and cut it into bite-sized cubes.
3. Place the cubed butternut squash on a baking sheet, spray with a bit of olive oil, salt, and pepper, and toss to coat evenly.
4. Roast the squash in the preheated oven for approximately 25-30 minutes, or until the squash is tender and lightly browned. You can check for doneness by piercing it with a fork; it should be easily pierced. Once roasted, remove the butternut squash from the oven and let it cool to room temperature.

Cook the quinoa to package instructions.

1. While the quinoa is simmering, prepare your dressing.

Prepare the Dressing:

1. In a small bowl, whisk together the extra-virgin olive oil, balsamic vinegar, honey, Dijon mustard, minced garlic, salt, and black pepper. Set the dressing aside.
2. Massage the Kale:
3. Remove the stems from the kale leaves and tear them into bite-sized pieces. Place the kale in a large bowl.
4. Drizzle a little bit of the dressing over the kale and use your hands to massage the kale leaves. This helps to tenderize them and infuse them with flavor.
5. Assemble the Salad:
6. Add the cooked quinoa, diced roasted butternut squash, chickpeas, dried cranberries, and crumbled feta cheese to the bowl with the massaged kale. Add the salad dressing and toss all of the ingredients together until they are well combined and coated. Season the salad with salt and pepper to taste, and enjoy!

CREAMY BROCCOLI MAC 'N' CHEESE

DIRECTIONS

1. Cook the einkorn wheat elbow macaroni according to package instructions, making sure to add salt to the boiling water. During the last 2 minutes of cooking, add the fresh broccoli florets to the boiling water. Reserve about 1/2 cup of pasta water before draining. Drain the pasta and broccoli and set aside.

2. In a large saucepan over low heat, melt the salted butter. Once melted, add the Greek yogurt, nutritional yeast, garlic powder, onion powder, paprika, salt and pepper to taste and a splash of the reserved pasta water. Whisk to combine. Slowly add the shredded cheddar cheese, stir continuously until the cheese is fully melted and the mixture is creamy. If needed, add more pasta water to reach your desired consistency.

3. Add the cooked macaroni and broccoli to the creamy cheese sauce. Stir to coat everything evenly. If the sauce becomes too thick, you can add a bit more pasta water.

4. Serve the Creamy Broccoli Mac 'n' Cheese hot, garnished with basil and a sprinkling of grated cheddar cheese. For a browned top, broil for a few minutes, or skip as the cheese will melt. Optionally, add panko crumbs before broiling for extra crunch. For extra flavor, consider topping with hot sauce and crushed red pepper flakes.

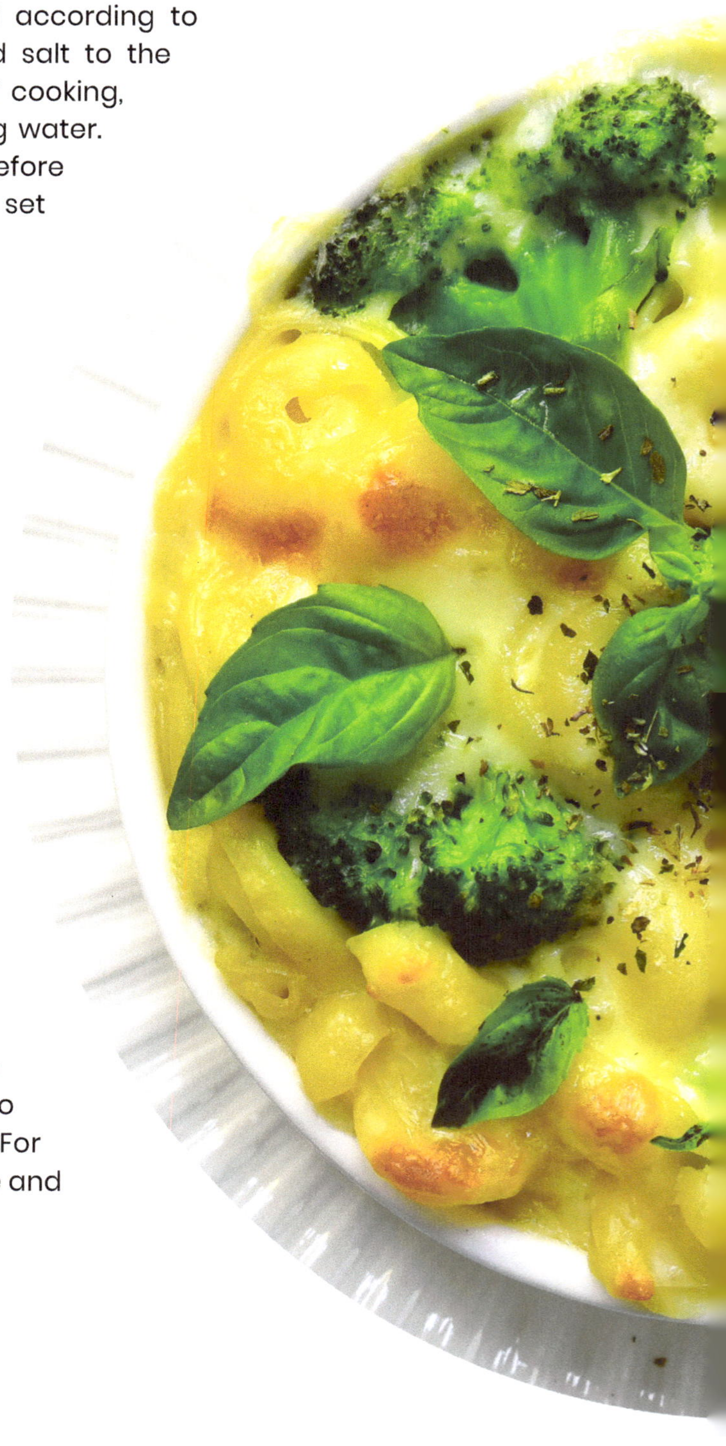

2 servings

16g P | 53g C 13g F

380 per serving

Prep Time: 10 minutes

Cooking Time: 10 minutes

Total Time: 20 minutes

INGREDIENTS

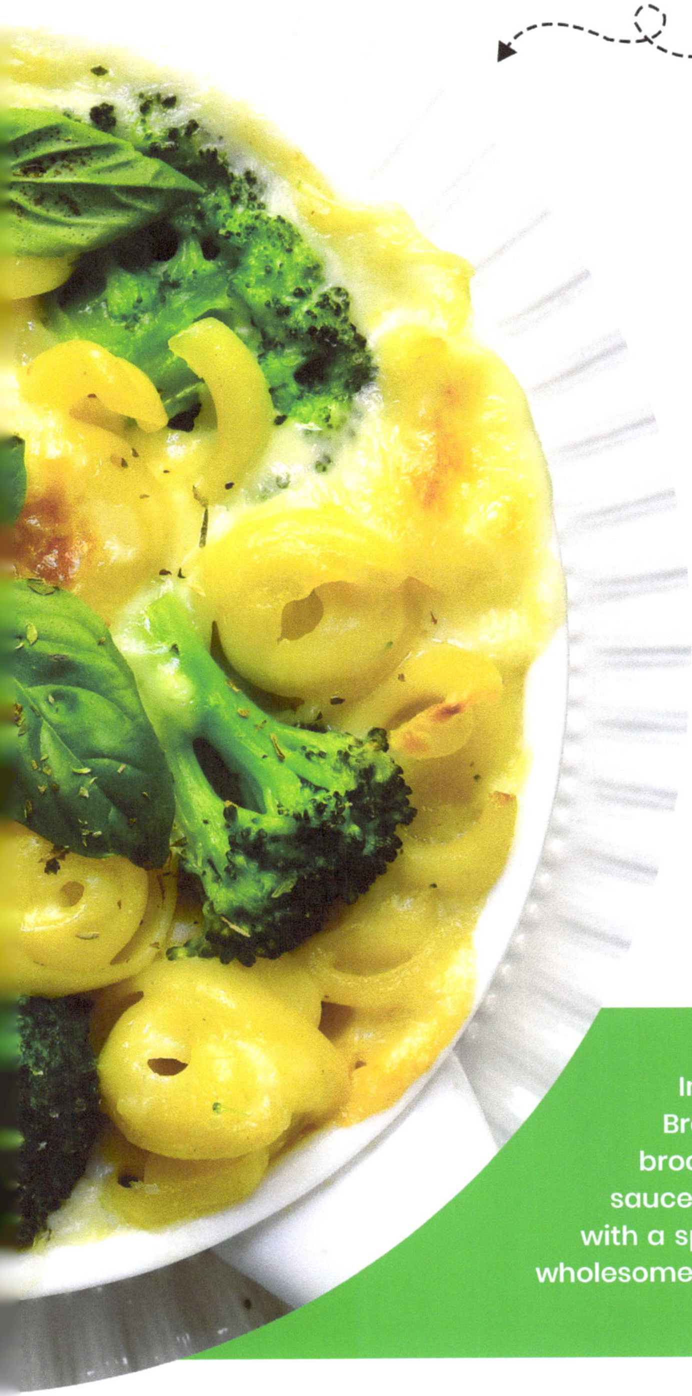

- 8 ounces elbow pasta by Jovial
- 2 cups broccoli florets
- 1/2 cup plain Greek yogurt
- 1 cup shredded low-fat cheddar cheese (or a dairy-free alternative)
- 1/4 cup nutritional yeast
- 2 tablespoons salted butter
- 1/2 teaspoon garlic powder
- 1/2 teaspoon onion powder
- 1/4 teaspoon paprika
- Salt and pepper to taste
- 2 tablespoons fresh basil for garnish (optional)
- Red pepper flakes and hot sauce (optional, for garnish)

Indulge in the comforting goodness of Creamy Broccoli Mac 'n' Cheese. Tender elbow pasta and broccoli florets are coated in a rich, creamy cheese sauce made with Greek yogurt and cheddar. Topped with a sprinkle of Parmesan and fresh basil, this dish is a wholesome and delicious take on a classic favorite.

VEGETABLE ZUCCHINI and PUMPKIN STEW

Warm up with this hearty and wholesome vegetable stew, featuring tender zucchini and sweet pumpkin simmered in a savory tomato broth. The combination of fresh vegetables, fragrant garlic, and a hint of paprika creates a comforting dish that's both nourishing and satisfying. Perfect for a cozy dinner, this stew brings the flavors of the garden to your table, providing a delicious way to enjoy a variety of seasonal vegetables.

INGREDIENTS

- 1 yellow zucchini, diced (or use yellow squash)
- 1 cup diced pumpkin or butternut squash
- 1/2 red onion, chopped
- 2 cloves garlic, minced
- 1 can (14 oz) diced tomatoes
- 2 cups vegetable broth
- 1 teaspoon paprika
- 1/2 teaspoon salt
- 1/8 teaspoon pepper
- Olive oil for sautéing
- Fresh parsley for garnish

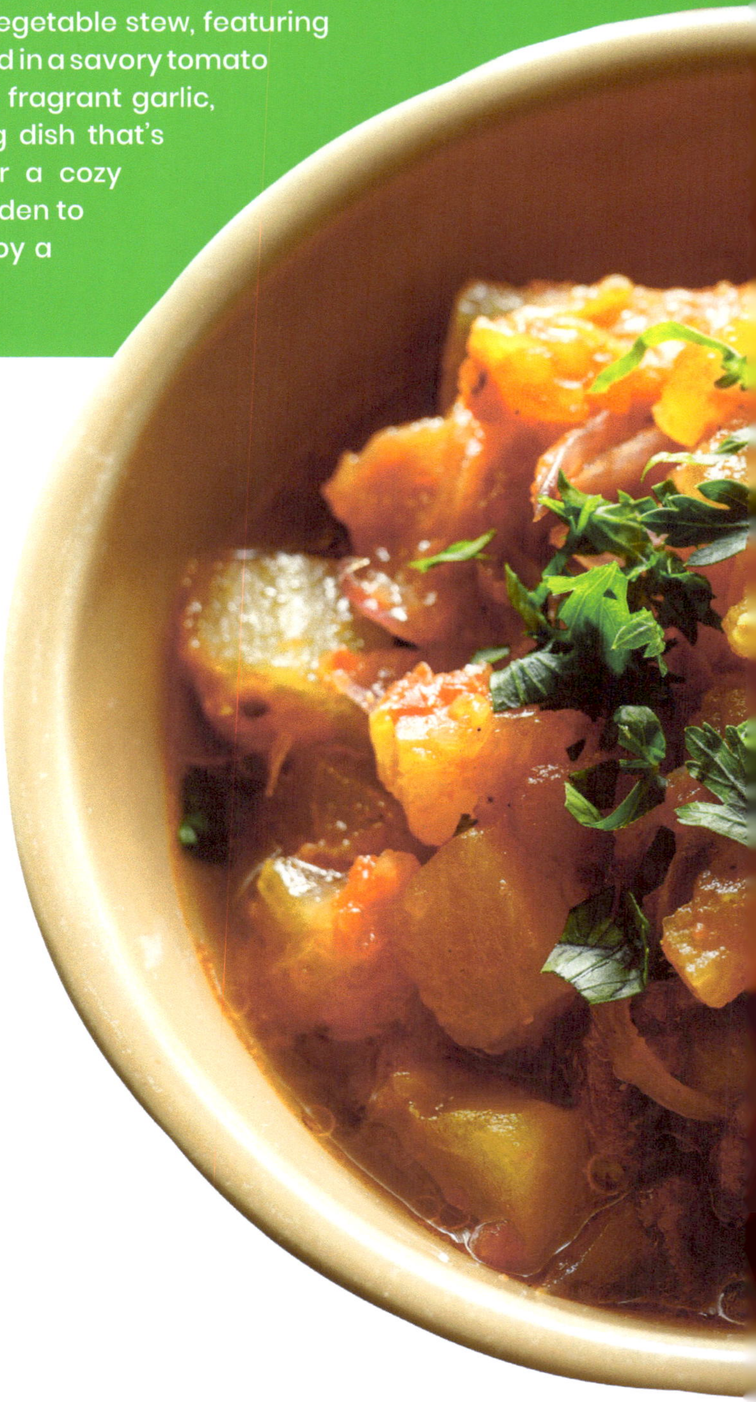

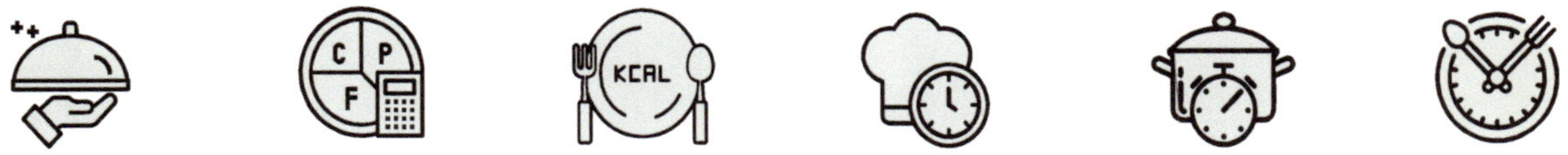

2 servings	2g P | 20g C 4g F	120 per serving	Prep Time: 15 minutes	Cooking Time: 20 minutes	Total Time: 35 minutes

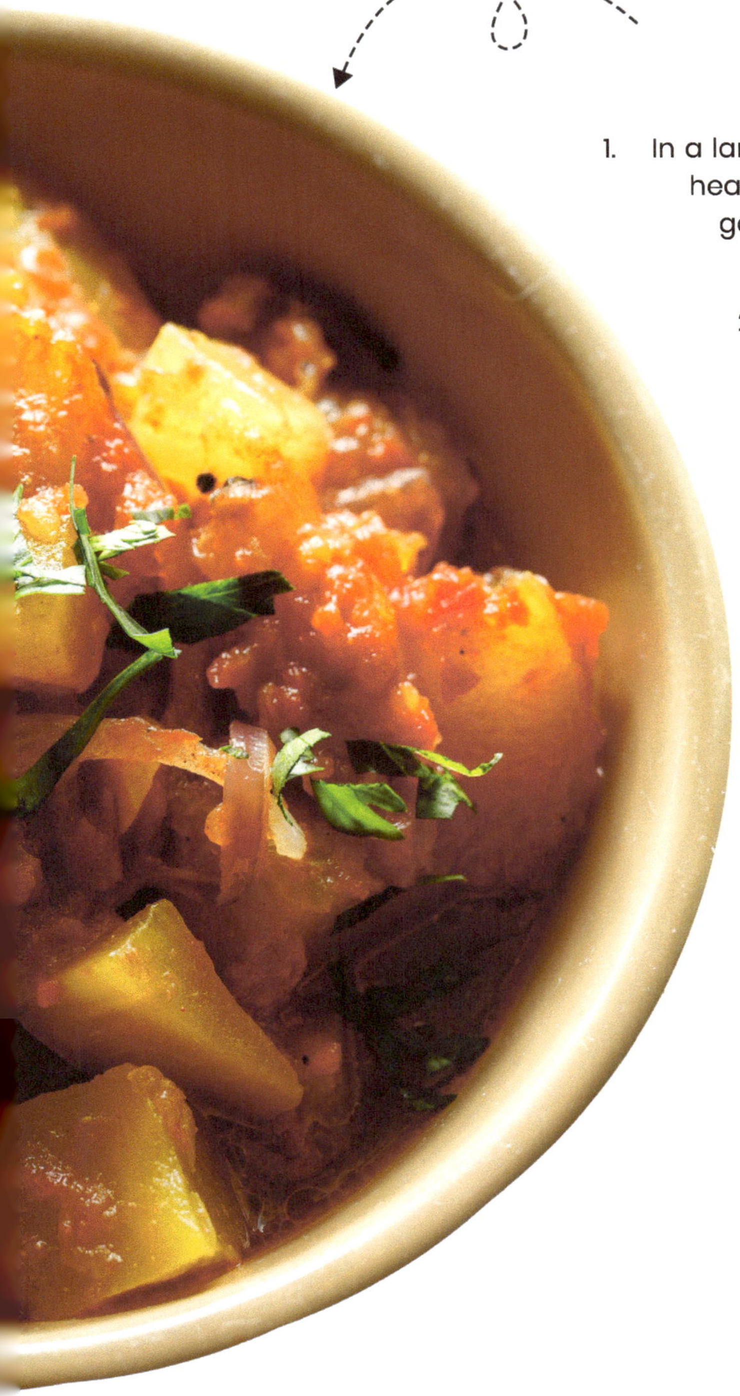

DIRECTIONS

1. In a large pot, heat a drizzle of olive oil over medium heat. Add the chopped red onion and minced garlic. Sauté for about 3-4 minutes until they become fragrant and translucent.
2. Add the diced zucchini and pumpkin to the pot. Sauté for another 3-4 minutes until they start to soften.
3. Pour in the diced tomatoes and vegetable broth. Stir well to combine.
4. Season the stew with paprika, salt, and pepper. Start with 1/2 teaspoon of salt and a pinch of pepper, then adjust as needed.
5. Bring the mixture to a boil, then reduce the heat to low, cover, and simmer for about 15-20 minutes or until the zucchini and pumpkin are tender.
6. Serve the Vegetable Zucchini and Pumpkin Stew hot and garnish with fresh parsley; add shredded parmesan if desired and a slice of crusty bread for dipping.

Beef

- Quick Low-Carb Beef Pho

Pork

- Sweet and Spicy Crispy Pork Stir Fry with Rice Noodles

Poultry

- Savory Lettuce Wraps with Peanut Sauce

Seafood

- Spicy Halibut in Creamy Coconut Curry

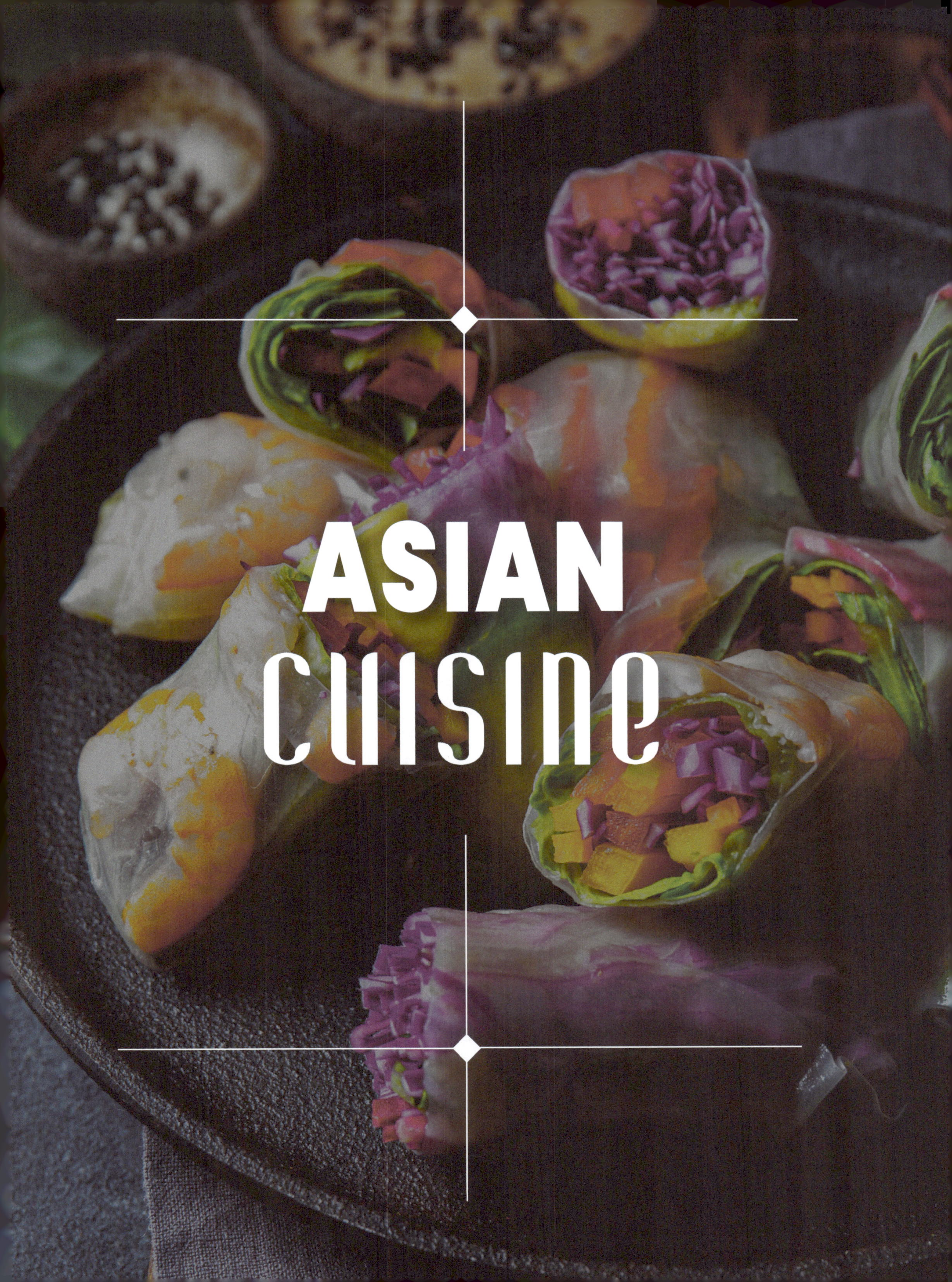
ASIAN
Cuisine

QUICK LOW-CARB BEEF PHO

2 servings

35g P | 20g C
10g F

350 per serving

Prep Time: 10 minutes

Cooking Time: 20 minutes

Total Time: 30 minutes

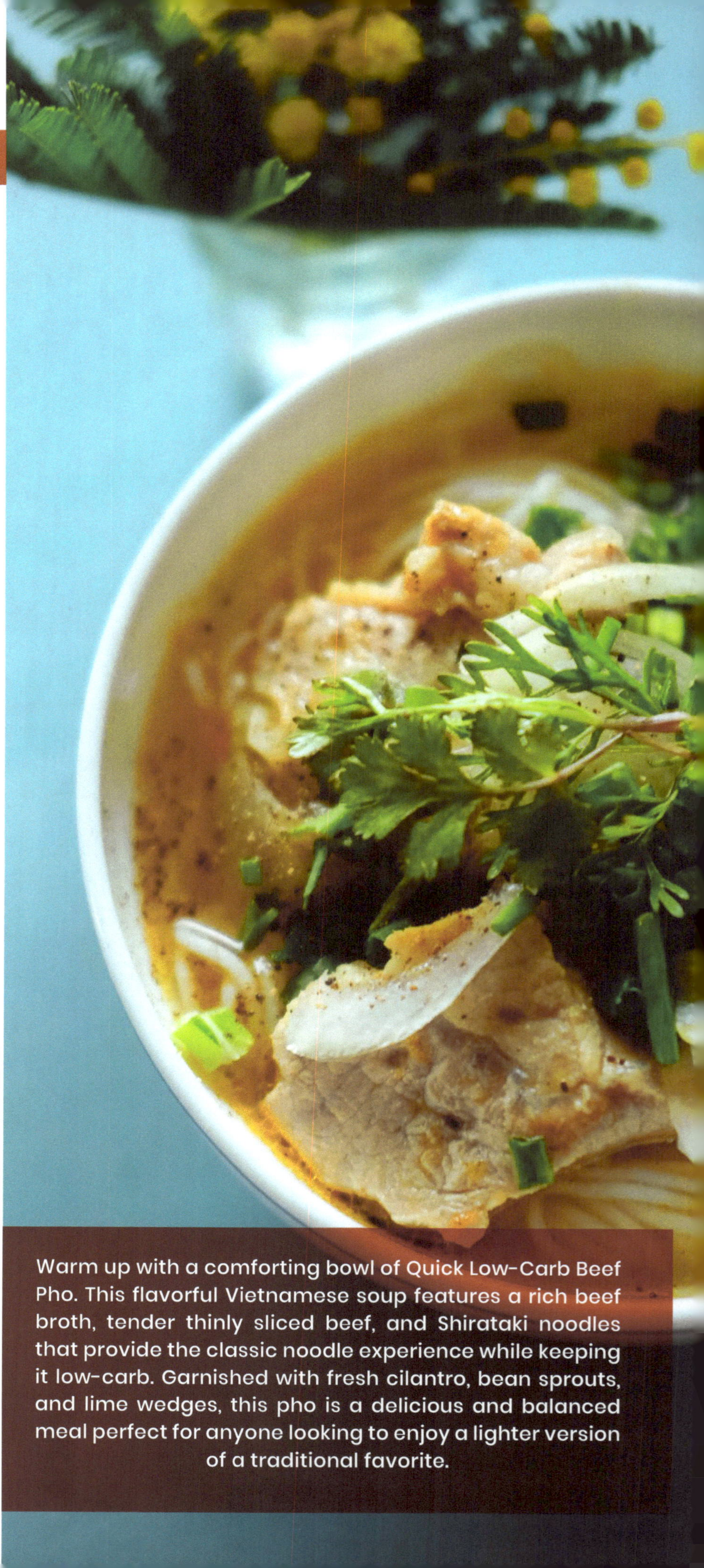

Warm up with a comforting bowl of Quick Low-Carb Beef Pho. This flavorful Vietnamese soup features a rich beef broth, tender thinly sliced beef, and Shirataki noodles that provide the classic noodle experience while keeping it low-carb. Garnished with fresh cilantro, bean sprouts, and lime wedges, this pho is a delicious and balanced meal perfect for anyone looking to enjoy a lighter version of a traditional favorite.

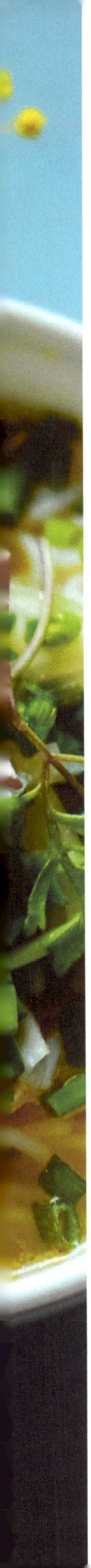

INGREDIENTS

For the Broth:

- 4 cups beef broth
- 1 small onion, thinly sliced
- 1-inch piece of ginger, thinly sliced
- 2 cloves garlic, minced
- 1 cinnamon stick
- 2-star anise
- 2 cloves
- 1 tablespoon fish sauce
- 1 tablespoon soy sauce
- 1 teaspoon sugar
- Salt to taste

For the Soup:

- 1/2 lb. beef sirloin or flank steak, very thinly sliced
- 1 cup fresh cilantro, chopped
- 1 cup green onions, thinly sliced
- 1 cup bean sprouts
- 1 lime, cut into wedges
- 2 packs of angel hair-style Shirataki noodles (drained and rinsed)
- Sriracha sauce (optional)
- Hoisin sauce (optional)
- Optional Protein Additions: boiled egg, shrimp, or tofu

DIRECTIONS

Prepare the Broth:

1. In a large pot, bring the beef broth to a boil.
2. Add the sliced onion, ginger, garlic, cinnamon stick, star anise, and cloves.
3. Reduce the heat and let it simmer for 15 minutes.
4. Add the fish sauce, soy sauce, sugar, and salt to taste. Simmer for an additional 5 minutes.
5. Strain the broth to remove the solids (cinnamon stick, star anise, cloves, onion, and ginger) and return the clear broth to the pot.

Prepare the Shirataki Noodles:

1. Drain and rinse the Shirataki noodles according to the package instructions.
2. Note: Shirataki noodles have a distinct smell when first opened, but it will disappear after rinsing and cooking.
3. Optionally, boil the noodles for 2-3 minutes to further reduce any remaining smell, then drain.

Assemble the Pho:

1. Divide the Shirataki noodles between two bowls.
2. Top with the thinly sliced beef and any additional protein (boiled egg, shrimp, or tofu).
3. Ladle the hot broth over the beef and noodles. The hot broth will cook the thin slices of beef.
4. Garnish with cilantro, green onions, and bean sprouts.
5. Serve with lime wedges, sriracha sauce, and hoisin sauce on the side.

SWEET and SPICY CRISPY PORK STIR FRY with RICE NOODLES

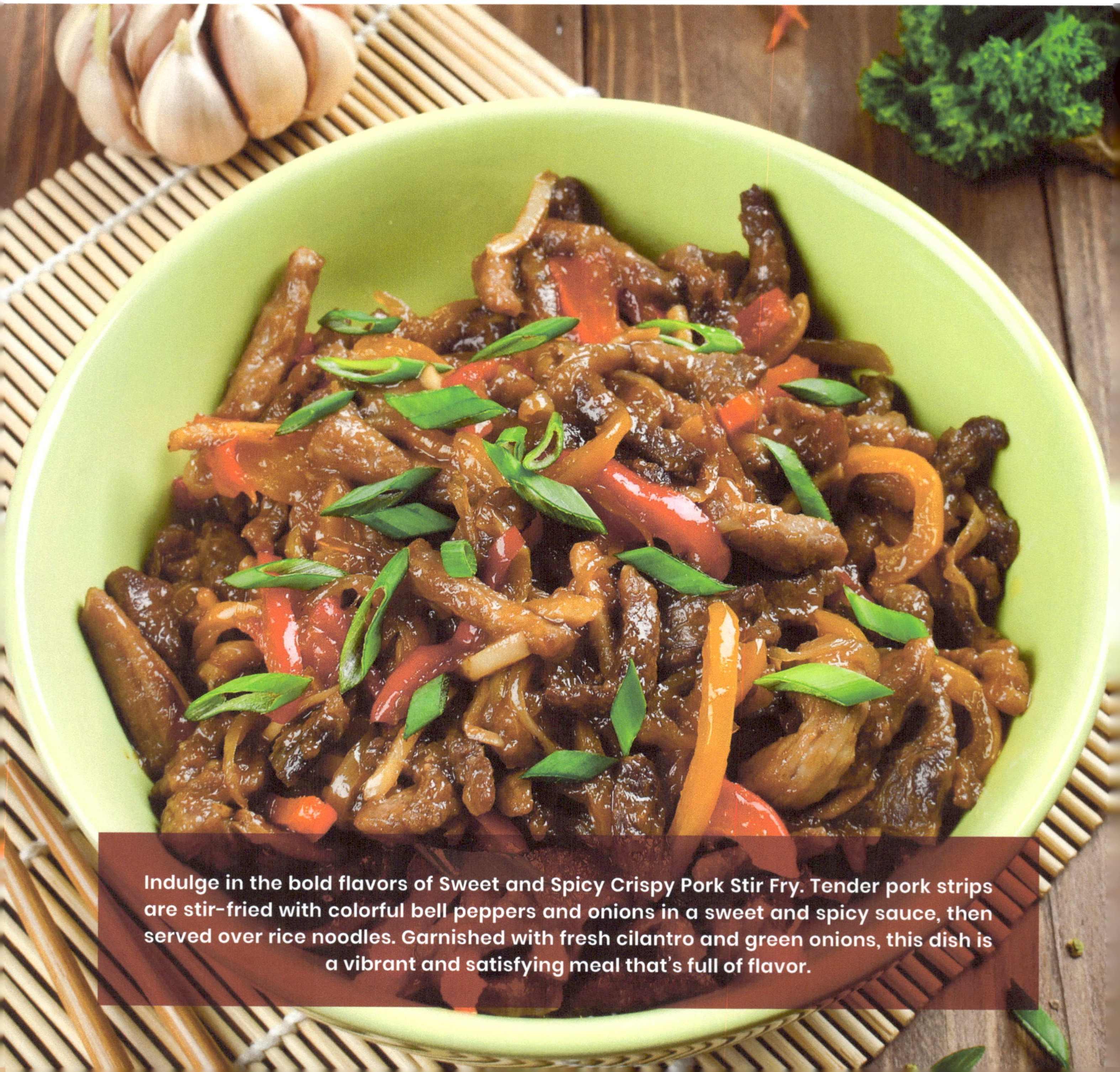

Indulge in the bold flavors of Sweet and Spicy Crispy Pork Stir Fry. Tender pork strips are stir-fried with colorful bell peppers and onions in a sweet and spicy sauce, then served over rice noodles. Garnished with fresh cilantro and green onions, this dish is a vibrant and satisfying meal that's full of flavor.

2 servings	25g P | 36g C 19g F	420 per serving	Prep Time: 15 minutes	Cooking Time: 15 minutes	Total Time: 30 minutes

INGREDIENTS

For the Stir Fry:

- 1 pound thinly sliced pork loin strips (or pork belly)
- 2 cups rice noodles
- 1 orange bell pepper, thinly sliced
- 1 red bell pepper, thinly sliced
- 1/2 white onion, thinly sliced
- 2 cloves garlic, minced
- 2 red chili peppers, sliced
- 2 green chili peppers, sliced
- 3 tablespoons olive oil
- Salt and pepper to taste
- Fresh cilantro leaves and chopped green onions for garnish

For Coating the Pork:

- 1 tablespoon all-purpose flour
- For the Sauce:
- 1 tablespoon low-sodium soy sauce
- 1 tablespoon oyster sauce
- 1 tablespoon honey
- 1 tablespoon rice wine vinegar
- 1 teaspoon sesame oil

DIRECTIONS

1. In a bowl, coat the thinly sliced pork strips with the all-purpose flour until it's evenly coated.
2. Cook the rice noodles according to the package instructions. Drain and set them aside.
3. In a small bowl, whisk together the soy sauce, oyster sauce, honey, rice vinegar, and sesame oil. Set aside.
4. Heat olive oil in a large skillet or wok over high heat.
5. Add the thinly sliced and coated pork to the hot skillet. Stir-fry for 2-3 minutes or until it becomes crispy and golden. Remove the crispy pork from the skillet and set it aside.
6. In the same skillet, add minced garlic, sliced onion, and both red and green chili peppers. Stir-fry for about 2 minutes until the onions become translucent.
7. Add the orange and red bell peppers to the skillet and continue to stir-fry for another 2-3 minutes until they start to soften.
8. Return the crispy pork to the skillet and pour the prepared sauce over the ingredients. Stir well to coat everything evenly. Cook for an additional 2-3 minutes until the sauce thickens slightly.
9. Season with salt and pepper to taste.
10. Place the cooked rice noodles on serving plates and top with the sweet and spicy crispy pork stir-fry.
11. Garnish with fresh, chopped, green onions and enjoy!

SAVORY LETTUCE WRAPS with PEANUT SAUCE

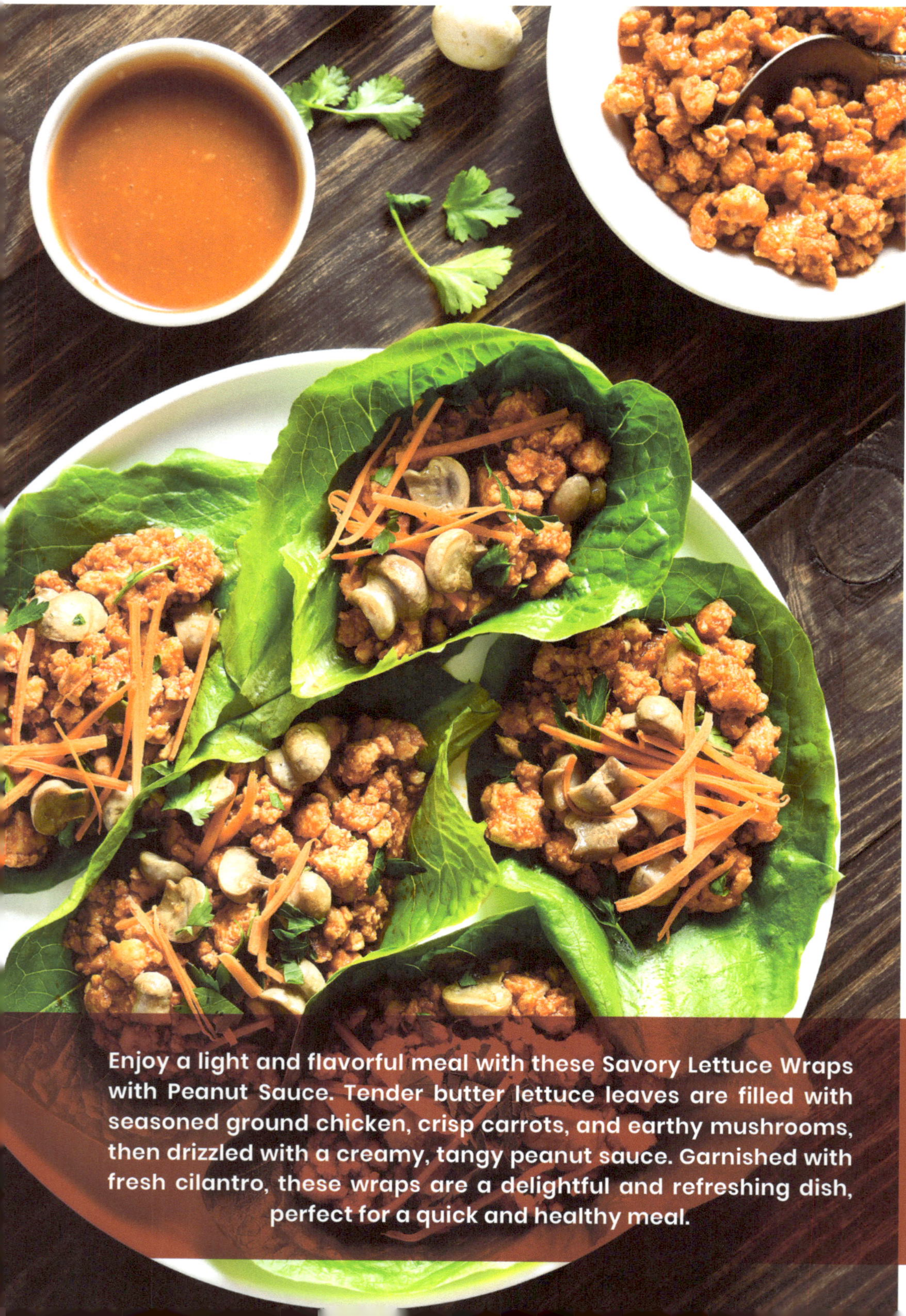

2 servings

25g P | 20g C
20g F

350 per serving

Prep Time:
15 minutes

Cooking Time:
15 minutes

Total Time:
30 minutes

Enjoy a light and flavorful meal with these Savory Lettuce Wraps with Peanut Sauce. Tender butter lettuce leaves are filled with seasoned ground chicken, crisp carrots, and earthy mushrooms, then drizzled with a creamy, tangy peanut sauce. Garnished with fresh cilantro, these wraps are a delightful and refreshing dish, perfect for a quick and healthy meal.

INGREDIENTS

For the Lettuce Wraps:

- 10 leaves of butter lettuce
- 1/2-pound ground chicken (or use ground pork, beef, turkey or tofu)
- 1/2 cup thinly sliced carrots
- 6 small button mushrooms, chopped
- 2 tablespoons low-sodium soy sauce or tamari (for a gluten-free option)
- 1 teaspoon sesame oil
- 1 teaspoon fresh ginger, minced
- 1 teaspoon garlic, minced
- Salt and pepper to taste
- Fresh cilantro leaves for garnish

For the Peanut Sauce:

- 1/4 cup natural organic peanut butter
- 2 tablespoons low-sodium soy sauce or tamari (for a gluten-free option)
- 1 tablespoon honey or maple syrup
- 1 tablespoon rice vinegar
- 1 teaspoon sesame oil
- 1/2 teaspoon fresh ginger, minced
- 1/2 teaspoon garlic, minced
- Water to adjust consistency

DIRECTIONS

Prepare the Lettuce Wraps:

1. Wash and carefully separate the butter lettuce leaves, keeping them whole. Pat them dry with a paper towel.

Cook the Protein:

1. In a large skillet over medium heat, add the ground chicken. Cook until browned and fully cooked.
2. Add the minced ginger and garlic, and cook for another 1-2 minutes until fragrant.
3. Stir in the soy sauce, sesame oil, chopped enoki mushrooms, and thinly sliced carrots. Cook for an additional 3-4 minutes, or until the vegetables are tender.
4. Season with salt and pepper to taste.

Prepare the Creamy Peanut Sauce:

1. Divide the Shirataki noodles between two bowls.
2. Top with the thinly sliced beef and any additional protein (boiled egg, shrimp, or tofu).
3. Ladle the hot broth over the beef and noodles. The hot broth will cook the thin slices of beef.
4. Garnish with cilantro, green onions, and bean sprouts.
5. Serve with lime wedges, sriracha sauce, and hoisin sauce on the side.

Assemble the Lettuce Wraps:

1. Lay out the butter lettuce leaves on a clean serving platter.
2. Spoon the cooked ground chicken filling evenly onto each lettuce leaf.

Garnish and Serve:

1. Serve the lettuce wraps with a side of peanut sauce, and generously drizzle the creamy peanut sauce over each one.
2. Garnish with fresh cilantro leaves.
3. Serve immediately and enjoy!

2 servings	27g P | 34g C 28g F	480 per serving	Prep Time: 10 minutes	Cooking Time: 20 minutes	Total Time: 30 minutes

DIRECTIONS

1. Prepare your rice or quinoa following the package instructions, as it will be ready to serve with your Spicy Halibut in Creamy Coconut Curry.
2. In a large skillet or pan, heat the olive oil over medium heat.
3. Add the minced garlic, diced white onion, and sliced red bell pepper. Sauté for about 3-4 minutes until they start to soften.
4. Add the red curry paste and minced ginger to the sautéed vegetables. Stir well to coat them with the spices. Continue to cook for another 2 minutes to toast the spices slightly.
5. Pour in the coconut milk and stir to combine. Bring the mixture to a gentle simmer.
6. Season the halibut fillets with salt and pepper to taste, then carefully place them into the simmering coconut milk.
7. Cover the skillet and let the fish cook for about 8-10 minutes, or until it's opaque and flakes easily with a fork.
8. During the last minute of cooking, add the chopped spinach to the skillet and let it wilt.
9. Squeeze the juice of one lime over the dish and gently stir.
10. Taste and adjust the seasoning with more salt and pepper if needed.
11. Serve the Spicy Halibut in Creamy Coconut Curry hot over cooked rice or quinoa, garnished with fresh cilantro.

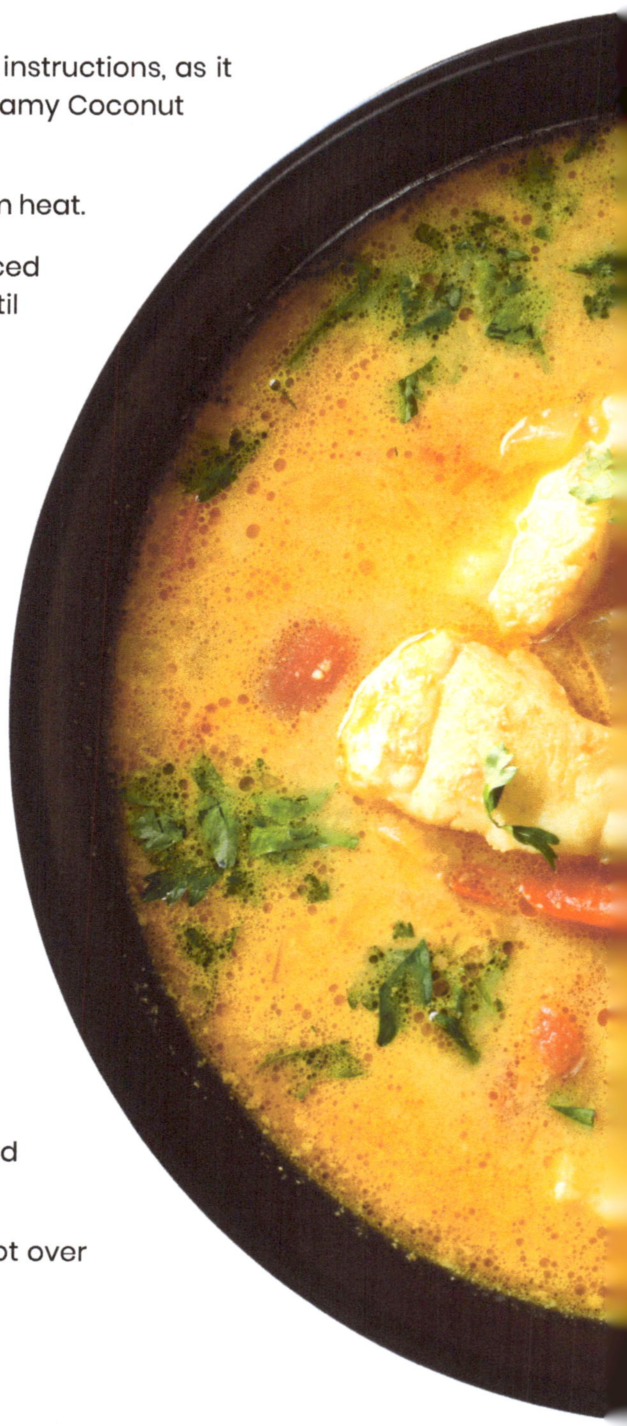

SPICY HALIBUT in CREAMY COCONUT CURRY

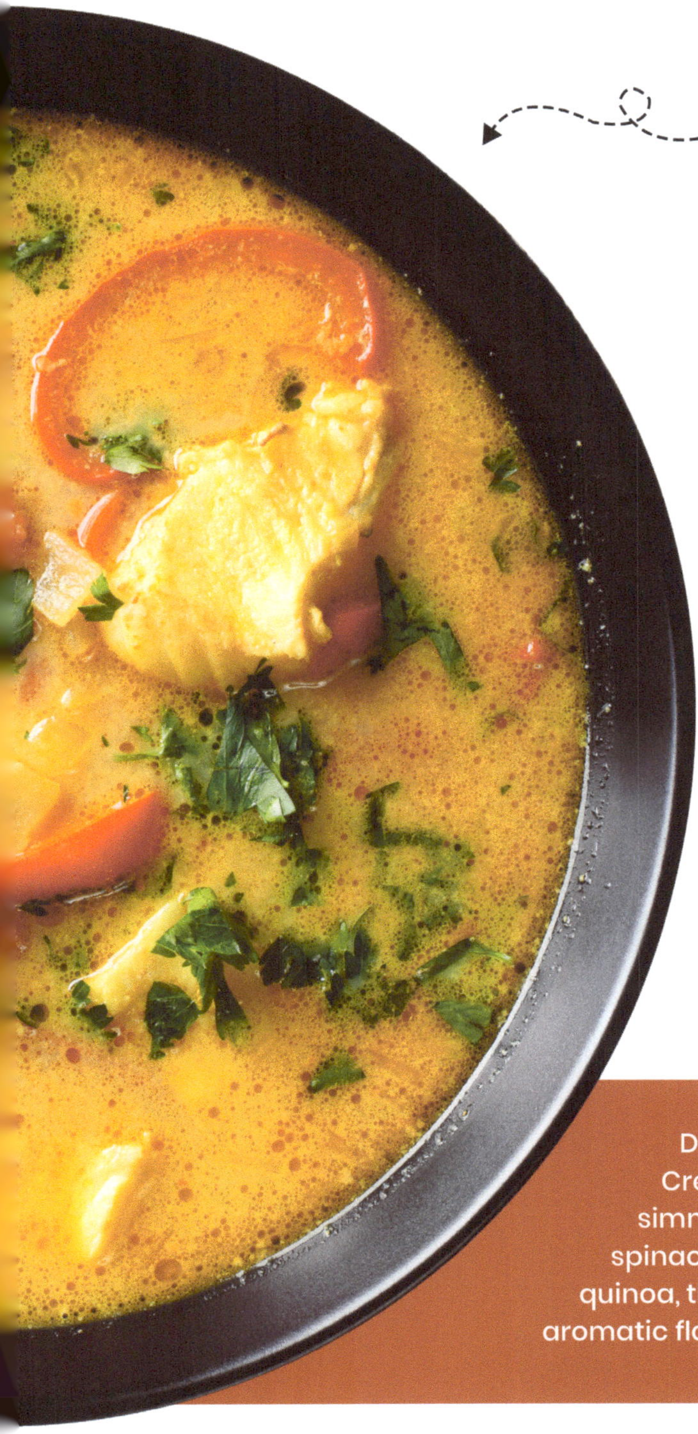

INGREDIENTS

- 2 halibut fish fillets (or any white fish fillets)
- 2 cups fresh spinach, roughly chopped
- 1/2 white onion, diced
- 1 red bell pepper, thinly sliced
- 1 can (14 oz) organic coconut milk by Trader Joe's (no additives; BPA-free can)
- 2 tablespoons red curry paste
- 2 cloves garlic, minced
- 1 teaspoon fresh ginger, minced
- 1 tablespoon olive oil
- Juice of 1 lime
- Salt and pepper to taste
- Fresh cilantro leaves for garnish
- Cooked rice or quinoa for serving

Dive into the exotic flavors of Spicy Halibut in Creamy Coconut Curry. Tender halibut fillets are simmered in a rich coconut curry sauce with fresh spinach and red bell pepper. Served over rice or quinoa, this dish is a delightful blend of spicy, creamy, and aromatic flavors, perfect for a special dinner.

Seafood

- Pesto Zucchini Noodles with Shrimp

ITALIAN INSPIRATIONS

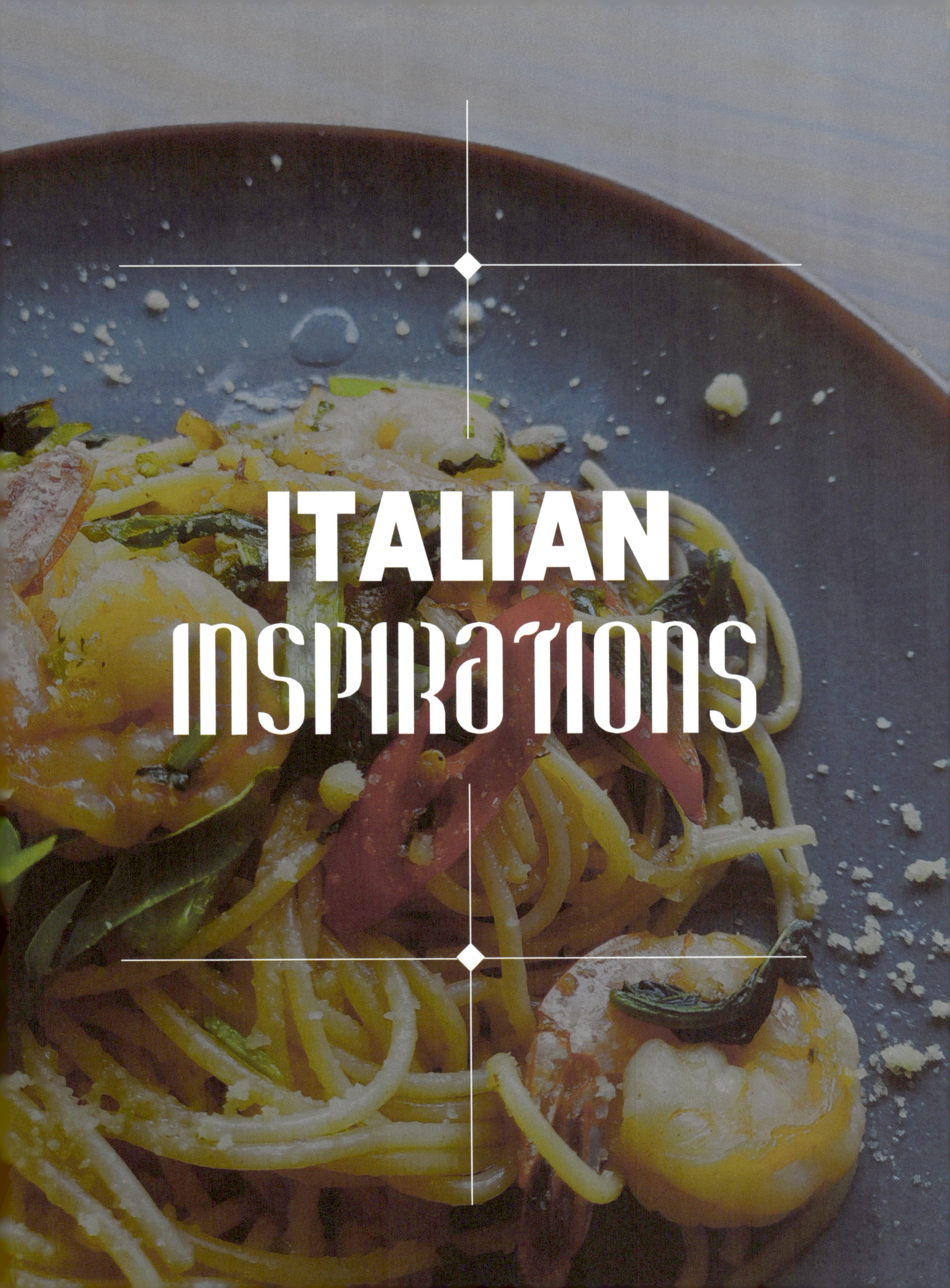

SEAFOOD

PESTO ZUCCHINI NOODLES with SHRIMP

2 servings

21g P | 14g C
38g F

485 per serving

Prep Time:
15 minutes

Cooking Time:
15 minutes

Total Time:
30 minutes

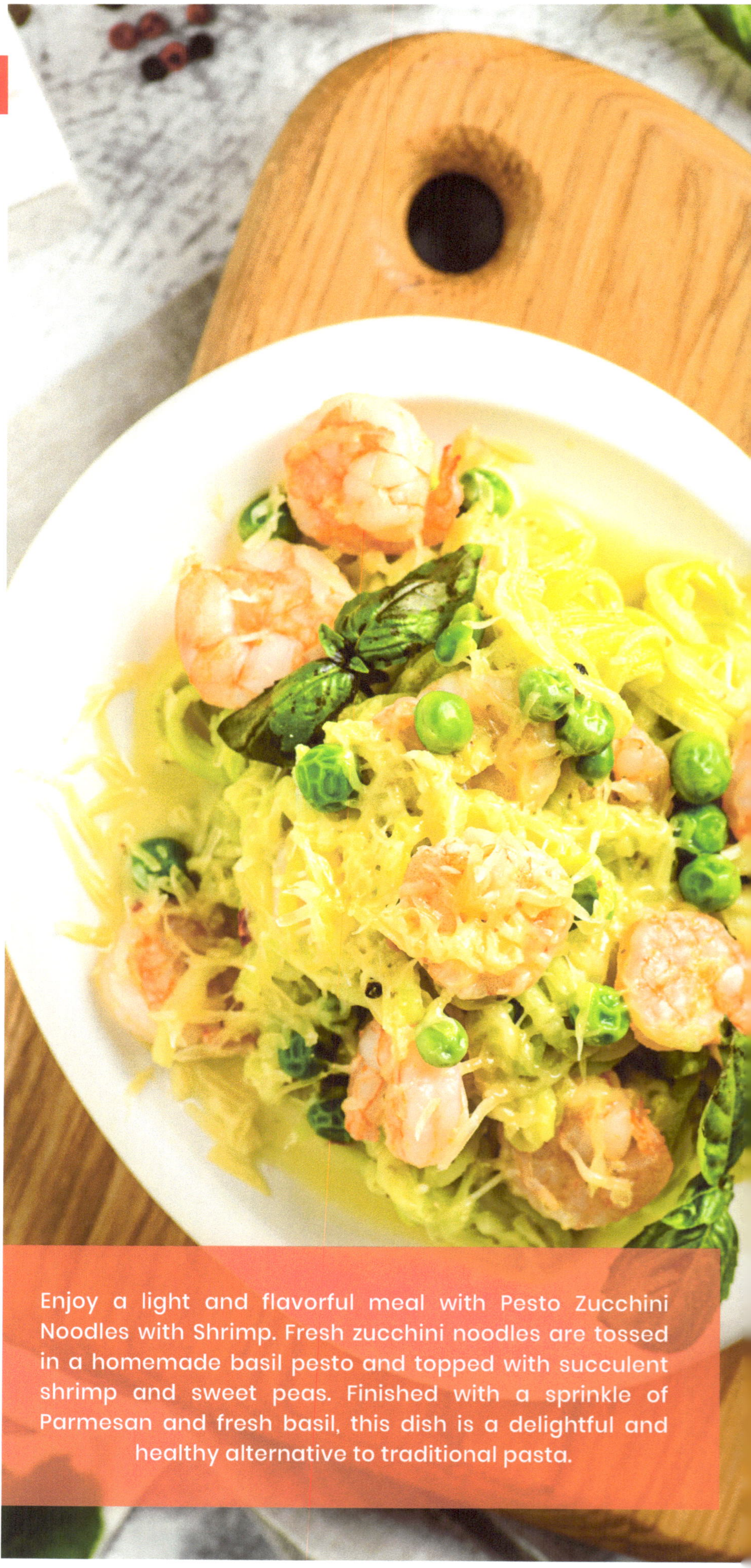

Enjoy a light and flavorful meal with Pesto Zucchini Noodles with Shrimp. Fresh zucchini noodles are tossed in a homemade basil pesto and topped with succulent shrimp and sweet peas. Finished with a sprinkle of Parmesan and fresh basil, this dish is a delightful and healthy alternative to traditional pasta.

INGREDIENTS

For the Pesto Sauce:

- 2 cups fresh basil leaves
- 1/2 cup grated Parmesan cheese
- 1/2 cup pine nuts
- 2 cloves garlic, minced
- 1/4 cup extra-virgin olive oil
- Juice of 1 lemon
- Salt and pepper to taste

For the Zucchini Noodles and Shrimp:

- 2 large zucchinis, spiralized into noodles (zoodles)
- 1 tablespoon olive oil
- 12 large shrimp, peeled and deveined
- 1/2 cup fresh or frozen peas
- 1/2 cup grated Parmesan cheese
- Fresh basil leaves for garnish

DIRECTIONS

Making Pesto Sauce:

1. In a food processor, combine fresh basil, grated Parmesan cheese, pine nuts, and minced garlic. Pulse until finely chopped.
2. While the processor is running, slowly drizzle in extra-virgin olive oil until the pesto reaches your desired consistency.
3. Add lemon juice, salt, and pepper; pulse to combine and adjust seasoning to taste.
4. Transfer the pesto to a bowl and set it aside.

Cooking Shrimp and Peas:

1. In a large skillet, heat olive oil over medium-high heat.
2. Add shrimp and cook for 2-3 minutes on each side until they turn pink and opaque.
3. Stir in peas and cook for an additional 2 minutes until heated through.
4. Remove shrimp and peas from the skillet and set aside

Preparing Zucchini Noodles:

1. In the same skillet, add zucchini noodles and cook for 2-3 minutes until just tender. Avoid overcooking.
2. Toss the cooked zoodles with 3/4 of the prepared pesto sauce until well coated, reserving the remaining pesto.

Assembling the Dish:

1. Divide the pesto-coated zucchini noodles between two serving plates.
2. Top with cooked shrimp and peas.
3. Sprinkle grated Parmesan cheese over the top.
4. Garnish with fresh basil leaves.

Serving:

1. Drizzle the remaining pesto sauce over each plate.
2. Serve your Pesto Zucchini Noodles with Shrimp immediately and enjoy!

Poultry

- Greek Chicken Souvlaki Wraps with Tzatziki Sauce
- Lavash Bread Pepperoni Pizza
- Mediterranean Sunshine Salad with Turmeric Chicken
- Savory Chicken & Spinach Tortilla Wrap
- Sundried Tomato and Mozzarella Stuffed Chicken

Seafood

- Baked Cod in Luscious Tomato Sauce
- Citrus Avocado Salmon Salad
- Grilled Salmon with Mango Salsa & Wilted Veggie Bed
- Mediterranean Salmon with Quinoa and Green Pea Puree
- Pan-Seared Salmon with Lemon Dill Sauce & Asparagus
- Savory Seafood Medley in Broth

Vegetarian

- Falafel Bowl with Zesty Tahini Dressing
- Mediterranean Orzo Pasta Salad
- Quinoa Bowl with Roasted Eggplant and Hummus
- Tomato and Red Lentil Soup with Homemade Croutons

MEDITERRANEAN Treasures

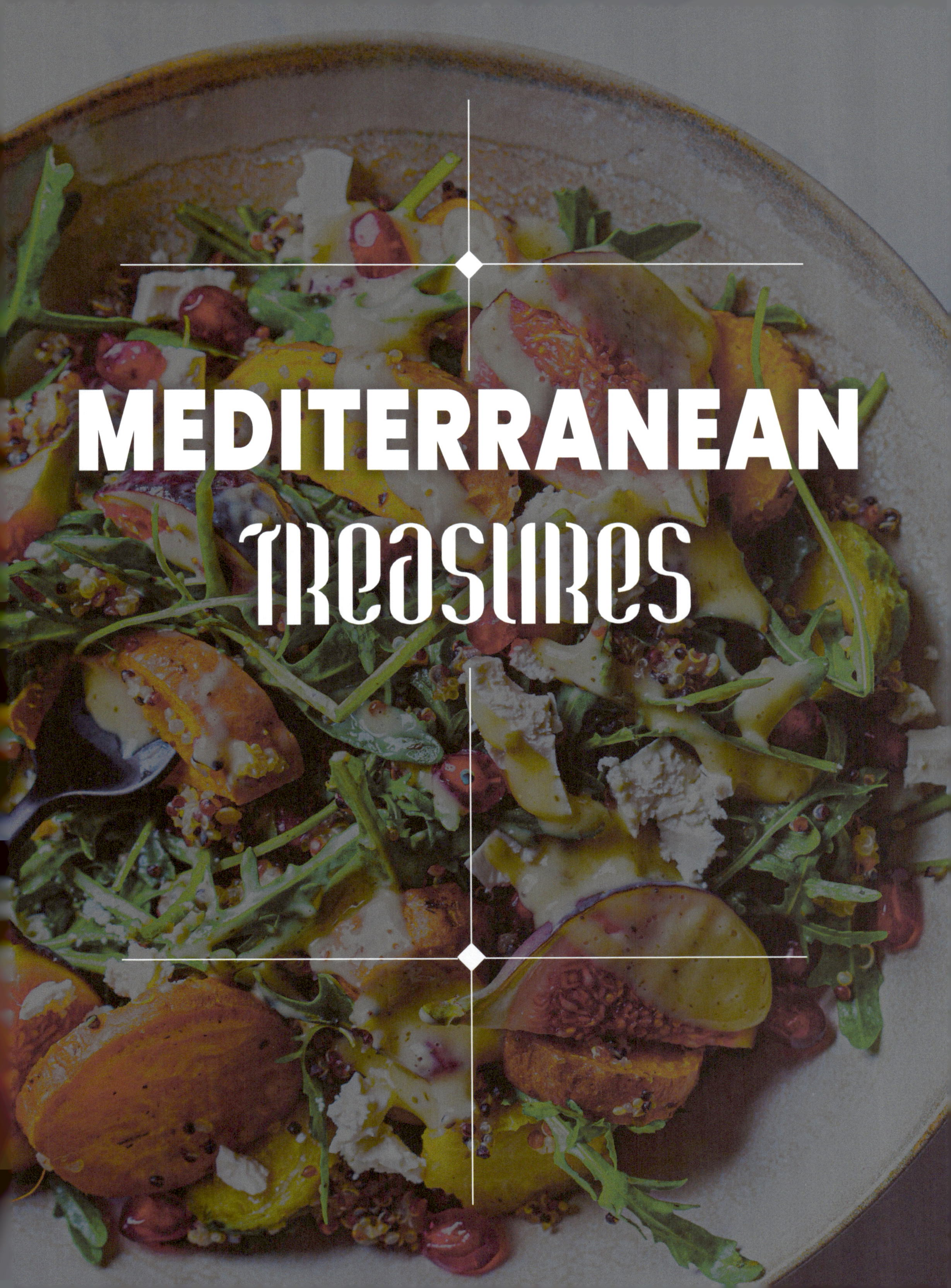

INGREDIENTS

For the Chicken Souvlaki:

- 1 lb. (about 450g) boneless, skinless chicken breasts, cut into bite-sized pieces
- 2 cloves garlic, minced
- Juice of 1 lemon
- 2 tablespoons olive oil
- 1 teaspoon dried oregano
- Salt and black pepper to taste
- Wooden skewers (soak in water for 30 minutes prior to preparing the meal to prevent from burning on grill)

For Assembling the Wraps:

- 2 pieces of Stonefire Organic Original Naan
- 1 cup romaine lettuce, chopped
- 1 large tomato, cut into wedges
- 1/2 red onion, thinly sliced
- Tzatziki sauce (store-bought or homemade, see below)
- Lemon wedges for garnish

For the Homemade Tzatziki Sauce:

- 1 cup Greek yogurt
- 1/2 cucumber, grated and squeezed to remove excess moisture
- 2 cloves garlic, minced
- 1 tablespoon fresh dill, chopped

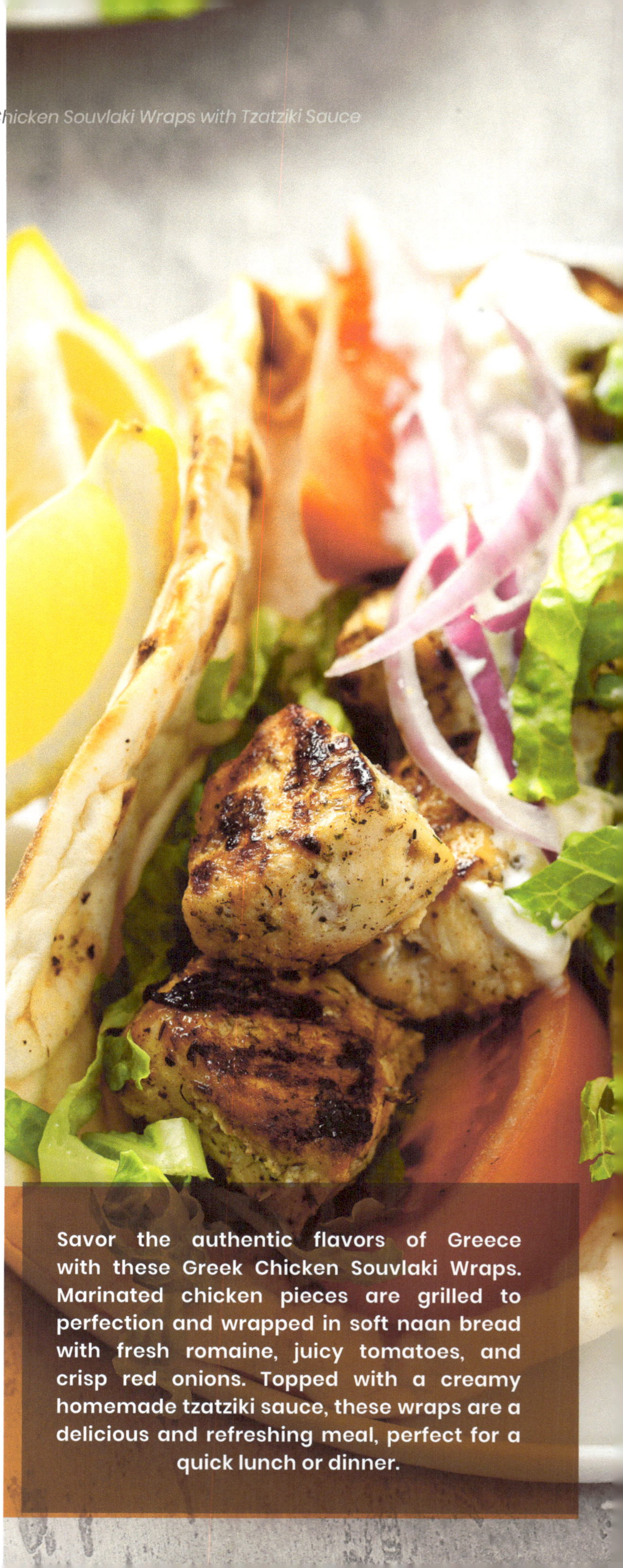

Savor the authentic flavors of Greece with these Greek Chicken Souvlaki Wraps. Marinated chicken pieces are grilled to perfection and wrapped in soft naan bread with fresh romaine, juicy tomatoes, and crisp red onions. Topped with a creamy homemade tzatziki sauce, these wraps are a delicious and refreshing meal, perfect for a quick lunch or dinner.

GREEK CHICKEN SOUVLAKI WRAPS with TZATZIKI SAUCE

2 servings	30g P | 35g C 15g F	360 per serving	Prep Time: 30 minutes	Cooking Time: 15 minutes	Total Time: 45 minutes

DIRECTIONS

Prepare the Chicken Souvlaki:

1. In a bowl, combine the minced garlic, lemon juice, olive oil, dried oregano, salt, and black pepper. Mix well to create the marinade.
2. Add the chicken pieces to the marinade and toss to coat. Cover and refrigerate for at least 30 minutes, allowing the flavors to infuse.
3. Skewer and Grill the Chicken:
4. Preheat a grill or grill pan over medium-high heat.
5. Thread the marinated chicken pieces onto wooden skewers that have been soaked in water for 30 minutes. This prevents them from burning on the grill.
6. Grill the chicken skewers for about 3-4 minutes per side or until they are cooked through, have grill marks, and are slightly charred.

Prepare the Tzatziki Sauce:

1. In a small bowl, combine the Greek yogurt, grated and squeezed cucumber, minced garlic, chopped fresh dill, chopped fresh mint, lemon juice, salt, and black pepper. Mix until well combined. Adjust the seasoning to taste.

Assemble the Greek Chicken Souvlaki Wraps:

1. Warm the round flatbreads or pita bread according to the package instructions.
2. Lay out each flatbread and spread a generous amount of tzatziki sauce on it.
3. Place a portion of grilled chicken skewers on each flatbread.
4. Add a generous handful of chopped romaine lettuce, tomato wedges, and thinly sliced red onion on top of the chicken.
5. Drizzle with extra tzatziki sauce if desired.

Garnish and Serve:

1. Garnish the wraps with lemon wedges.
2. Fold the flatbreads over the fillings and secure them with toothpicks if needed.
3. Serve the Greek Chicken Souvlaki Wraps immediately and enjoy!

1 servings

30g P | 16g C
15g F

375 per
serving

Prep Time:
10 minutes

Cooking Time:
15 minutes

Total Time:
25 minutes

Enjoy a healthier twist on a classic favorite with this Lavash Bread Pepperoni Pizza. Crisp and golden lavash bread serves as the perfect base for a generous layer of marinara, a blend of savory cheeses, and zesty turkey pepperoni. Finished with a touch of fresh arugula, this pizza is a delightful balance of flavors and textures, offering a satisfying meal that's both delicious and nutritious.

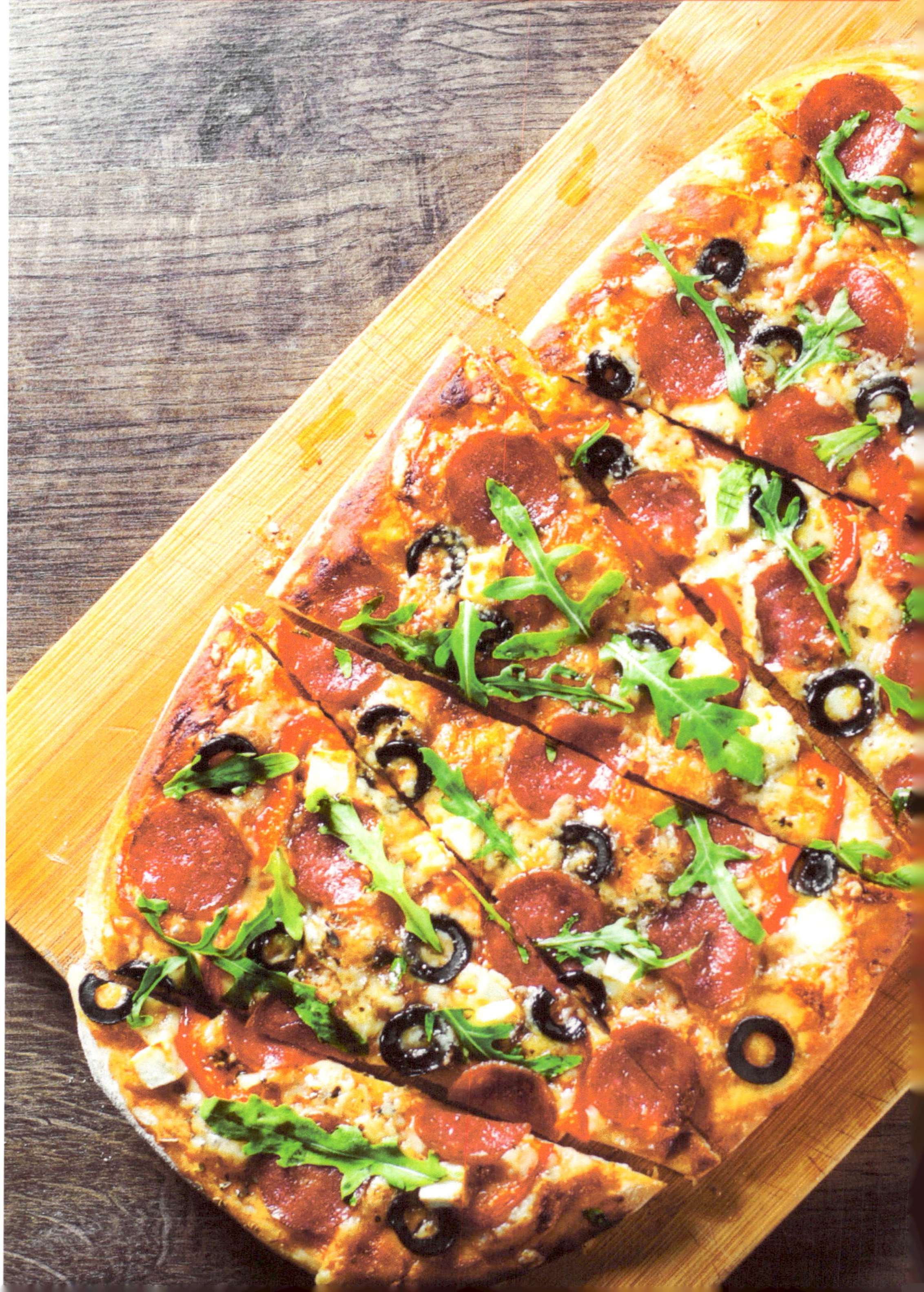

LAVASH BREAD PEPPERONI PIZZA

INGREDIENTS

- 1 sheet of Joseph's flax, oat bran & whole wheat lavash bread
- Olive oil cooking spray
- 2-3 tablespoons marinara sauce
- Italian seasoning blend (to taste)
- 17 pieces of Hormel turkey pepperoni (70g less fat)
- 1/4 cup shredded white cheese blend
- 1 tablespoon grated Parmesan cheese
- Black olives, sliced
- Handful of fresh arugula
- Red pepper flakes (optional, for garnish)

DIRECTIONS

1. Preheat your oven to 400°F (200°C).
2. Place the lavash bread on a baking sheet and lightly spray it with olive oil cooking spray. Bake in the preheated oven for 5 minutes or until it becomes slightly golden and crispy.
3. Remove the lavash bread from the oven and let it cool slightly.
4. Assembling Your Pizza:
5. Spread 2-3 tablespoons of marinara sauce evenly over the lavash bread, leaving a small border around the edges. Sprinkle Italian seasoning blend over the sauce.
6. Lay 15 slices of pepperoni evenly over the sauce.
7. Sprinkle a quarter cup of shredded white cheese blend over the pepperoni.
8. Add a tablespoon of grated Parmesan cheese.
9. Scatter sliced black olives and a small sprinkling of crumbled feta cheese over the cheese.
10. Place the lavash pizza back in the oven for 7-8 minutes, or until the cheese is melted and bubbly, and the edges of the lavash are golden brown.
11. Remove the pizza from the oven and let it cool for a minute.
12. Garnish with a handful of fresh arugula for a peppery, fresh kick.
13. If you like a bit of heat, sprinkle red pepper flakes over the pizza as desired.
14. Slice and enjoy your delicious Lavash Bread Pepperoni Pizza! Note: The nutritional information is approximate and can vary based on specific brands and ingredient quantities. Enjoy your healthy pizza!

MEDITERRANEAN Sunshine SALAD with GRILLED TURMERIC CHICKEN

DIRECTIONS

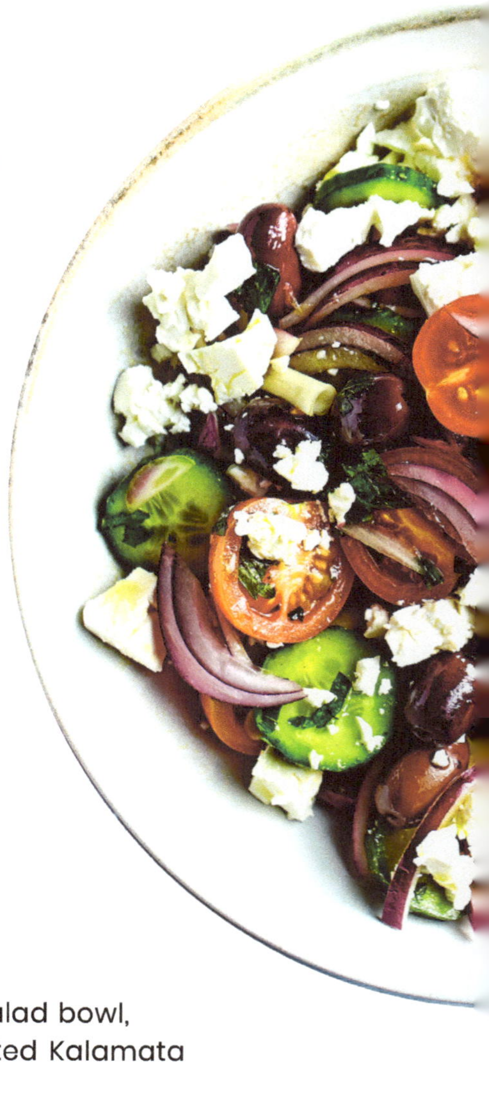

Marinate the Chicken:

1. In a small bowl, whisk together the Greek yogurt, ground turmeric, paprika, garlic powder, salt, and black pepper. Place the chicken breasts in a resealable plastic bag or a shallow dish and pour the marinade over them. Seal the bag or cover the dish and refrigerate for at least 10 minutes, or longer if time allows.

Prepare the Vinaigrette:

1. In a small bowl, whisk together the extra-virgin olive oil, lemon juice, dried oregano, dried basil, honey, salt, and black pepper. Set aside.

Grill the Chicken:

1. Preheat your grill or grill pan over medium-high heat. Remove the chicken from the marinade, allowing any excess to drip off.
2. Grill the chicken breasts for about 4-5 minutes per side, or until they are cooked through and have a golden-yellow color. Cooking time may vary based on the thickness of the chicken breasts.

Assemble the Salad:

1. While the chicken is grilling, prepare the salad. In a large salad bowl, combine the diced cucumber, halved grape tomatoes, pitted Kalamata olives, thinly sliced red onion, and crumbled feta cheese.
2. Once the chicken is done, remove it from the grill and let it rest for 2-3 minutes. Then, slice it into thin strips.
3. Drizzle the lemon-honey-based vinaigrette over the salad and toss gently to combine.
4. Divide the salad between two plates and top with the grilled turmeric chicken slices and enjoy!

2 servings

35g P | 14g C
20g F

370 per serving

Prep Time: 15 minutes

Cooking Time: 10 minutes

Total Time: 25 minutes

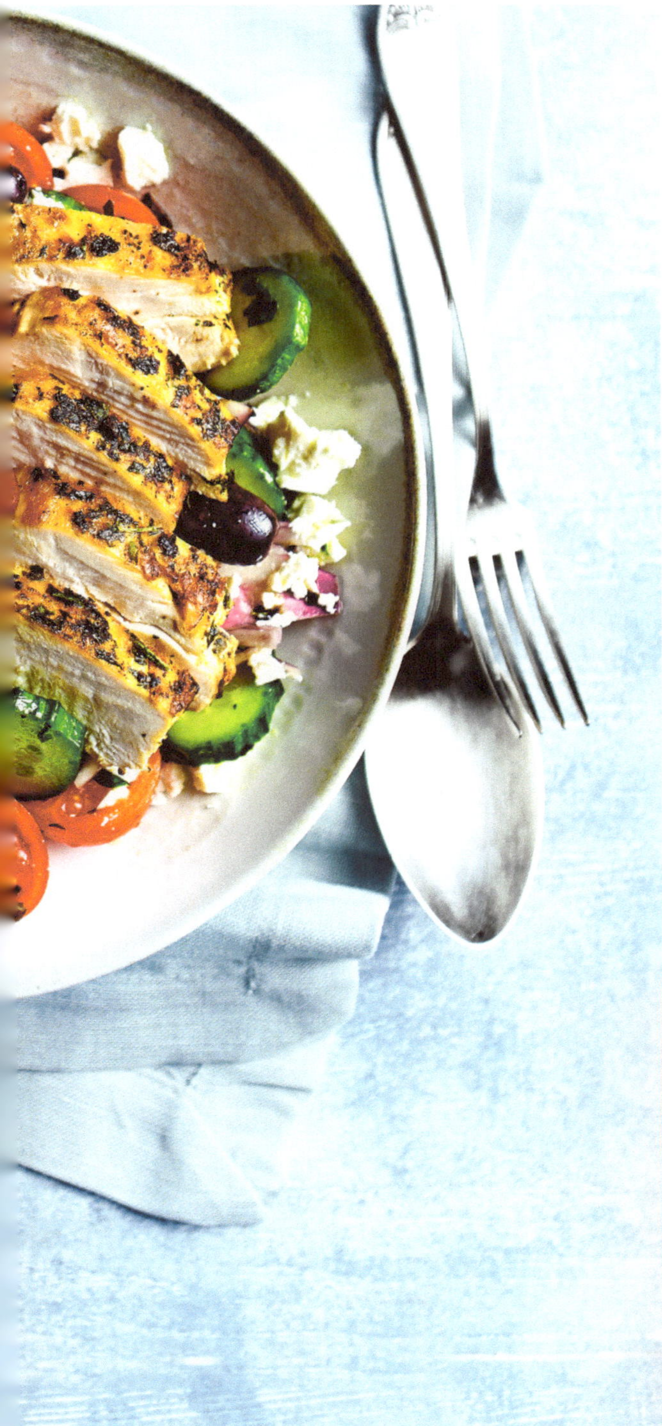

INGREDIENTS

For the Salad:

- 2 boneless, skinless chicken breasts
- 1 English cucumber, diced
- 1 cup grape tomatoes, halved
- 1/2 cup pitted Kalamata olives
- 1/4 red onion, thinly sliced
- 1/2 cup crumbled feta cheese

For the Chicken Marinade:

- 1/2 cup plain Greek yogurt
- 1 teaspoon ground turmeric
- 1 teaspoon paprika
- 1 teaspoon garlic powder
- Salt and black pepper to taste

For the Lemon-Honey-Based Vinaigrette:

- 3 tablespoons extra-virgin olive oil
- Juice of 1 lemon
- 1 teaspoon dried oregano
- 1/2 teaspoon dried basil
- 2 teaspoons honey
- Salt and black pepper to taste

Brighten your day with the Mediterranean Sunshine Salad with Grilled Turmeric Chicken. Juicy, marinated chicken breast is grilled to a golden hue and served atop a fresh salad of cucumbers, tomatoes, olives, and feta cheese. Drizzled with a zesty lemon-honey vinaigrette, this salad is a burst of vibrant flavors and wholesome goodness.

2 servings	25g P | 30g C 20g F	400 per serving	Prep Time: 15 minutes	Cooking Time: 10 minutes	Total Time: 25 minutes

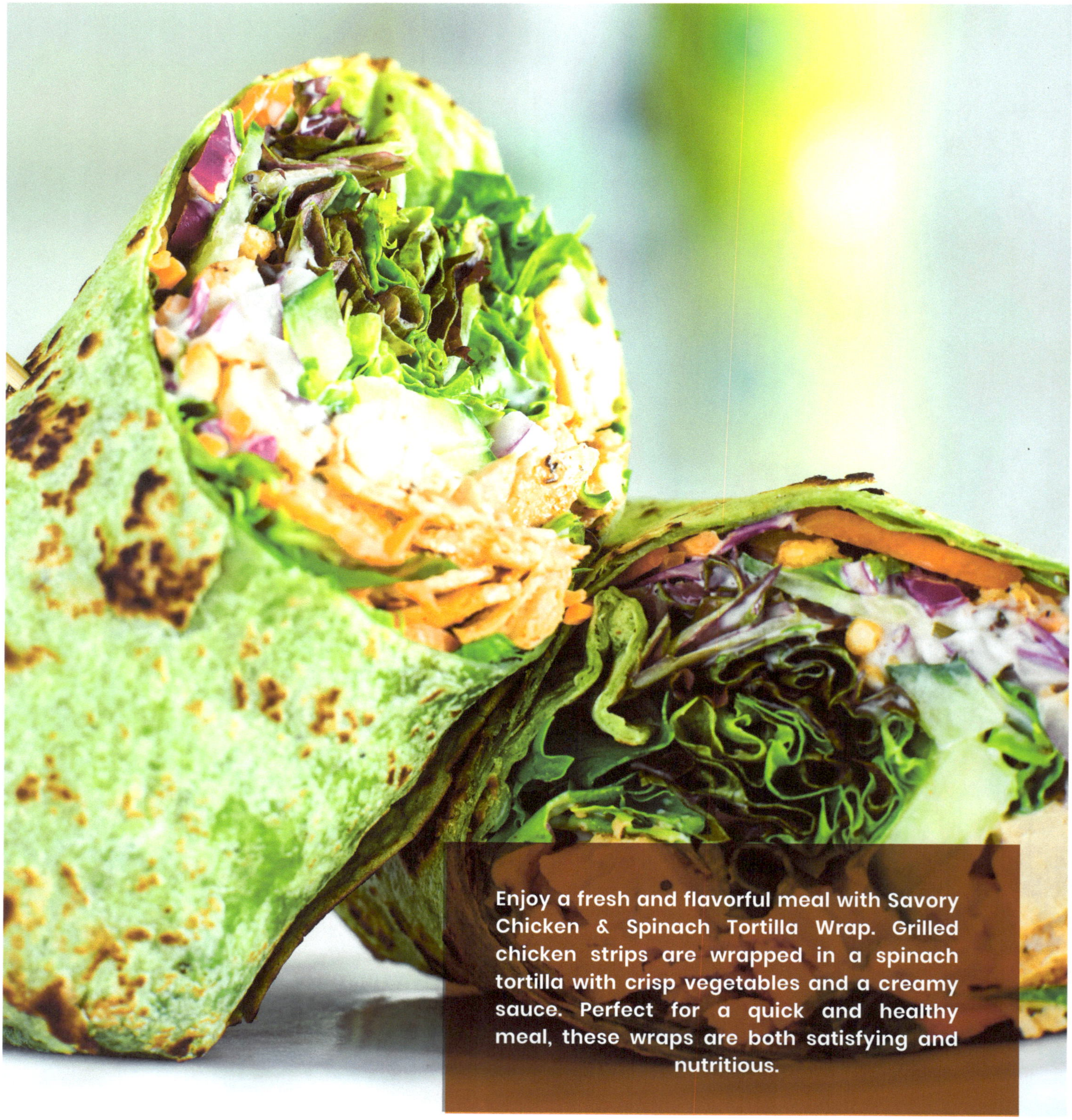

Enjoy a fresh and flavorful meal with Savory Chicken & Spinach Tortilla Wrap. Grilled chicken strips are wrapped in a spinach tortilla with crisp vegetables and a creamy sauce. Perfect for a quick and healthy meal, these wraps are both satisfying and nutritious.

SAVORY CHICKEN & SPINACH TORTILLA WRAP

INGREDIENTS

For the Chicken:

- 1 boneless, skinless chicken breast
- 1 tablespoon olive oil
- Salt and black pepper to taste
- 1/4 teaspoon garlic powder
- 1/4 teaspoon paprika
- 1/4 teaspoon dried oregano (optional)

For the Wraps:

- 2 spinach tortilla wraps
- 1 cup spring mix greens
- 1/2 cup shredded carrot
- 1/2 cup thinly sliced red cabbage
- 1/2 cup shaved cucumber
- 1/4 cup thinly sliced red onion

For the Creamy Sauce:

- 2 tablespoons Greek yogurt
- 1 tablespoon mayonnaise
- 1 tablespoon Dijon mustard
- 1 clove garlic, minced
- 1/4 teaspoon honey
- Salt and black pepper to taste

DIRECTIONS

Prepare the Chicken:

1. Season the chicken breast with salt, black pepper, garlic powder, paprika, and dried oregano (if using).
2. Heat olive oil in a pan over medium-high heat. Add the seasoned chicken breast and cook for about 5-6 minutes per side or until fully cooked and no longer pink in the center. The internal temperature should reach 165°F (74°C) to ensure it's fully cooked and safe to eat. You can use a meat thermometer to check the internal temperature of the chicken breast.
3. Remove the chicken from the pan and let it rest for a few minutes. Slice it into thin strips.

Prepare the Creamy Sauce:

1. In a small bowl, whisk together Greek yogurt, mayonnaise, Dijon mustard, minced garlic, honey, salt, and black pepper until smooth.

Assembly:

1. Lay out the spinach tortilla wraps.
2. Spread the creamy sauce evenly over each tortilla.
3. Divide the sliced chicken, spring mix greens, shredded carrot, red cabbage, shaved cucumber, and red onion slices between the two tortillas.
4. Carefully fold in the sides of each tortilla, then roll it up tightly from the bottom to create a wrap.
5. Slice in half and serve immediately or wrap them in foil for an on-the-go meal.

SUNDRIED TOMATO AND MOZZARELLA STUFFED CHICKEN

2 servings

42g P | 2g C
23g F

410 per serving

Prep Time: 10 minutes

Cooking Time: 20 minutes

Total Time: 30 minutes

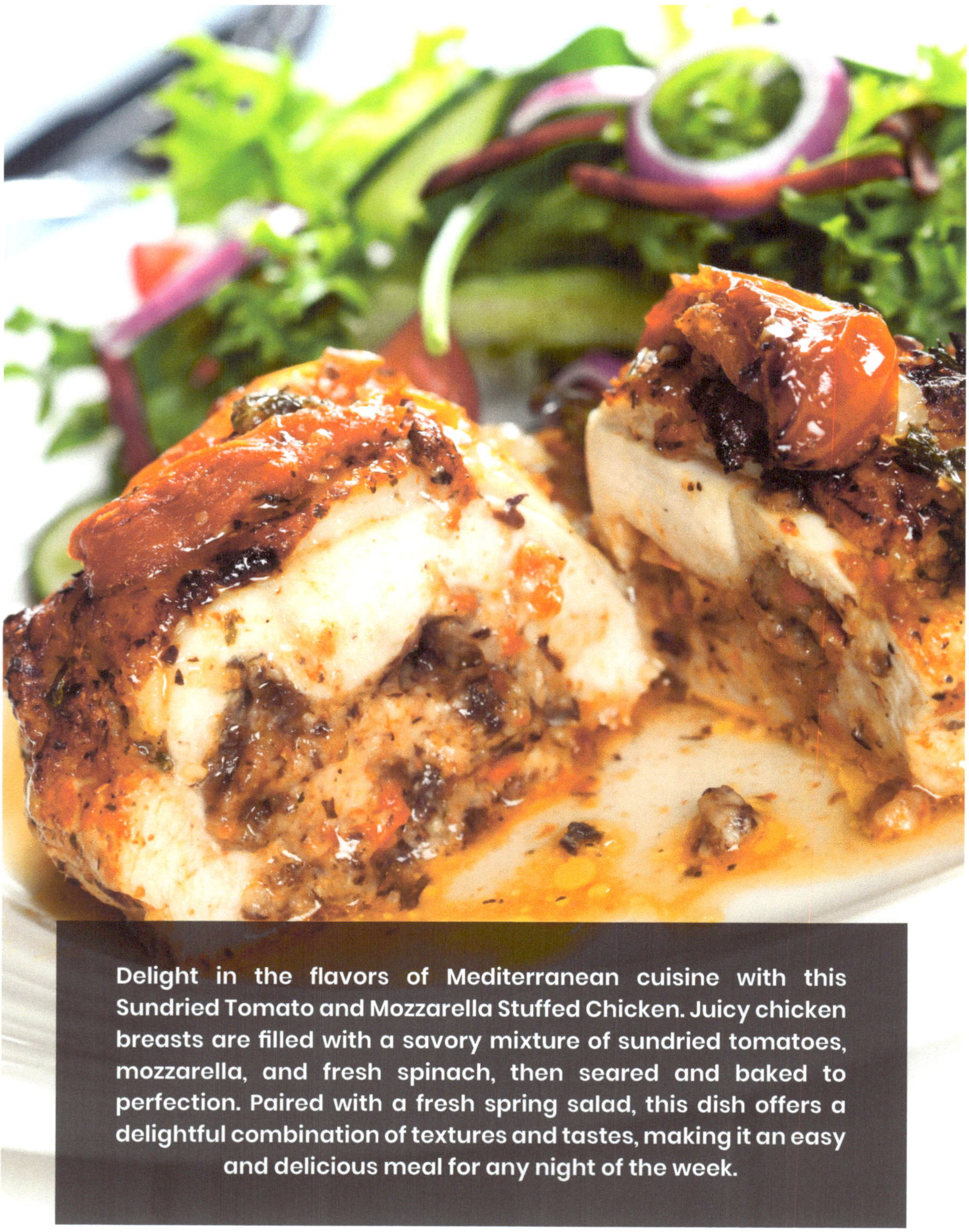

Delight in the flavors of Mediterranean cuisine with this Sundried Tomato and Mozzarella Stuffed Chicken. Juicy chicken breasts are filled with a savory mixture of sundried tomatoes, mozzarella, and fresh spinach, then seared and baked to perfection. Paired with a fresh spring salad, this dish offers a delightful combination of textures and tastes, making it an easy and delicious meal for any night of the week.

INGREDIENTS

For the Chicken:

- 2 boneless, skinless chicken breasts
- 1/2 cup shredded mozzarella cheese
- 1/4 cup sundried tomatoes, chopped
- 1/2 cup fresh spinach, chopped
- 1 clove garlic, minced
- 1 tablespoon olive oil
- 1 tablespoon fresh basil, chopped (or 1 teaspoon dried basil)
- 1/2 teaspoon dried oregano
- Salt and pepper to taste
- Toothpicks or kitchen twine
- 1/2 cup cherry or grape tomatoes, halved

For the Spring Salad:

- 2 cups mixed spring greens
- 1/4 red onion, thinly sliced
- 1/2 cucumber, thinly sliced
- 1/4 cup cherry or grape tomatoes, halved
- 2 tablespoons olive oil
- 1 tablespoon balsamic vinegar
- Salt and pepper to taste

DIRECTIONS

1. Preheat your oven to 375°F (190°C).
2. In a bowl, mix the shredded mozzarella, chopped sundried tomatoes, and half of the chopped spinach.
3. Using a sharp knife, make a horizontal cut along the side of each chicken breast to create a pocket, being careful not to cut all the way through.
4. Stuff each chicken breast with the mozzarella, sundried tomato, and spinach mixture. Secure with toothpicks or kitchen twine if necessary.
5. In a small bowl, mix the minced garlic, olive oil, chopped basil, dried oregano, salt, and pepper. Brush this mixture over the stuffed chicken breasts.
6. Heat an oven-safe skillet over medium-high heat and sear the chicken breasts for 2-3 minutes on each side until golden brown.
7. Transfer the skillet to the preheated oven and bake for 15-20 minutes, or until the chicken is cooked through and reaches an internal temperature of 165°F (74°C).
8. In the last 5 minutes of baking, top each chicken breast with the remaining chopped spinach and halved cherry or grape tomatoes.
9. Remove the toothpicks or twine before serving.

Spring Salad:

1. In a large bowl, combine mixed spring greens, thinly sliced red onion, cucumber, and halved cherry or grape tomatoes.
2. In a small bowl, whisk together olive oil, balsamic vinegar, salt, and pepper.
3. Drizzle the dressing over the salad and toss to combine.

Serving Suggestion:

1. Serve the stuffed chicken breasts with the fresh spring salad on the side for a light and flavorful meal.

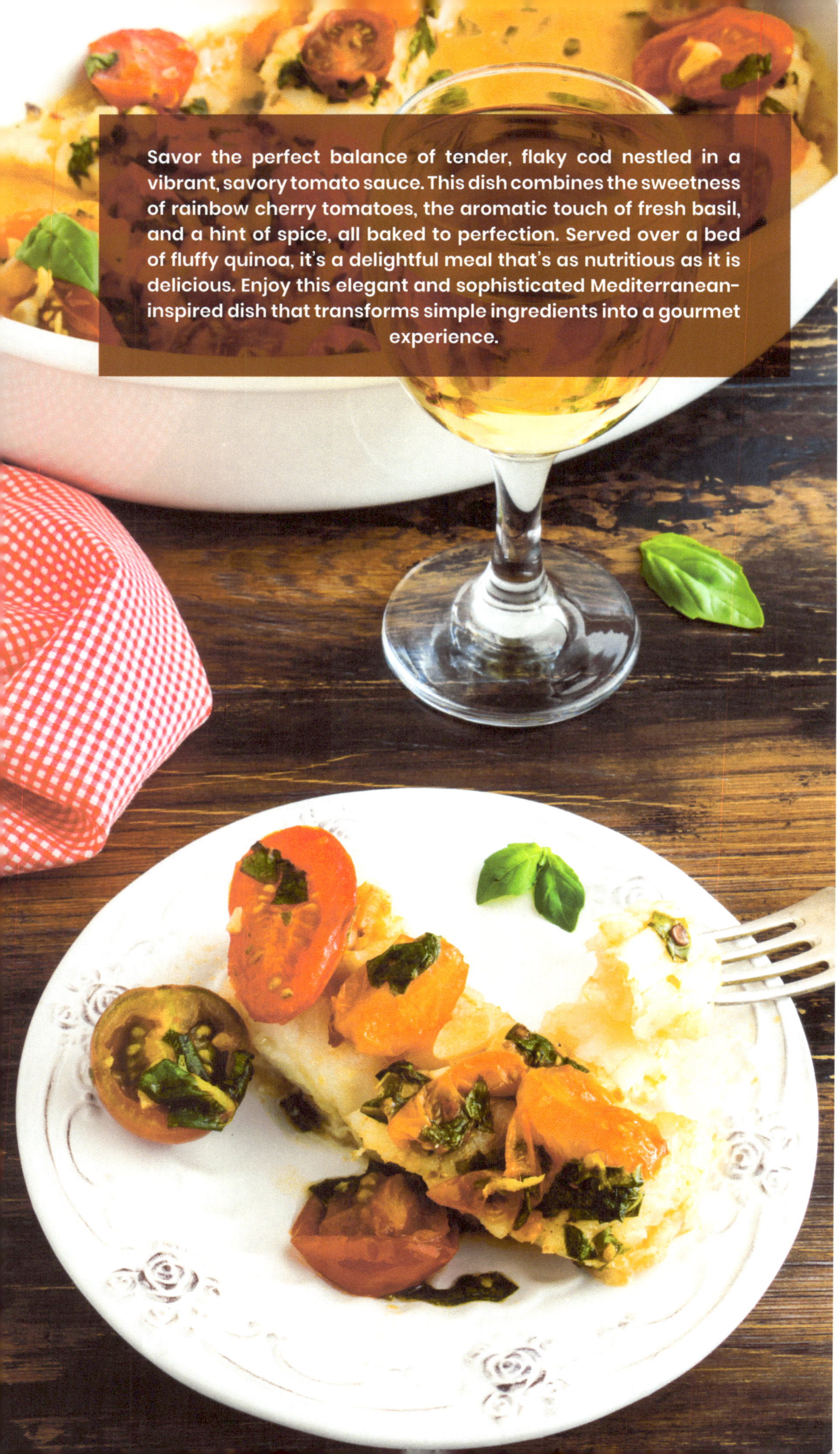

Savor the perfect balance of tender, flaky cod nestled in a vibrant, savory tomato sauce. This dish combines the sweetness of rainbow cherry tomatoes, the aromatic touch of fresh basil, and a hint of spice, all baked to perfection. Served over a bed of fluffy quinoa, it's a delightful meal that's as nutritious as it is delicious. Enjoy this elegant and sophisticated Mediterranean-inspired dish that transforms simple ingredients into a gourmet experience.

2 servings

30g P | 28g C
14g F

350 per serving

Prep Time:
15 minutes

Cooking Time:
15 minutes

Total Time:
30 minutes

SEAFOOD

BAKED COD in LUSCIOUS TOMATO SAUCE

INGREDIENTS

- 2 cod fillets (6-8 ounces each)
- 1 cup rainbow cherry tomatoes, halved
- 1/2 cup diced onion
- 2 cloves garlic, minced
- 1/4 cup fresh basil leaves, chopped
- 2 tablespoons olive oil
- 1 teaspoon dried oregano
- 1 teaspoon dried basil
- Salt and pepper to taste
- 1/2 teaspoon red pepper flakes
- 1 teaspoon honey
- 2 tablespoons salted butter
- 1/2 cup chicken stock
- 1 Lemon cut into four wedges
- Fresh basil leaf for garnish
- *Cooked quinoa, for serving*

DIRECTIONS

1. Preheat your oven to 375°F (190°C).
2. Prepare quinoa according to instructions on package.
3. Place the cod fillets in a baking dish and season them with 1 tablespoon of olive oil, salt, pepper, and the juice of half a lemon. Bake in the preheated oven for 15-20 minutes or until the cod is cooked through and flakes easily with a fork.
4. In a skillet, heat the 1 tablespoon of olive oil over medium heat. Add the diced onion and minced garlic, and sauté until the onion turns translucent, about 2-3 minutes.
5. Add the cherry tomatoes to the skillet and cook for an additional 3-4 minutes, or until they begin to soften and release their juices.
6. Add chicken stock and stir in salt, pepper, red pepper flakes, honey. Cook for another 1-2 minutes.
7. Stir in the salted butter until the sauce slightly thickens.
8. While the cod is baking, continue simmering the tomato sauce until it reaches your desired consistency. You will add the dried oregano and dried basil to the tomato sauce just as the cod has finished baking.
9. Once the cod is done, pour the tomato sauce over the fillets in the baking dish.
10. To serve, place a portion of cooked quinoa on each plate. Top with the tomato sauce and a cod fillet. Garnish with fresh basil leaves and lemon wedge.

CITRUS AVOCADO SALMON SALAD

DIRECTIONS

Prepare the Salmon:

1. Season the salmon fillets with salt, pepper, minced garlic, and dried oregano.
2. Heat a non-stick skillet over medium-high heat. Add 1 teaspoon of olive oil.
3. Cook the salmon fillets for about 4-6 minutes per side, or until they are cooked through and have a nice golden crust. Remove from heat and let rest.

Make the Balsamic Vinaigrette:

1. In a small bowl, whisk together the olive oil, balsamic vinegar, Dijon mustard, honey, minced garlic, salt, and pepper until well combined.

Assemble the Salad:

1. Divide the spring greens mix evenly between two plates.
2. Arrange the blood orange slices, avocado slices, and lime wedges on top of the greens.
3. Sprinkle each salad with 1 tablespoon of pine nuts.
4. Optionally, add 1/2 cup of cooked quinoa to each plate under the greens.
5. Place a cooked salmon fillet atop each salad.
6. Drizzle 2 tablespoons of balsamic vinaigrette over each salad.
7. Serve immediately.

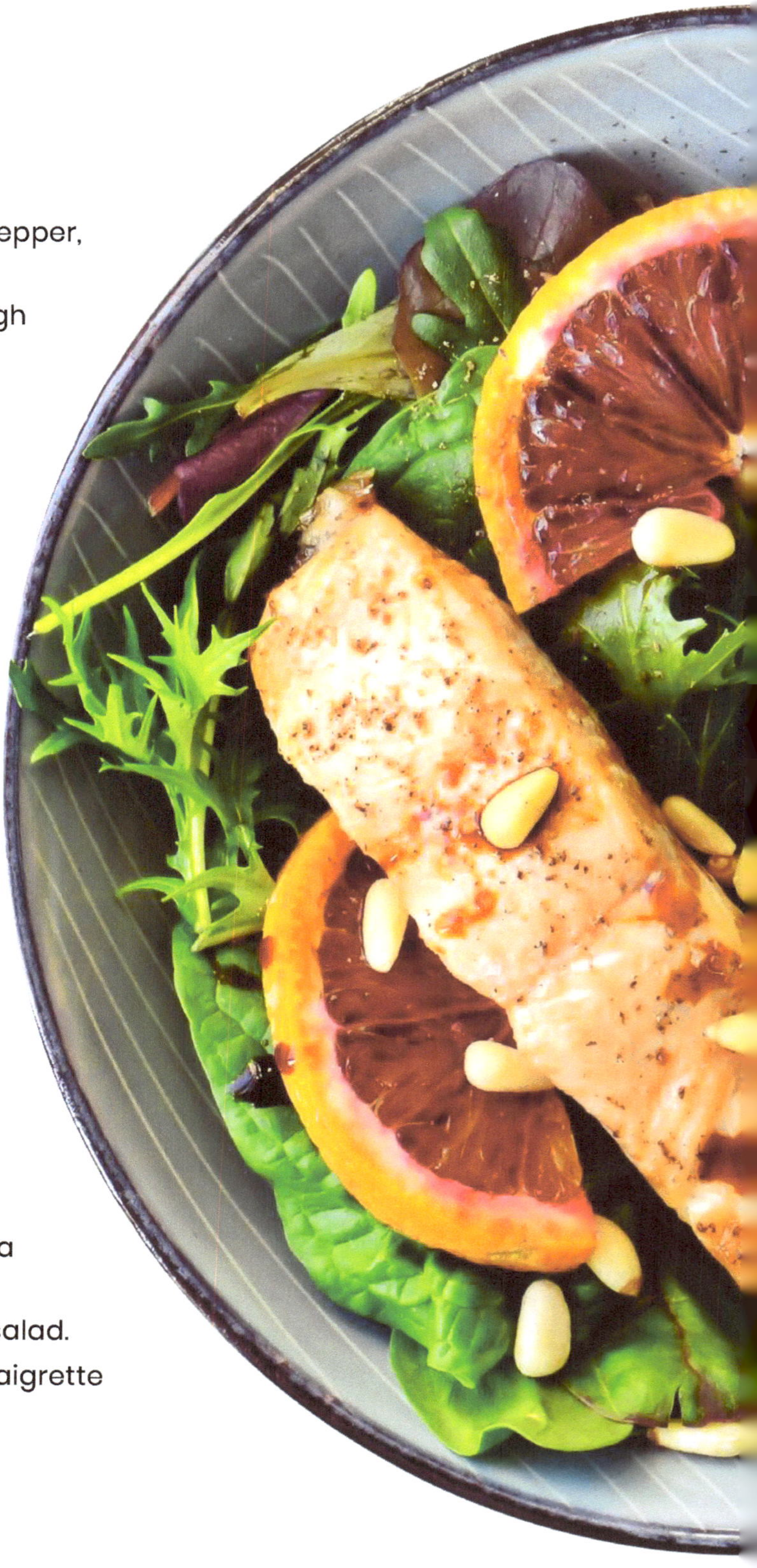

2 servings

35g P | 20g C
25g F

450 per
serving

Prep Time:
10 minutes

Cooking Time:
15 minutes

Total Time:
25 minutes

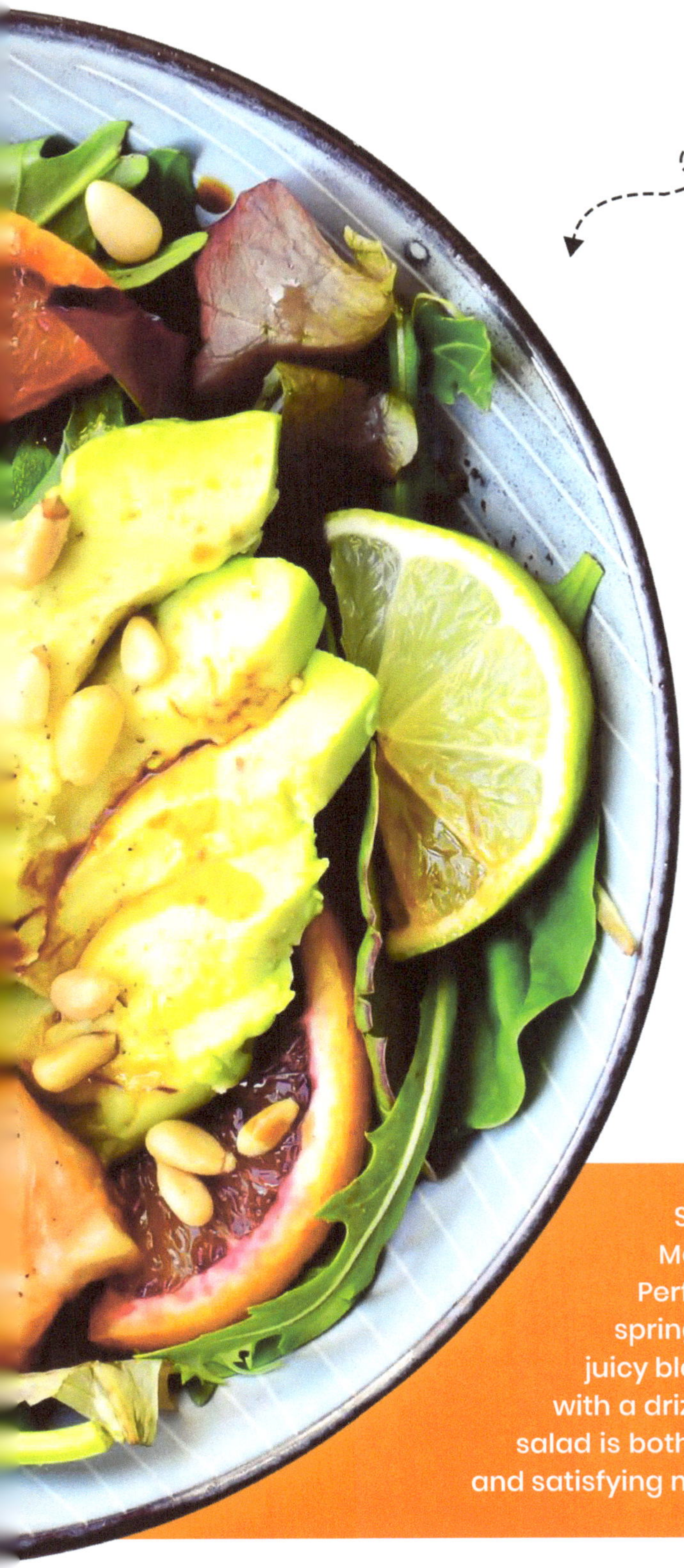

INGREDIENTS

For the Salad:

- 2 salmon fillets (about 6 oz each)
- Salt and pepper to taste
- 2 cloves garlic, minced
- 1 teaspoon dried oregano
- 1 teaspoon olive oil
- 4 cups spring greens mix
- 1 avocado, sliced
- 6 slices of blood orange (about 1 small blood orange)
- 1 lime, cut into wedges
- 2 tablespoons pine nuts
- 4 tablespoons balsamic vinaigrette (recipe below)

For the Balsamic Vinaigrette:

- 1/4 cup extra-virgin olive oil
- 2 tablespoons balsamic vinegar
- 1 teaspoon Dijon mustard
- 1 teaspoon honey
- 1 small garlic clove, minced
- Salt and pepper to taste

Optional:

- 1 cup cooked quinoa (to serve under the greens)

Savor the fresh and vibrant flavors of the Mediterranean with this exquisite Salmon Salad. Perfectly grilled salmon fillets rest on a bed of crisp spring greens, accompanied by creamy avocado, juicy blood orange slices, and crunchy pine nuts. Finished with a drizzle of zesty homemade balsamic vinaigrette, this salad is both nutritious and delicious—perfect for a refreshing and satisfying meal.

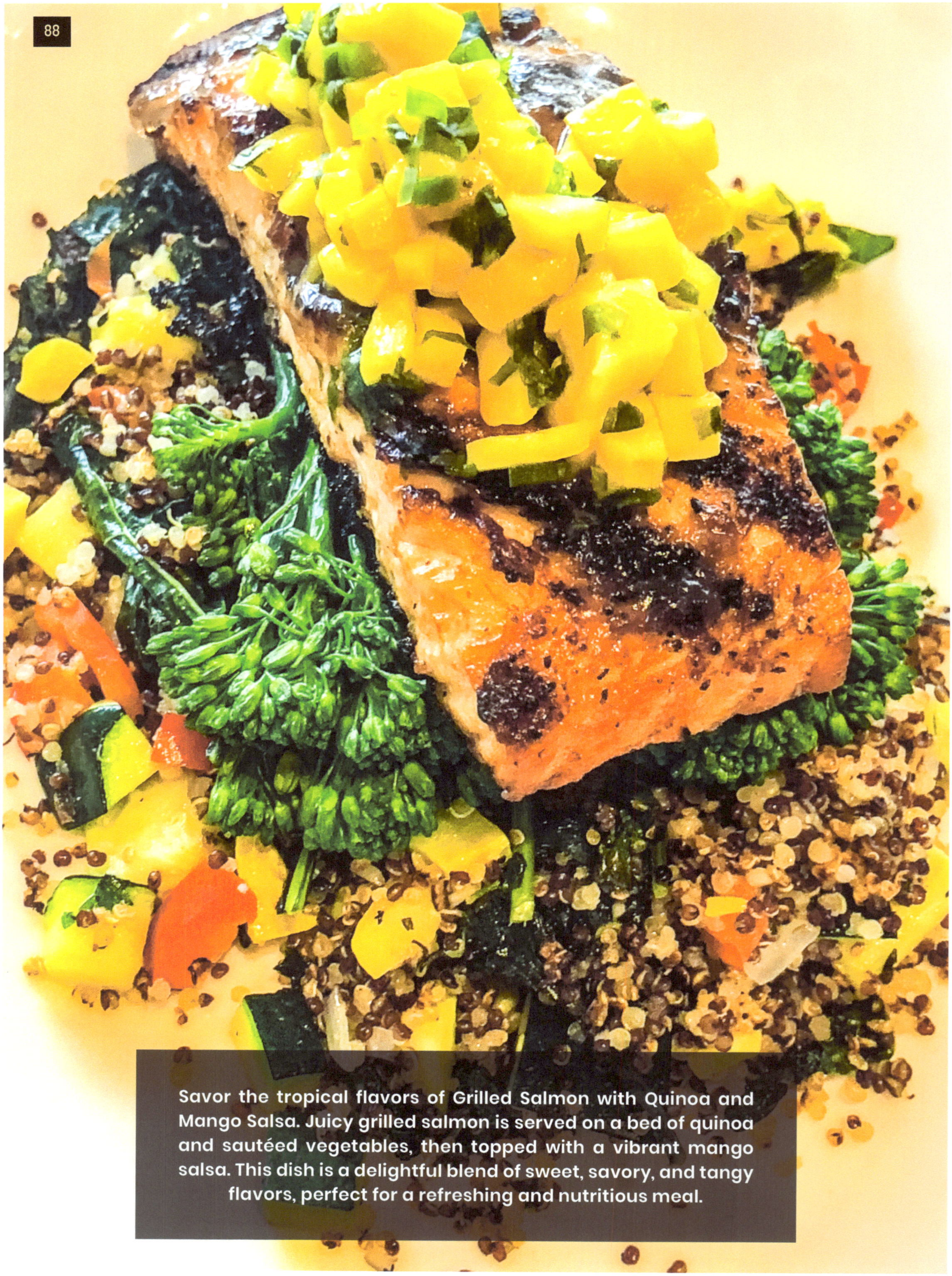

Savor the tropical flavors of Grilled Salmon with Quinoa and Mango Salsa. Juicy grilled salmon is served on a bed of quinoa and sautéed vegetables, then topped with a vibrant mango salsa. This dish is a delightful blend of sweet, savory, and tangy flavors, perfect for a refreshing and nutritious meal.

GRILLED SALMON with MANGO SALSA & WILTED VEGGIE BED

2 servings	32g P | 45g C 20g F	475 per serving	Prep Time: 20 minutes	Cooking Time: 15 minutes	Total Time: 35 minutes

INGREDIENTS

For the Grilled Salmon:

- 2 salmon fillets (about 6 ounces each)
- 1 tablespoon olive oil
- Salt and pepper to taste
- Lemon wedges for garnish (optional)

For the Cooked Veggie Bed:

- 2 cups mixed greens (such as arugula or baby kale)
- 1/2 cup diced red bell pepper
- 1/2 cup diced green zucchini
- 1 cup cooked quinoa
- 1 cup blanched broccolini

For the Mango Salsa:

- 1 ripe mango, diced
- 2 green spring onions, thinly sliced
- 1 tablespoon lime juice
- 1/2 teaspoon red pepper flakes (optional)
- Salt and pepper to taste

DIRECTIONS

1. Preheat your grill to medium-high heat.
2. Season the salmon fillets with olive oil, salt, and pepper.
3. Grill the salmon fillets for about 3-4 minutes per side, or until the salmon flakes easily with a fork and has grill marks. Cooking time may vary depending on the thickness of your salmon fillets. Remove from the grill and set aside.
4. In a large skillet, heat a bit of olive oil over medium heat. Add the diced red bell pepper, diced green zucchini, and blanched long broccoli florets. Sauté for about 4-5 minutes or until they are tender-crisp and slightly charred.
5. In a large bowl, mix together the mixed greens, cooked quinoa, and the sautéed vegetables.
6. In a separate bowl, prepare the mango salsa by mixing diced mango, thinly sliced green spring onions, lime juice, red pepper flakes (if using), salt, and pepper.
7. To serve, place a portion of the cooked veggie bed on each plate, top with a grilled salmon fillet, and then spoon the mango salsa over the salmon.

MEDITERRANEAN SALMON with QUINOA & GREEN PEA PURÉE

DIRECTIONS

Start by preparing the Green Pea Purée:

1. If using frozen peas, cook them according to the package instructions. If using fresh peas, blanch them in boiling water for 2-3 minutes, then drain.
2. In a blender or food processor, combine the cooked peas, minced garlic, fresh mint leaves, extra-virgin olive oil, salt, and black pepper. Blend until smooth. Set aside.

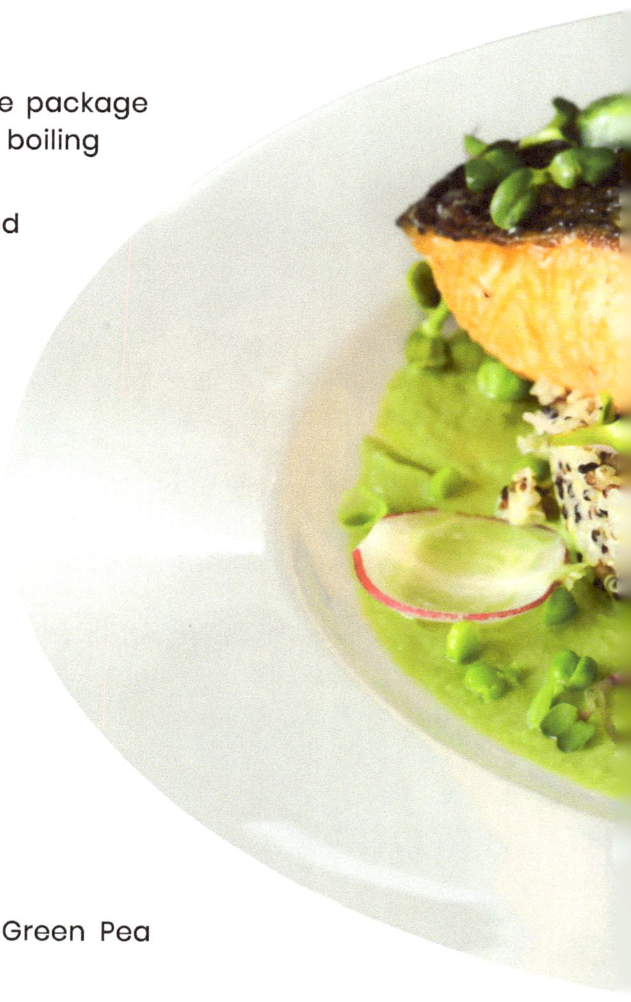

Next, Prepare the Salmon:

1. Season the salmon fillets with salt and pepper. Grill or bake them until they reach your desired level of doneness. This usually takes around 4 minutes per side for medium-rare. Once done, set the salmon aside.

Steam the Asparagus Spears:

1. Steam the asparagus spears until they are tender but still crisp, about 2-3 minutes. Set aside.

Assemble the Plate:

1. Start by spreading a generous spoonful of the Green Pea Purée at the bottom of each serving bowl.
2. Place 4 thin slices of crisp radish on top of the pea puree.
3. Add a layer of multigrain quinoa over the vegetable slices.
4. Carefully place a grilled or baked salmon fillet on top of the quinoa.
5. Top the salmon with the additional radish slices and the steamed asparagus spears.
6. Garnish the Mediterranean Salmon Bowl with pea shoot microgreens for a burst of freshness.
7. Serve with lemon wedges on the side for squeezing over the salmon and enjoy this restaurant-worthy meal in the comfort of your home.

2 servings	38g P | 41g C 20g F	460 per serving	Prep Time: 15 minutes	Cooking Time: 20 minutes	Total Time: 35 minutes

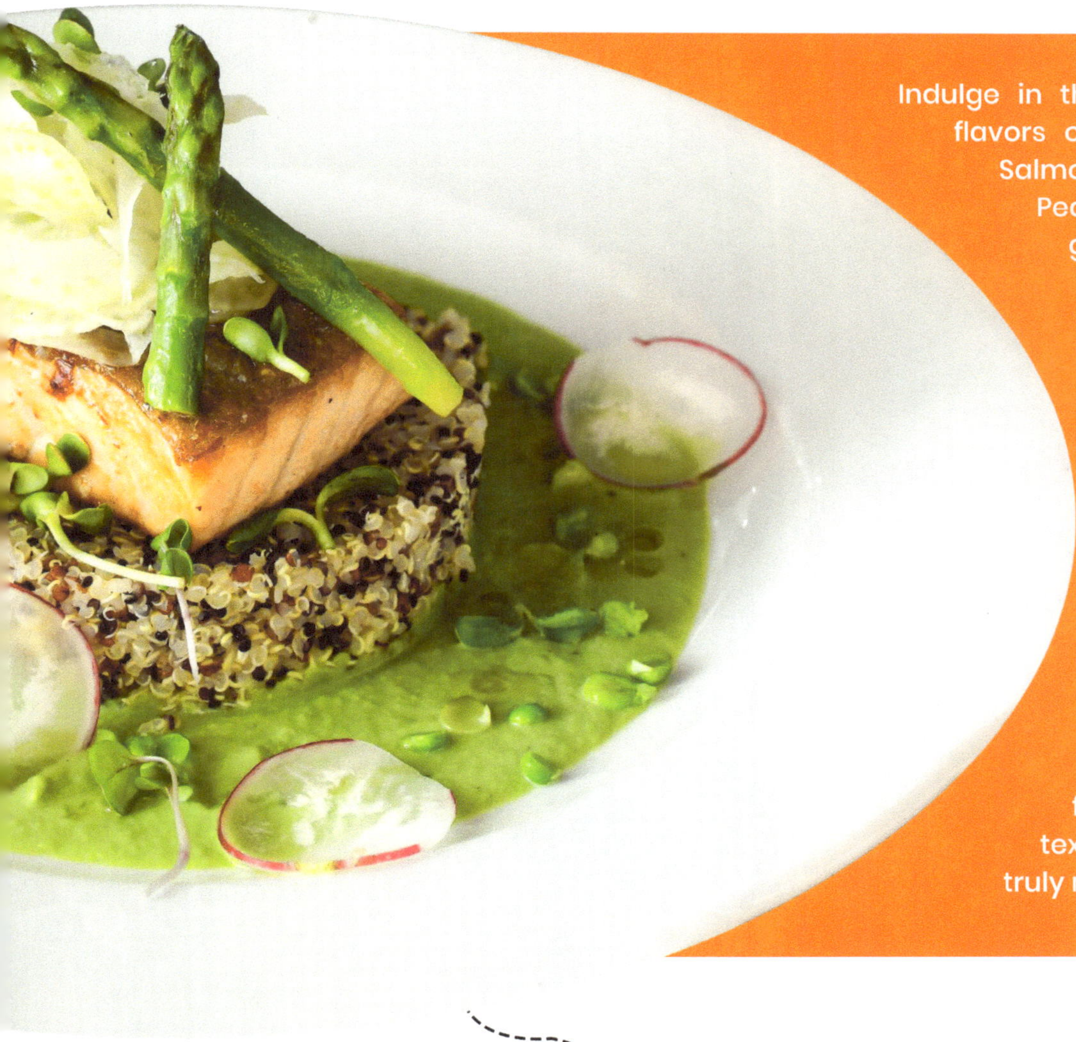

Indulge in the fresh and vibrant flavors of this Mediterranean Salmon with Quinoa & Green Pea Purée. Perfectly grilled salmon fillets rest atop a bed of nutritious quinoa, complemented by a smooth green pea purée infused with mint and garlic. Served with steamed asparagus and garnished with pea shoot microgreens, this dish is a delightful fusion of flavors and textures, making for a truly memorable meal.

INGREDIENTS

For the Green Pea Purée:

- 1 cup fresh or frozen green peas
- 1 clove garlic, minced
- 2 tablespoons fresh mint leaves
- 1 tablespoon extra-virgin olive oil
- Salt and black pepper to taste

For the Plates:

- 4 thin slices of radish
- 1 cup cooked multigrain quinoa
- 2 (6-ounce) salmon fillets, grilled or baked
- 4 asparagus spears, steamed
- Handful of pea shoot microgreens for garnish
- Lemon wedges, for serving

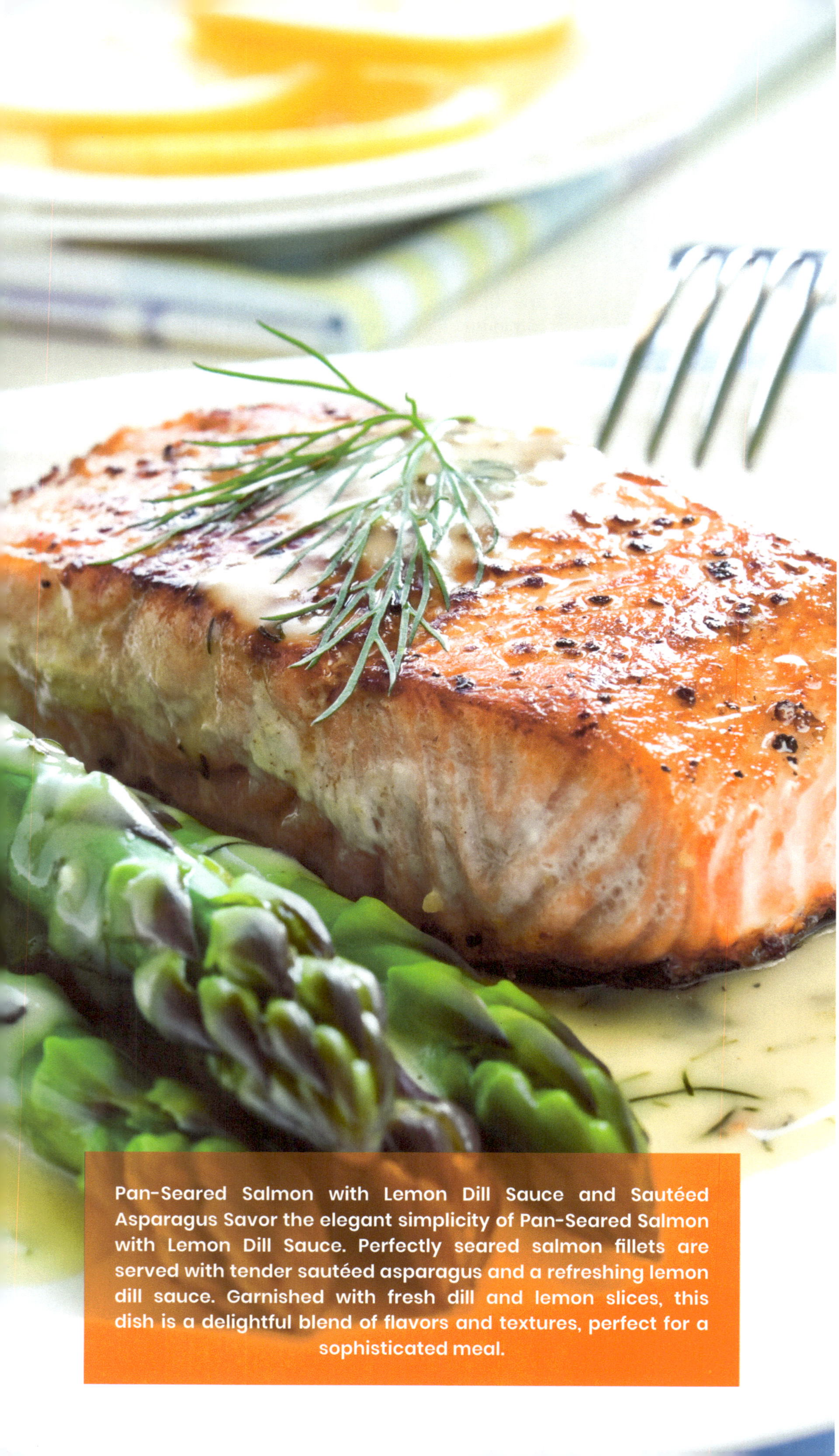

Pan-Seared Salmon with Lemon Dill Sauce and Sautéed Asparagus Savor the elegant simplicity of Pan-Seared Salmon with Lemon Dill Sauce. Perfectly seared salmon fillets are served with tender sautéed asparagus and a refreshing lemon dill sauce. Garnished with fresh dill and lemon slices, this dish is a delightful blend of flavors and textures, perfect for a sophisticated meal.

2 servings

35g P | 10g C
20g F

350 per
serving

Prep Time:
15 minutes

Cooking Time:
15 minutes

Total Time:
30 minutes

PAN-SEARED SALMON with LEMON DILL SAUCE and SAUTÉED ASPARAGUS

INGREDIENTS

For the Salmon:

- 2 salmon fillets (6-8 ounces each)
- 1 tablespoon olive oil, divided
- Salt and black pepper to taste
- Fresh dill sprigs for garnish
- 1 lemon, sliced for garnish

For the Sautéed Asparagus:

- 1 bunch of asparagus, trimmed
- 1 tablespoon olive oil
- Salt and black pepper to taste
- Zest of 1 lemon (for garnish)

For the Lemon Dill Sauce:

- Juice of 1 lemon
- 2 tablespoons fresh dill, chopped
- 1/4 cup plain Greek yogurt
- Salt and black pepper to taste

DIRECTIONS

1. Preheat your oven to 375°F (190°C).
2. In a small bowl, prepare the lemon dill sauce by whisking together the lemon juice, fresh dill, plain Greek yogurt, salt, and black pepper. Set aside.
3. In a skillet, heat 1/2 tablespoon of olive oil over medium-high heat. Add the trimmed asparagus, season with salt and black pepper, and sauté for about 5-7 minutes, or until the asparagus is tender and lightly charred. Remove from heat.
4. Season the salmon fillets with salt and black pepper. In a separate skillet, heat the remaining 1/2 tablespoon of olive oil over medium-high heat. Add the salmon fillets, skin-side down, and sear for about 4-5 minutes, or until the skin is crispy and golden. Flip the fillets and cook for an additional 3-4 minutes, or until the salmon is cooked to your desired level of doneness.
5. Divide the sautéed asparagus between two plates, place a pan-seared salmon fillet on each plate, and drizzle the lemon dill sauce over the salmon. Garnish with fresh dill sprigs, lemon slices, and lemon zest.

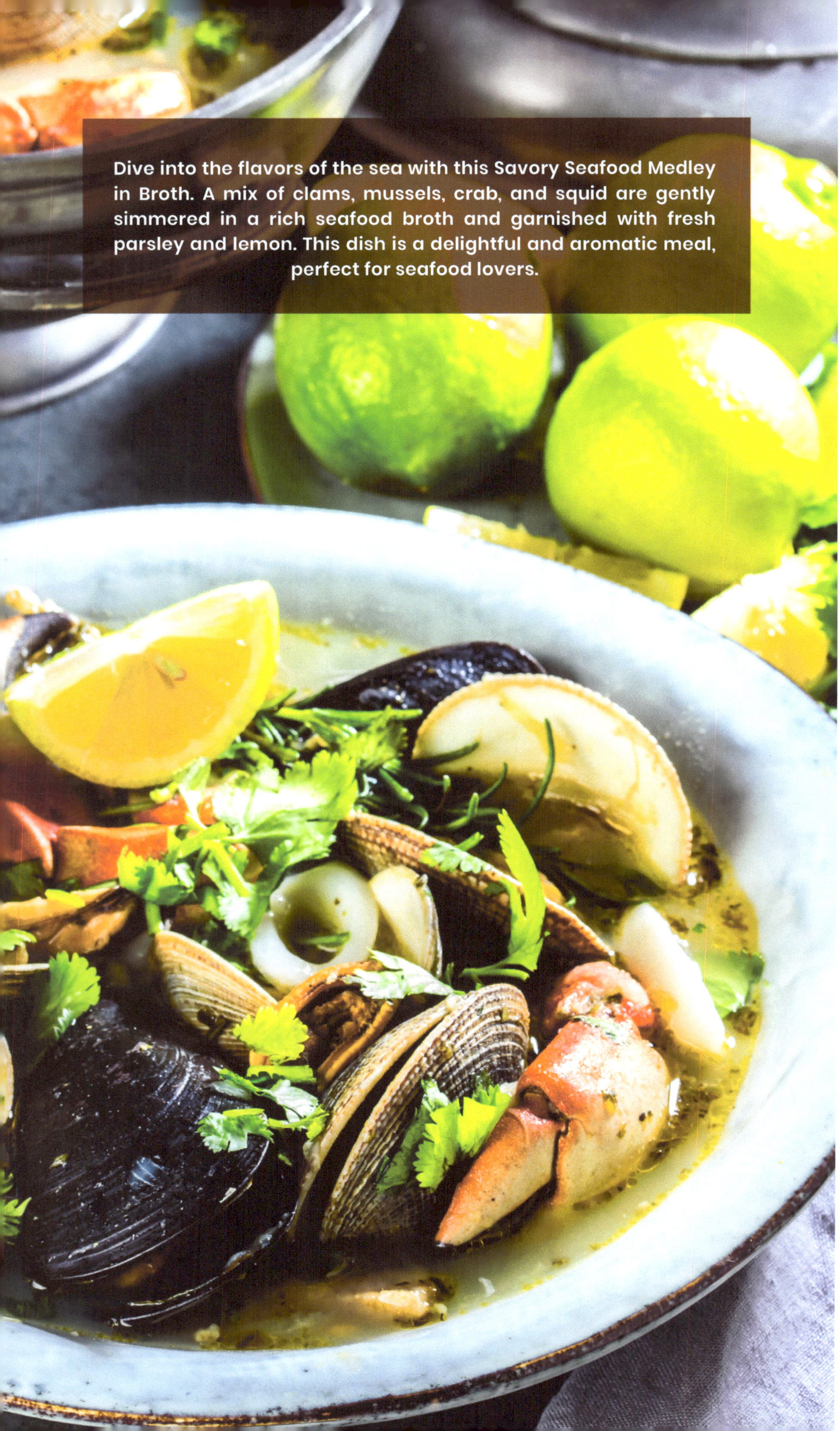

Dive into the flavors of the sea with this Savory Seafood Medley in Broth. A mix of clams, mussels, crab, and squid are gently simmered in a rich seafood broth and garnished with fresh parsley and lemon. This dish is a delightful and aromatic meal, perfect for seafood lovers.

2 servings

30g P | 16g C
20g F

375 per serving

Prep Time:
15 minutes

Cooking Time:
20 minutes

Total Time:
35 minutes

SAVORY SEAFOOD MEDLEY in BROTH

INGREDIENTS

- 20 small clams, scrubbed and rinsed cleaned
- 10 mussels, cleaned and debearded
- 1 cup fresh lump crab meat
- 4-6 crab claws, cleaned
- 1 small squid tube, sliced into rings
- 4 cups seafood broth
- 1 tablespoon green herb oil (you can use a combination of olive oil and finely chopped herbs like parsley, chives, and dill)
- 1 Lemon cut into wedges
- Fresh parsley leaves for garnish
- Salt and black pepper to taste

DIRECTIONS

1. In a large pot, bring the seafood broth to a gentle simmer over medium heat.
2. While the broth is heating, prepare the squid tube by slicing it into rings.
3. In a large pot, heat the seafood broth over medium heat.
4. Add both the cleaned crab claws, clams, and mussels to the pot together. Cover and simmer for 5-7 minutes or until the clams and mussels have opened up, and the crab claws have turned red or orange and opaque. Discard any clams or mussels that do not open.
5. While the crab claws, clams, and mussels are cooking, season the broth with salt and black pepper to taste. Adjust the seasoning according to your preference.
6. Gently fold in the sliced squid rings or strips and lump crab meat. Cook for an additional 2-3 minutes to heat through, being careful not to overcook the squid.
7. Ladle the savory seafood medley, including the broth, crab claws, clams, mussels, squid, and lump crab meat, into serving bowls.
8. Garnish with fresh parsley leaves and serve hot with lemon wedges on the side.
9. Just before serving, drizzle each serving with a tablespoon of green herb oil for added flavor.

Note on the Seafood:

1. For the clams and mussels, ensure that you purchase ones that are sealed and not opened. It's a good idea to buy extra, as some may not open during cooking, and you'll want to discard those.
2. When it comes to lump crab meat, you have the option to use canned lump crab meat. If you choose canned crab meat, make sure to drain it from any liquid before adding it to the dish for a quick and easy option.
3. To savor the crab claws, use a crab cracker or a seafood fork to gently crack the shells, revealing the delicious meat inside. Enjoy!

VEGETARIAN

FALAFEL BOWL with ZESTY TAHINI DRESSING

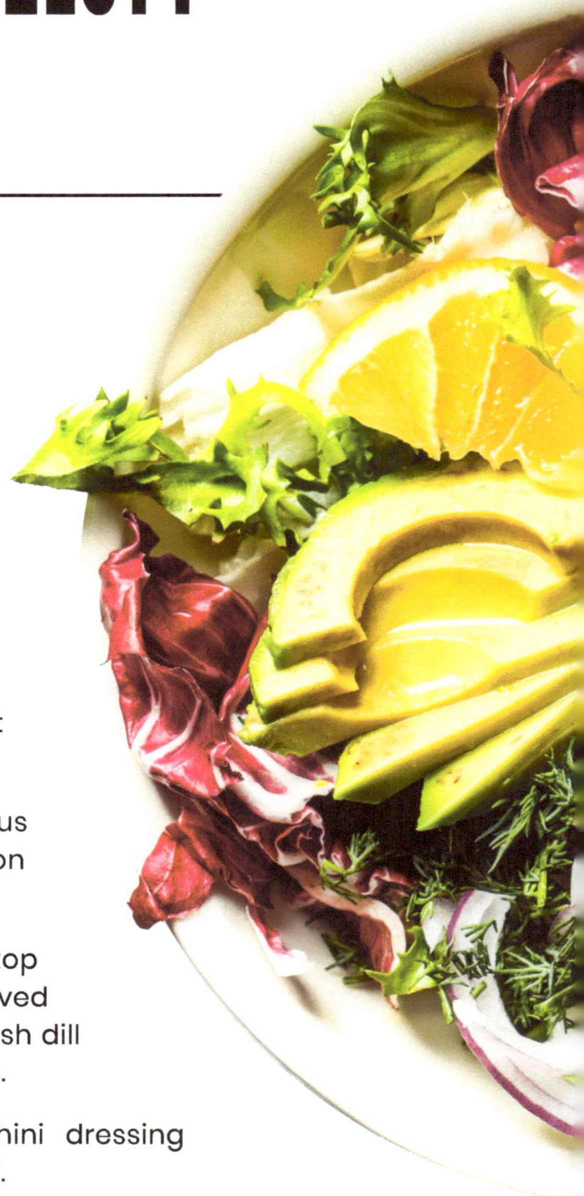

DIRECTIONS

1. Cook the Falafel: Heat the store-bought falafel patties according to the package instructions. Typically, this involves baking them in the oven or heating them in a skillet over medium heat for about 5-7 minutes per side until they are heated through and have a golden crust.
2. Prepare the Tahini Dressing: In a small bowl, whisk together the tahini paste, lemon juice, minced garlic, olive oil, salt, and black pepper until smooth. Adjust the consistency by adding a bit of water if needed.
3. Assemble the Falafel Bowl: Start by placing a generous bed of spring mix greens in two serving bowls or on plates.
4. Add the Toppings: Place 4 cooked falafel patties on top of the greens in each bowl. Surround them with halved heirloom grape tomatoes, thinly sliced red onion, fresh dill sprigs, fresh mint leaves, and creamy avocado slices.
5. Drizzle with Tahini Dressing: Drizzle the zesty tahini dressing generously over the falafel and veggies in each bowl.
6. Garnish with Lemon Wedges: Serve the bowls with lemon wedges on the side for an extra burst of citrusy flavor.
7. Enjoy Your Quick Falafel Bowl with Zesty Tahini Dressing: Dive into this delectable and vibrant falafel bowl that combines the convenience of store-bought falafel with a medley of fresh Mediterranean flavors. The creamy tahini dressing ties it all together for a sensational meal, perfect for sharing with a loved one.

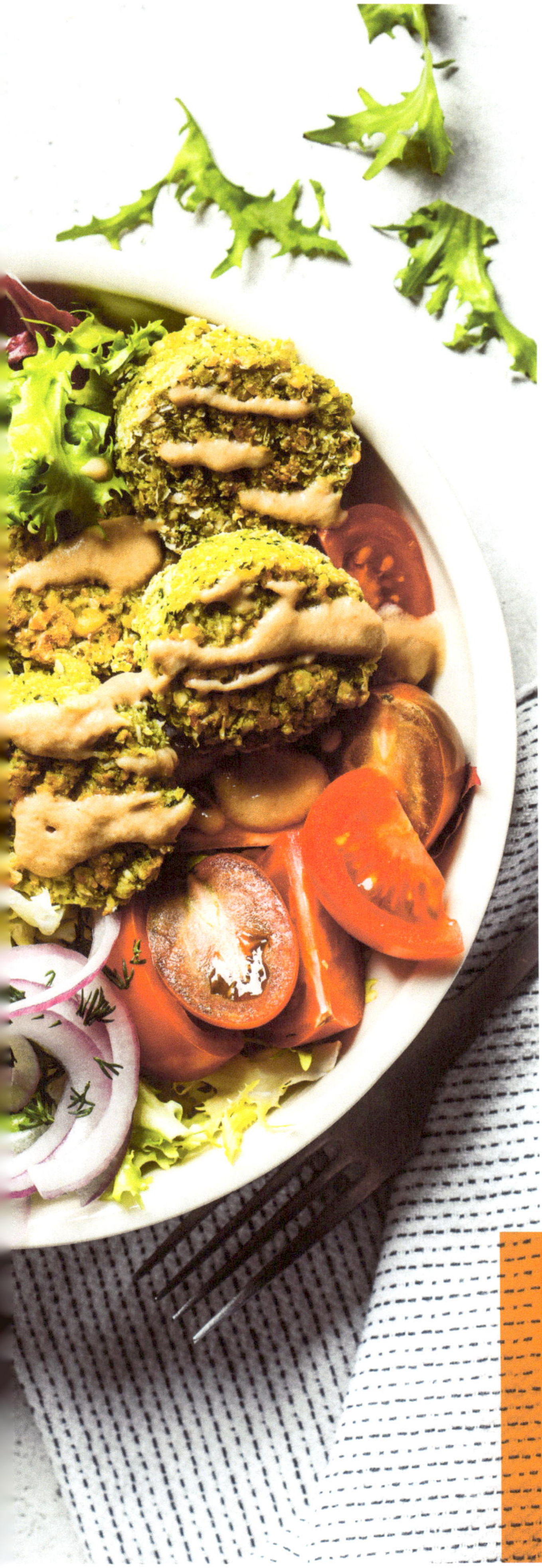

2 servings

10g P | 18g C
34g F

400 per serving

Prep Time:
10 minutes

Cooking Time:
10 minutes

Total Time:
20 minutes

INGREDIENTS

For the Bowl:

- 8 store-bought falafel patties (available in the frozen food section)
- 8 cups spring mix greens
- Fresh dill sprigs
- Fresh mint leaves
- Heirloom grape tomatoes, halved
- Red onion, thinly sliced
- Avocado slices
- Lemon wedges

For the Tahini Dressing:

- 4 tablespoons tahini paste
- Juice of 1/2 lemon
- 1 clove garlic, minced
- 2 tablespoons olive oil
- Salt and black pepper to taste

Enjoy a taste of the Mediterranean with this Falafel Bowl with Zesty Tahini Dressing. Crispy falafel patties are served on a bed of fresh greens, tomatoes, and red onions, then drizzled with a tangy tahini dressing. Garnished with fresh herbs and lemon wedges, this bowl is a delicious and wholesome meal that's full of flavor.

Refresh your palate with the Mediterranean Orzo Pasta Salad. Al dente orzo pasta is tossed with tangy sundried tomatoes, sweet bell peppers, and briny olives, then dressed with a light and zesty red wine vinaigrette. Topped with crumbled feta and fresh basil, this salad is a vibrant and satisfying dish, perfect as a main course or a side. For a heartier meal, add your choice of grilled chicken, shrimp, or beef.

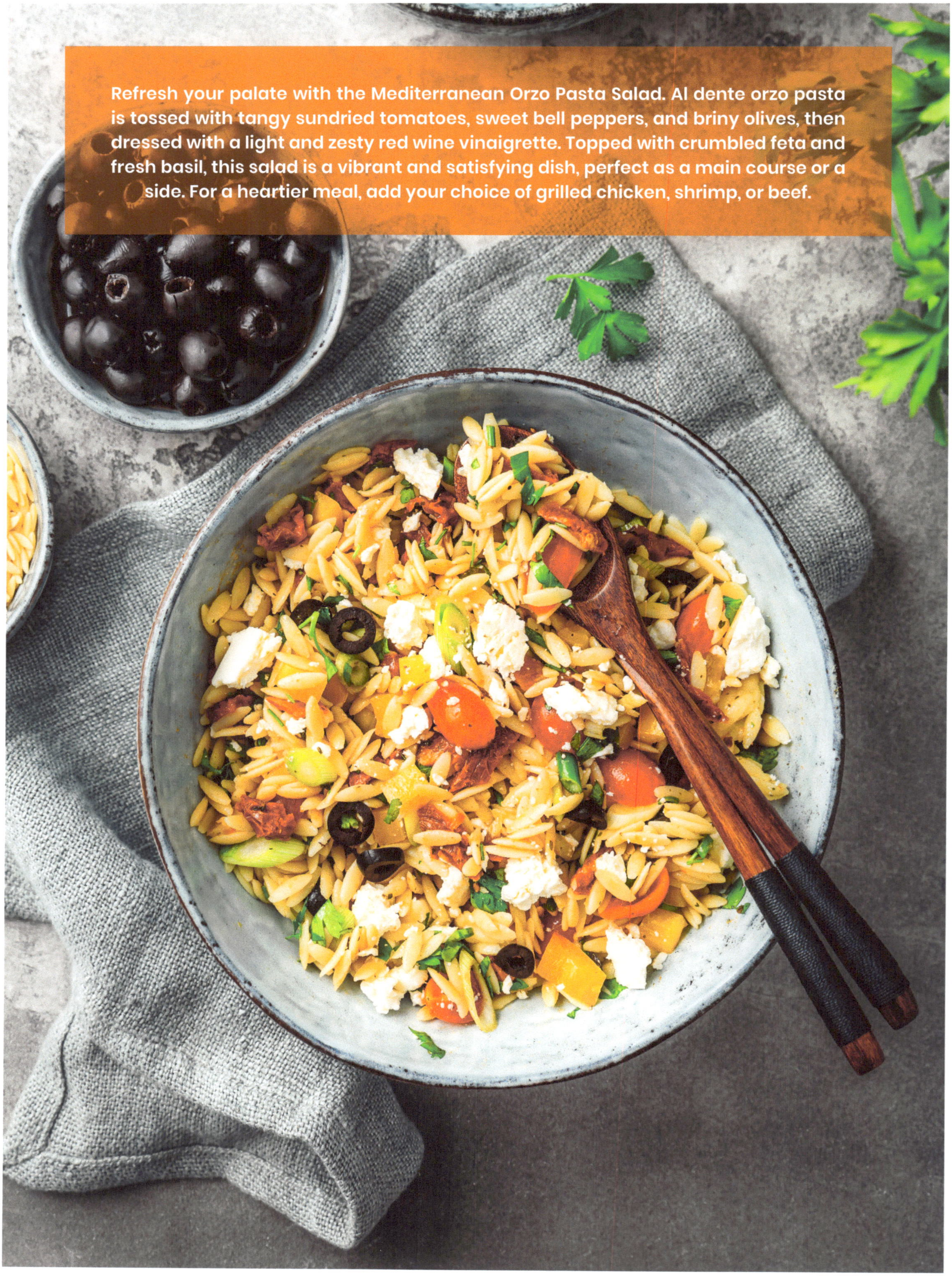

MEDITERRANEAN ORZO PASTA SALAD

2 servings	6g P | 45g C 15g F	350 per serving	Prep Time: 10 minutes	Cooking Time: 15 minutes	Total Time: 25 minutes

INGREDIENTS

- 4 oz. organic dry orzo pasta by Montebello brand
- 1/2 cup crumbled feta cheese
- 1/4 cup sundried tomatoes, chopped
- 1/2 yellow bell pepper, diced
- 1 cup grape tomatoes, halved
- 2 green scallions, thinly sliced
- 1/4 cup sliced black olives

For the Red Wine Vinaigrette:

- 2 tablespoons extra-virgin olive oil
- 2 tablespoons red wine vinegar
- 1 clove garlic, minced
- 1 teaspoon dried oregano
- Salt and black pepper to taste
- Fresh basil leaves for garnish (optional)

DIRECTIONS

1. In a large pot of salted boiling water, cook the orzo pasta according to the package instructions until al dente. Drain and keep warm in pot.
2. In a small bowl, whisk together the extra-virgin olive oil, red wine vinegar, minced garlic, dried oregano, salt, and black pepper to create the dressing. Set it aside.
3. In a large mixing bowl, combine the warm orzo pasta, chopped sundried tomatoes, diced yellow bell pepper, halved grape tomatoes, sliced green scallions, and sliced black olives.
4. Pour the prepared dressing over the salad ingredients in the bowl and gently toss all the ingredients together until they are well coated. Serve immediately while it's warm.
5. Before serving, top with crumbled feta cheese and garnish the Mediterranean Orzo Pasta Salad with fresh basil leaves, if desired. Serve as a light and refreshing main course or as a side dish. You can also add a meat of your choice, such as grilled chicken, shrimp, or beef, for additional protein and flavor.

QUINOA BOWL with ROASTED EGGPLANT and HUMMUS

DIRECTIONS

1. Preheat your oven to 400°F (200°C)

Next, Prepare the Quinoa:

1. Rinse the quinoa thoroughly under cold water.
2. Prepare the quinoa according to package instructions. When done, remove from heat and let it sit, covered, for 5 minutes. Fluff with a fork before serving.

Roast the Eggplant and Chickpeas:

1. Place the eggplant slices and chickpeas on a baking sheet side by side.
2. Drizzle them with olive oil and season with salt and pepper.
3. Roast in the preheated oven for 15-20 minutes, or until the eggplant slices are tender and golden brown. Halfway through, flip the eggplant slices and stir the chickpeas.

Make the Hummus:

1. In a food processor, combine the chickpeas, minced garlic, tahini, fresh lemon juice, olive oil, ground cumin, salt, and pepper.
2. Blend until smooth, adding water as needed for your desired consistency. Adjust seasonings to taste.

Assemble the Bowl:

1. Divide the cooked quinoa between two bowls.
2. Top with roasted eggplant slices, chickpeas, cherry tomato halves, and baby spinach leaves.
3. If making your own hummus, add a generous scoop on top of each bowl.
4. Drizzle with extra olive oil if desired.
5. Enjoy!

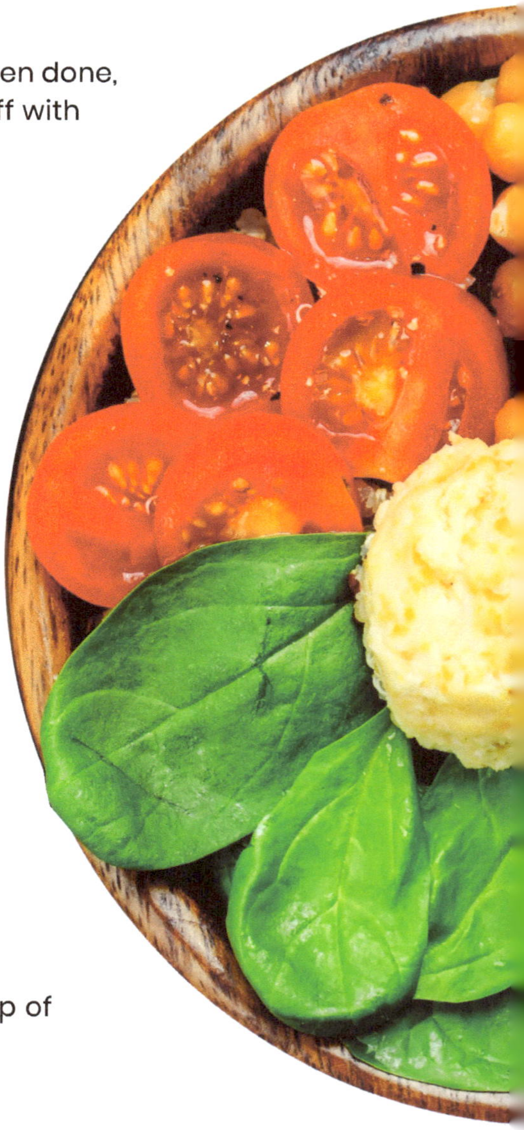

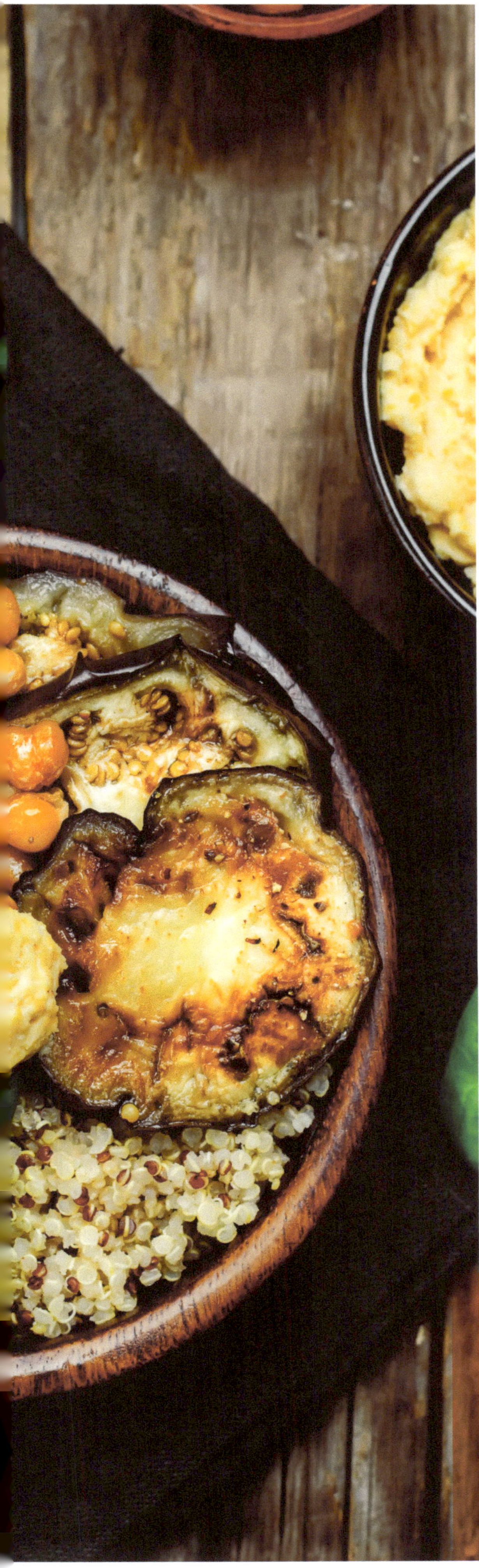

2 servings	16g P | 67g C 11g F	425 per serving
Prep Time: 10 minutes	Cooking Time: 20 minutes	Total Time: 30 minutes

INGREDIENTS

For the Quinoa Bowl:

- 1/2 cup dry organic tri-color quinoa
- 1 small eggplant, sliced into rounds
- 1 can (15 ounces) chickpeas, drained and rinsed
- 6 cherry tomatoes, halved
- 2 cups baby spinach leaves
- Olive oil for roasting
- Salt and pepper to taste

For the Hummus:

- 1 can (15 ounces) chickpeas, drained and rinsed
- 2 cloves garlic, minced
- 3 tablespoons tahini
- 2 tablespoons fresh lemon juice
- 2 tablespoons extra-virgin olive oil
- 1/2 teaspoon ground cumin
- Salt and pepper to taste
- Water, as needed for consistency

Enjoy a nourishing and flavorful meal with the Quinoa Bowl with Roasted Eggplant and Hummus. Nutty quinoa is paired with tender roasted eggplant, sweet cherry tomatoes, and baby spinach, all topped with a dollop of creamy hummus. Drizzled with olive oil, this bowl is a wholesome and satisfying dish that's perfect for any meal.

TOMATO AND and LENTIL SOUP with HOMEMADE CROUTONS

DIRECTIONS

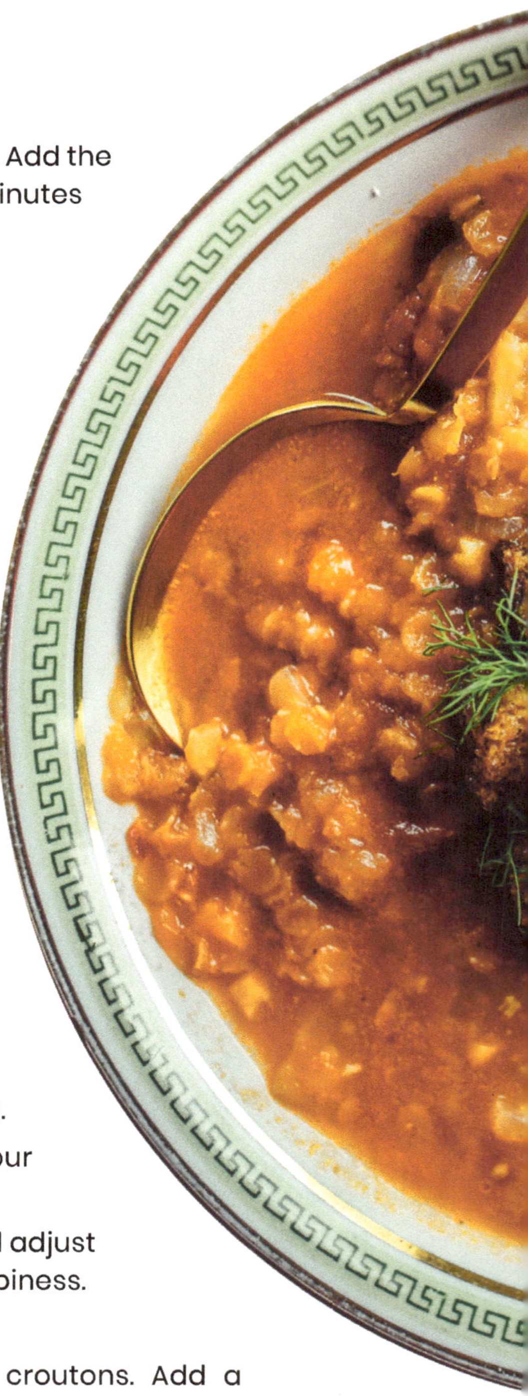

For the Lentil Soup:

1. In a large pot, heat a drizzle of olive oil over medium heat. Add the chopped onion and minced garlic. Sauté for about 3-4 minutes until they become fragrant and translucent.
2. Rinse the red lentils thoroughly under cold water.
3. Add the red lentils, diced tomatoes, vegetable broth, cumin, and paprika to the pot. Stir well to combine.
4. Season the soup with salt and pepper. Start with 1/2 teaspoon of salt and a pinch of pepper, then adjust as needed.
5. Bring the mixture to a boil, then reduce the heat to low, cover, and simmer for about 15-20 minutes or until the lentils are tender.

Prepare the Homemade Croutons:

1. Preheat your oven to 350°F (175°C).
2. In a mixing bowl, combine the cubed bread, olive oil, garlic powder, thyme, salt, and pepper. Toss everything together until the bread cubes are evenly coated with the oil and seasonings.
3. Spread the seasoned bread cubes on a baking sheet in a single layer.
4. Bake in the preheated oven for about 5 minutes, then check the croutons. Depending on your desired level of crispiness, they may need an additional 2-5 minutes. Be sure to keep a close eye on them to prevent overcooking.
5. Once the croutons are golden brown and crispy to your liking, remove them from the oven and let them cool.
6. Note: Check the croutons after 5 minutes in the oven, and adjust the baking time according to your preferred level of crispiness.

Serve the Tomato and Red Lentil Soup:

1. Serve hot, garnished with fresh dill and homemade croutons. Add a sprinkling of parmesan cheese if desired.

2 servings

14g P | 47g C 7g F

360 per serving

Prep Time: 10 minutes

Cooking Time: 25 minutes

Total Time: 35 minutes

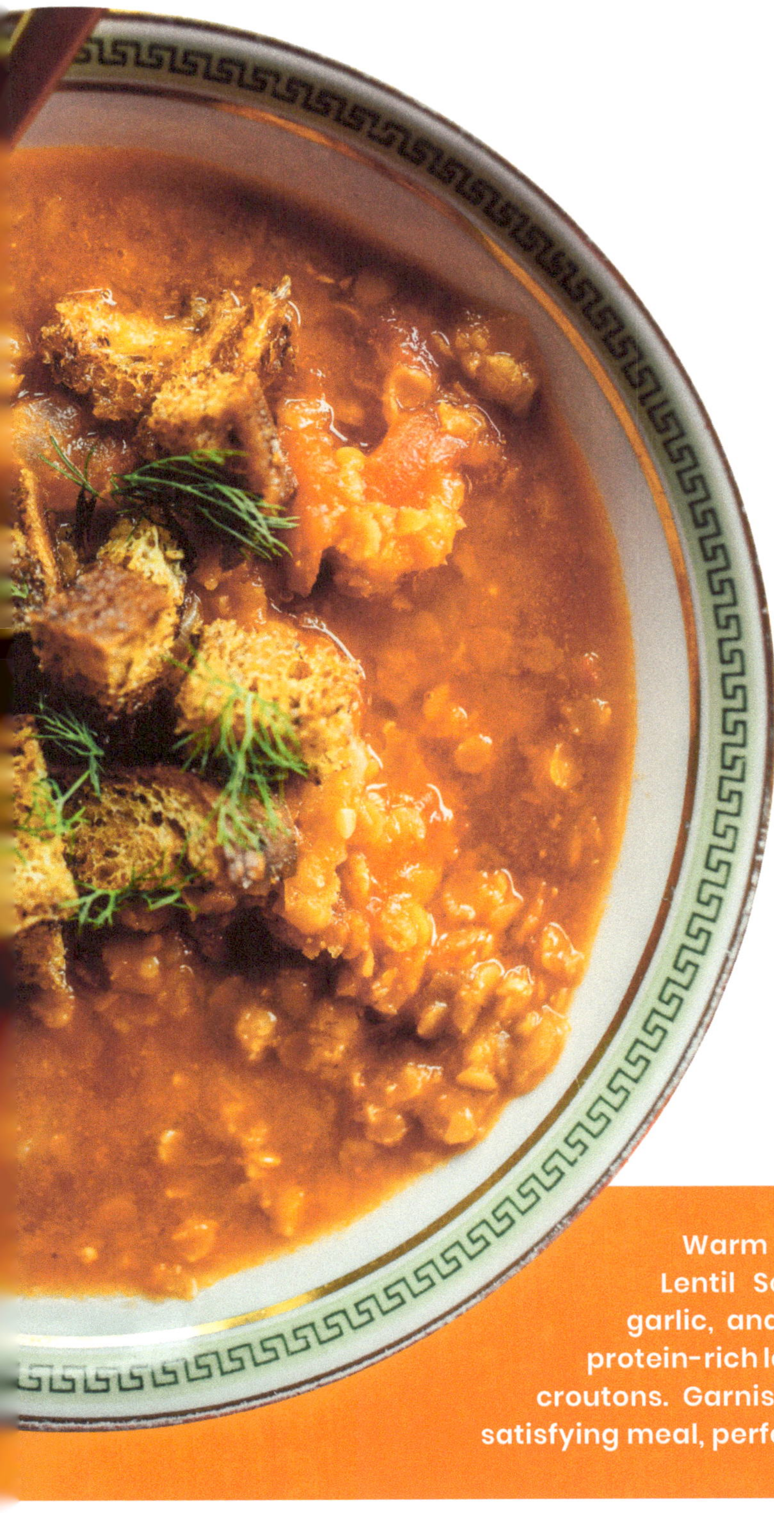

INGREDIENTS

For the Soup:

- 1 cup red lentils
- 1 can (14 oz) diced tomatoes
- 1 onion, chopped
- 2 cloves garlic, minced
- 4 cups vegetable broth
- 1/8 teaspoon cumin
- 1/2 teaspoon paprika
- 1/2 teaspoon salt
- 1/8 teaspoon pepper
- Olive oil for sautéing
- Fresh dill for garnish

For the Homemade Croutons:

- 2 slices of Artisanal Einkorn Bread (see the recipe), cubed
- 1 tablespoons olive oil
- 1/2 teaspoon garlic powder
- 1/2 teaspoon dried thyme
- Salt and pepper to taste

Warm up with this comforting Tomato and Red Lentil Soup. Rich with the flavors of tomatoes, garlic, and spices, this hearty soup is packed with protein-rich lentils and topped with crunchy homemade croutons. Garnished with fresh dill, it's a nourishing and satisfying meal, perfect for any day of the week.

Beef

- Traditional Albondigas Soup

Poultry

- Chipotle Chicken Salad Bowl
- White Bean & Chicken Tortilla Soup with Cassava Strips

Seafood

- Golden Seafood and Chicken Paella
- Shrimp Tacos with Creamy Citrus Sauce

SPANISH and MEXICAN FLAVORS

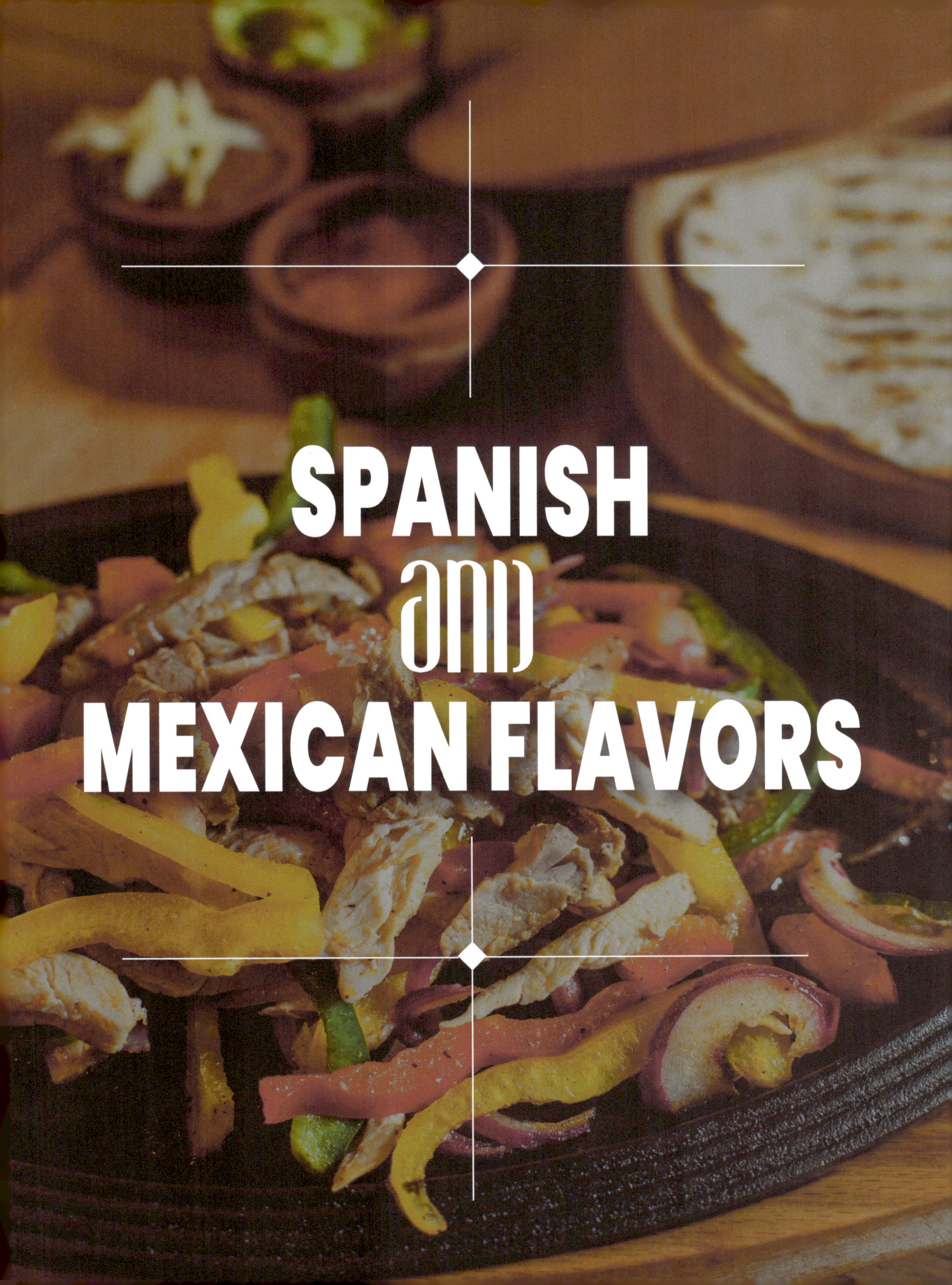

TRADITIONAL ALBONDIGAS SOUP

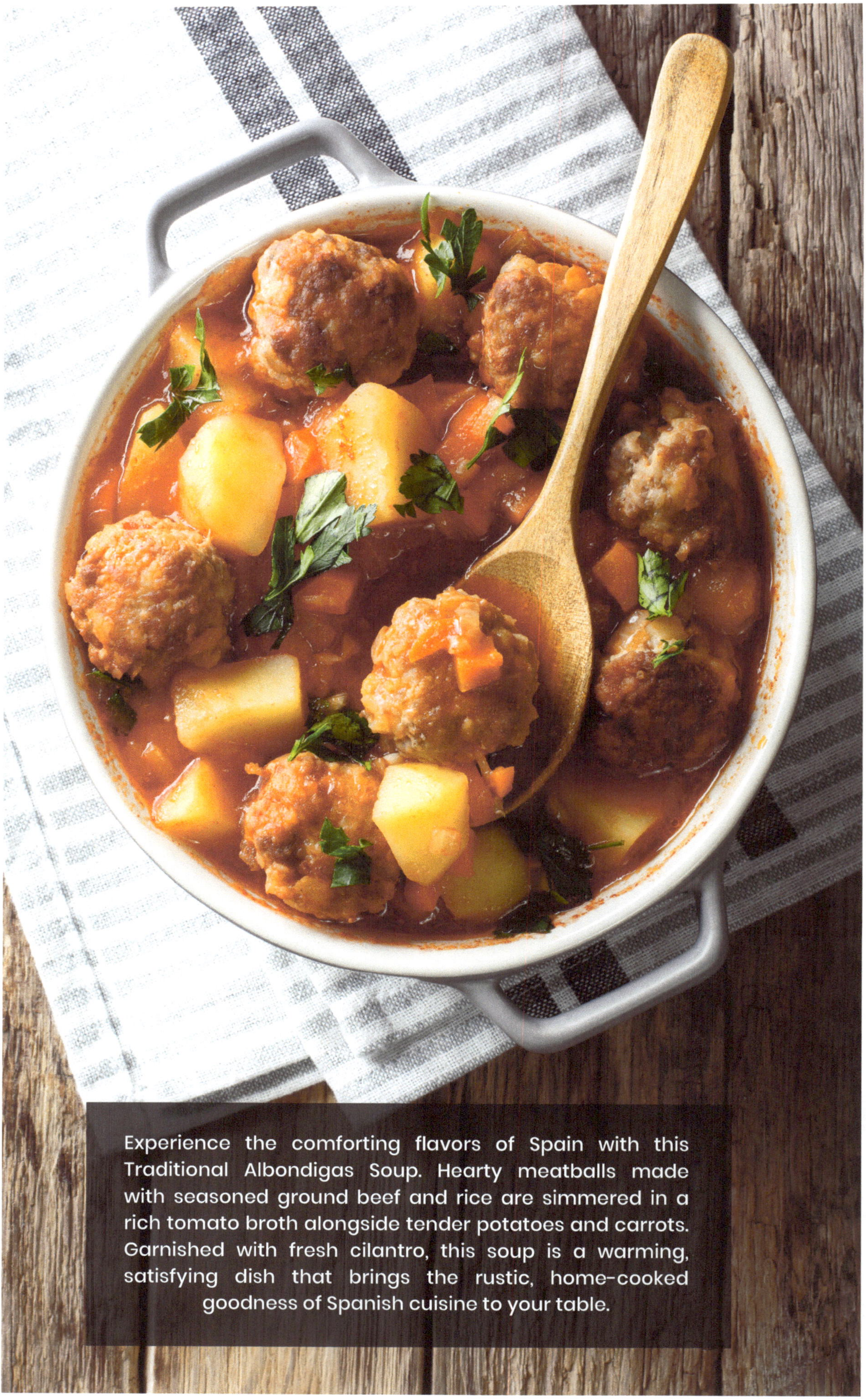

Experience the comforting flavors of Spain with this Traditional Albondigas Soup. Hearty meatballs made with seasoned ground beef and rice are simmered in a rich tomato broth alongside tender potatoes and carrots. Garnished with fresh cilantro, this soup is a warming, satisfying dish that brings the rustic, home-cooked goodness of Spanish cuisine to your table.

BEEF

2 servings	19g P | 34g C 17g F	370 per serving	Prep Time: 15 minutes	Cooking Time: 20 minutes	Total Time: 35 minutes

INGREDIENTS

- 1/2 lb. ground beef (or other ground meat of your liking)
- 1/4 cup long-grain white rice
- 1/2 small onion, finely chopped
- 2 cloves garlic, minced
- 1/2 teaspoon dried oregano
- 1/4 teaspoon ground cumin
- Salt and pepper to taste
- 2 medium Yukon Gold potatoes, peeled and diced
- 1 medium carrot, finely diced
- 1 can (14 oz) diced tomatoes
- 4 cups beef or vegetable broth
- Fresh cilantro leaves for garnish
- Olive oil for sautéing

DIRECTIONS

1. In a mixing bowl, combine the ground beef, uncooked rice, chopped onion, minced garlic, dried oregano, ground cumin, salt, and pepper. Mix until well combined, then form the mixture into small meatballs, about 1-inch in diameter. The rice grains will cook with the meatballs as they simmer in the soup.
2. Heat a drizzle of olive oil in a large pot over medium heat. Add the meatballs and cook for about 4-5 minutes, turning occasionally until they are browned on all sides. Remove the meatballs from the pot and set them aside.
3. In the same pot, add the diced potatoes and carrots. Sauté for about 3-4 minutes until they start to soften.
4. Pour in the diced tomatoes and broth. Stir well to combine.
5. Return the meatballs to the pot. Bring the mixture to a boil, then reduce the heat to low, cover, and simmer for about 20 minutes or until the potatoes are tender and the meatballs are fully cooked.
6. Taste and adjust the seasoning with salt and pepper as needed.
7. Serve the Albondigas Stew hot, dividing it between two bowls. Garnish with fresh cilantro leaves and enjoy this hearty Spanish classic.

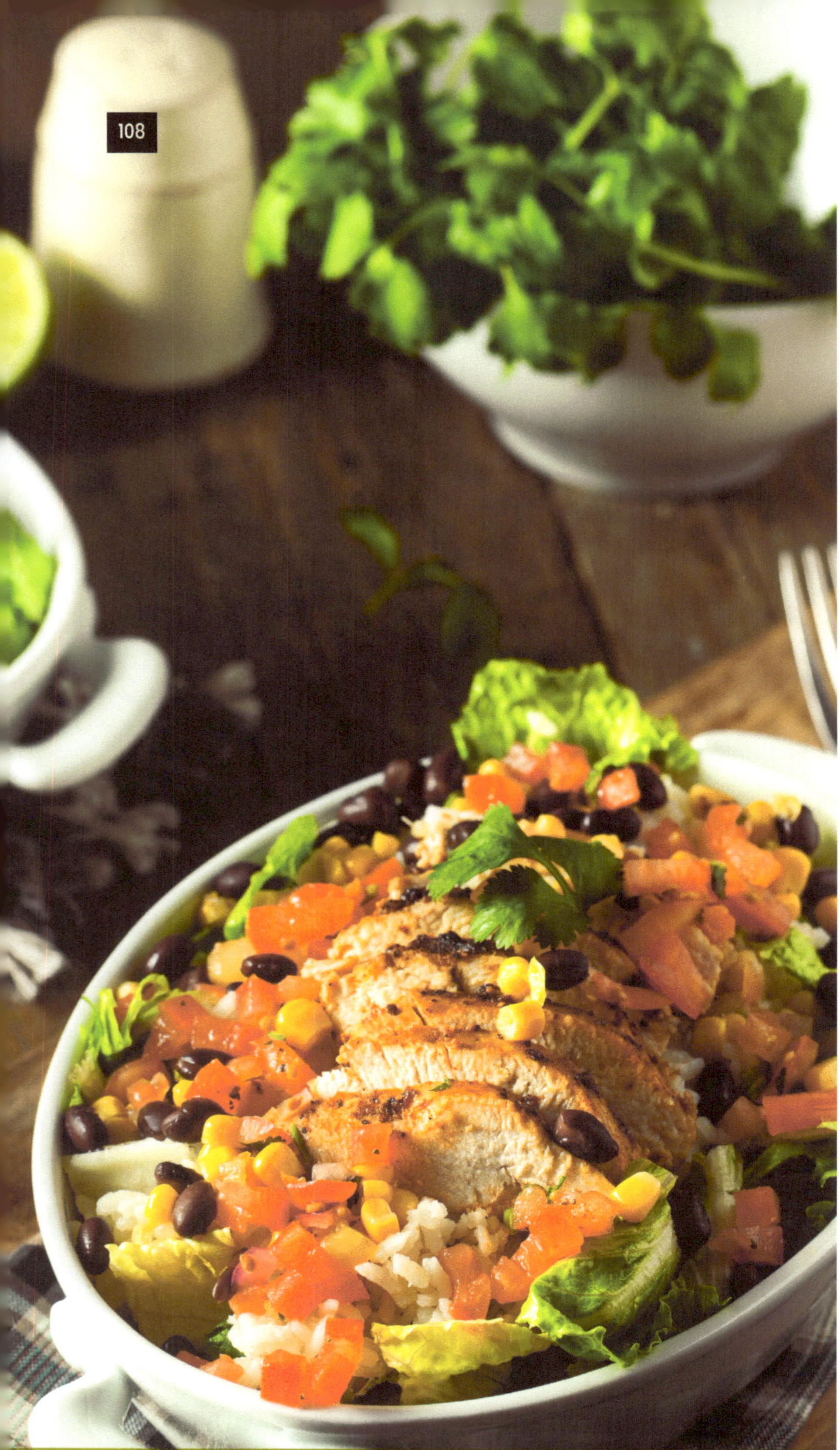

Spice up your meal with the Chipotle Chicken Salad Bowl. Grilled chipotle-marinated chicken is served over a bed of romaine lettuce, rice, corn, and black beans, then drizzled with a zesty lemon honey vinaigrette. Garnished with fresh cilantro and lime wedges, this salad is a flavorful and hearty dish that's both satisfying and nutritious.

INGREDIENTS

For the Salad:

- 2 boneless, skinless chicken breasts
- 2 cups romaine lettuce, chopped
- 1 cup cooked white or brown rice
- 1/2 cup corn kernels (fresh, frozen, or canned)
- 1/2 cup black beans, drained and rinsed
- 1 medium tomato, finely diced
- Fresh cilantro leaves for garnish
- Fresh lime wedges for garnish
- Olive oil for cooking
- Salt and pepper to taste

For the Lemon Honey Olive Oil Vinaigrette:

- 4 tablespoons olive oil
- Juice of 1 lemon
- 1 tablespoon honey
- 1 teaspoon dried oregano
- Salt and pepper to taste

For the Chicken Marinade:

- For the Chicken Marinade:
- 2 tablespoons olive oil
- 2 teaspoons chipotle chili powder
- 1/4 teaspoon ground cumin
- 1 teaspoon smoked paprika
- 1/8 teaspoon cayenne chili powder
- 1/2 teaspoon garlic powder
- Juice of 1 lime
- 1/2 teaspoon salt

For the Cilantro Lime Rice:

- 1 cup cooked white or brown rice
- Juice of 1 lime
- 2 tablespoons fresh cilantro, finely chopped
- Salt to taste

POULTRY

CHIPOTLE CHICKEN SALAD BOWL

2 servings	31g P | 41g C 24g F	498 per serving	Prep Time: 30 minutes	Cooking Time: 15 minutes	Total Time: 45 minutes

DIRECTIONS

Marinate the Chicken:

1. Mix olive oil, chipotle chili powder, ground cumin, smoked paprika, garlic powder, lime juice, salt, and pepper in a bowl.
2. Place chicken breasts in a resealable bag or shallow dish, pour marinade, and refrigerate for at least 30 minutes (or overnight).

Prepare the Cilantro Lime Rice:

1. Combine cooked rice, lime juice, chopped cilantro, and a pinch of salt in a bowl. Mix well and set aside.
2. Grill or Cook the Chicken:
3. Preheat grill or skillet over medium-high heat.
4. Grill chicken for about 6-8 minutes per side or until fully cooked (internal temp: 165°F (75°C)).
5. Remove from grill and let the chicken rest for a few minutes, then slice into thin strips.

Prepare the Lemon Honey Olive Oil Vinaigrette:

1. Whisk olive oil, lemon juice, honey, dried oregano, salt, and pepper in a small bowl until well combined.

Assemble the Salad Bowl:

1. Divide chopped romaine lettuce into two serving bowls.
2. Add a portion of cooked rice to each bowl.
3. Top with corn, black beans, diced tomato, and sliced chipotle-marinated chicken.

Drizzle and Garnish:

1. Drizzle vinaigrette over each salad bowl.
2. Garnish with fresh cilantro leaves and lime wedges.
3. Serve your Chipotle Chicken Salad Bowl immediately and enjoy!

WHITE BEAN & CHICKEN TORTILLA SOUP with CASSAVA STRIPS

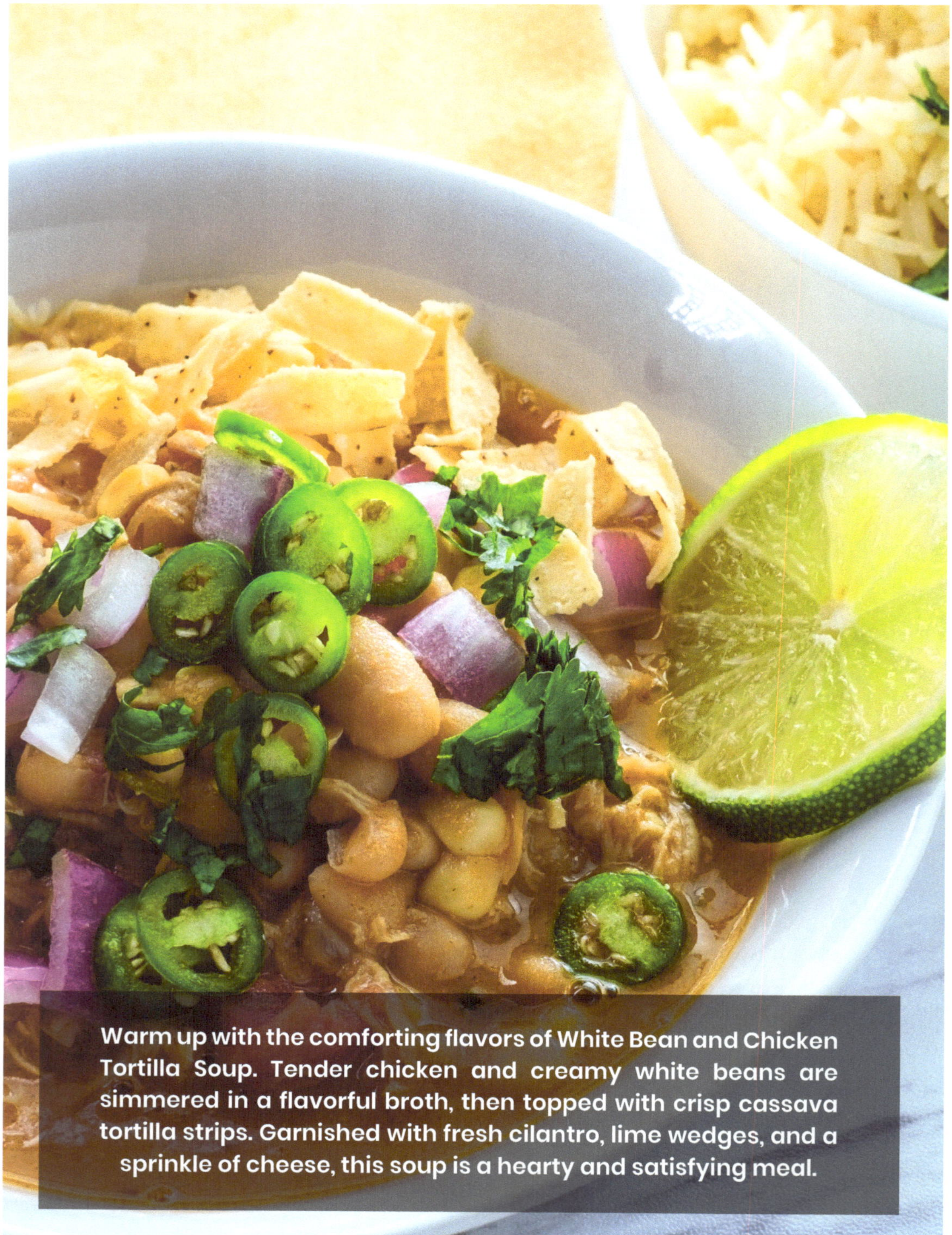

Warm up with the comforting flavors of White Bean and Chicken Tortilla Soup. Tender chicken and creamy white beans are simmered in a flavorful broth, then topped with crisp cassava tortilla strips. Garnished with fresh cilantro, lime wedges, and a sprinkle of cheese, this soup is a hearty and satisfying meal.

2 servings

31g P | 25g C
15g F

360 per serving

Prep Time: 15 minutes

Cooking Time: 10 minutes

Total Time: 25 minutes

INGREDIENTS

For the Soup:

- 1 1/2 cups cooked and shredded white chicken meat (use leftover roasted, poached or canned)
- 1/2 can (7.5 oz) white beans, drained and rinsed
- 1/4 cup white corn kernels (frozen or canned)
- 1/4 cup diced red onion (reserve a tablespoon for garnish)
- 1/4 can (3.6 oz) diced tomatoes (preferably no-salt-added)
- 3 1/2 cups low-sodium chicken broth (adjust as needed for desired consistency)
- 2 tablespoons Monterey Jack or white cheese blend
- 2 tablespoons fresh cilantro leaves, chopped
- 1/2 lime, cut into wedges
- Salt and pepper to taste

For the Cassava Flour Tortilla Strips:

- 1 cassava flour tortilla (or use store bought cassava flour tortilla chips by Siete)
- Olive oil spray
- Salt to taste
- Garnish:
- Thinly sliced green chilies
- Diced red onion
- Shredded cheese of your choice
- Cilantro
- Cheese

DIRECTIONS

1. In a small pot, optionally heat a small amount of olive oil over medium heat. Add the diced red onion and sauté for about 3-4 minutes until it becomes translucent.
2. Pour in 3.5 cups of chicken broth and 1/4 can of diced tomatoes. Bring the mixture to a boil, then reduce the heat to low and let it simmer for about 10 minutes to allow the flavors to meld.
3. Add the shredded chicken, white beans, and white corn to the pot. Simmer for an additional 5-7 minutes until everything is heated through. Adjust the amount of chicken broth as needed for your desired consistency.
4. Season the soup with salt and pepper to taste. Adjust the seasoning as needed.
5. For Cassava Flour Tortilla Strips: Preheat your oven to 350°F (175°C). Brush both sides of the cassava flour tortilla with olive oil or use olive oil spray and sprinkle with salt. Cut the tortilla into thin strips. Place the strips on a baking sheet and bake for about 5-7 minutes until they are crisp and golden brown. Keep an eye on them to prevent burning.
6. To serve, ladle the soup into two bowls. Top each bowl with a handful of cassava flour tortilla strips.
7. Garnish each bowl with thinly sliced green chilies, shredded cheese, and chopped cilantro.
8. Serve with lime wedges on the side for squeezing over the soup.

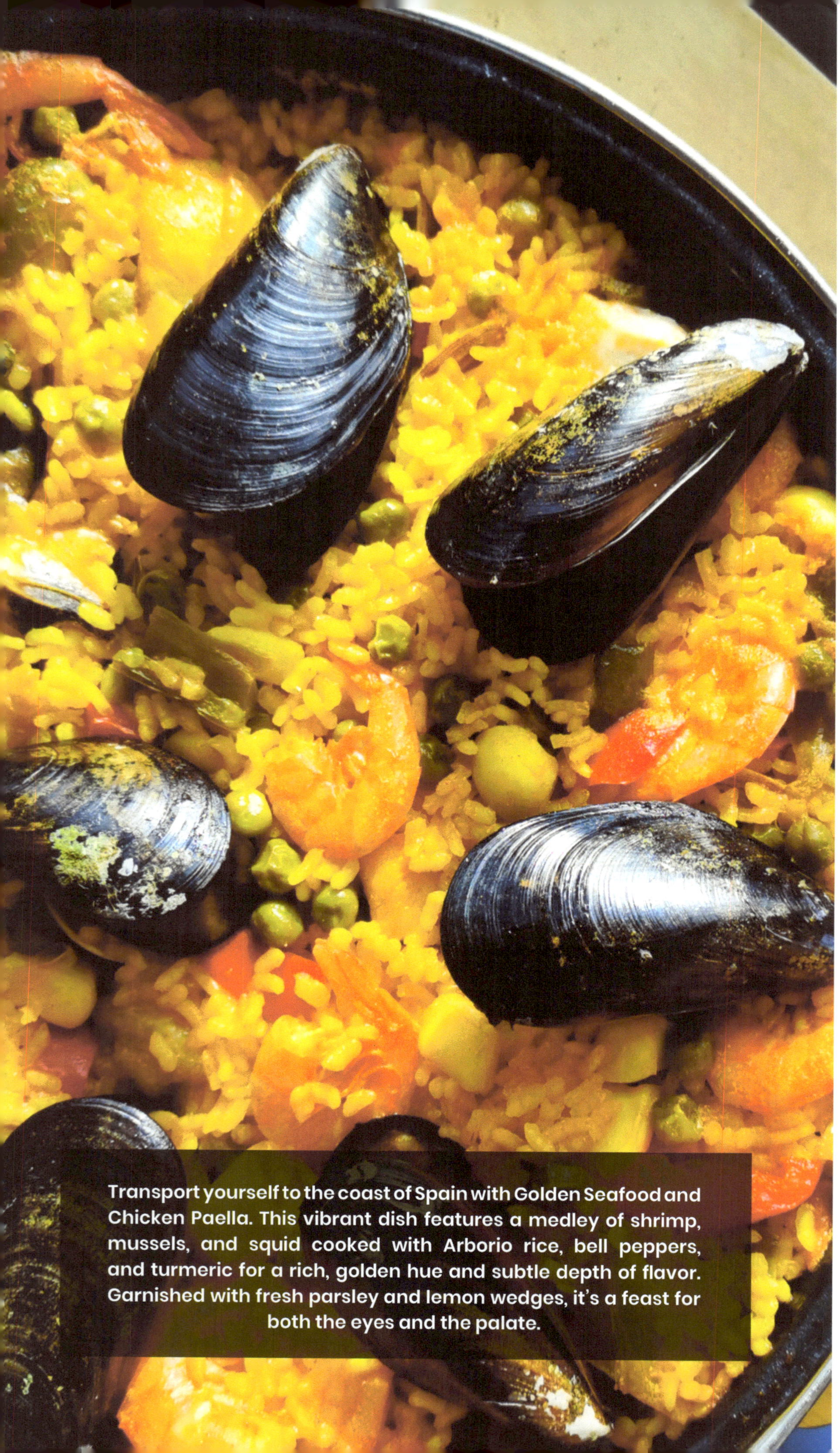

Transport yourself to the coast of Spain with Golden Seafood and Chicken Paella. This vibrant dish features a medley of shrimp, mussels, and squid cooked with Arborio rice, bell peppers, and turmeric for a rich, golden hue and subtle depth of flavor. Garnished with fresh parsley and lemon wedges, it's a feast for both the eyes and the palate.

2 servings

27g P | 63g C
16g F

470 per serving

Prep Time:
15 minutes

Cooking Time:
35 minutes

Total Time:
50 minutes

SEAFOOD

GOLDEN SEAFOOD AND CHICKEN PAELLA

INGREDIENTS

- 1 1/2 cups Arborio rice (or any short-grain rice)
- 1 lb. fresh mussels, cleaned and debearded (small to medium)
- 1/2 lb. large shrimp, peeled and deveined
- 1/4 lb. squid, cleaned and sliced into rings or strips
- 1/2 cup frozen green peas, thawed
- 1/2 red bell pepper, diced
- 1/2 green bell pepper, diced
- 1/2 small white onion, finely chopped
- 2 cloves garlic, minced
- 1/2 teaspoon ground turmeric
- 1 1/2 cups chicken or vegetable broth (preferably low-sodium)
- 1 tablespoon olive oil
- Salt and pepper to taste
- Lemon wedges for garnish
- Fresh parsley for garnish

DIRECTIONS

1. In a small bowl, mix the ground turmeric with a few tablespoons of warm water to create a turmeric paste. Set it aside.
2. Add the diced onion, red and green bell peppers and sauté for about 2-3 minutes until the onion becomes translucent and the peppers begin to soften.
3. Add the minced garlic and cook for an additional 1-2 minutes until fragrant.
4. Stir in the Arborio rice, chicken chunks and add the turmeric paste. Cook for 2-3 minutes, stirring frequently, until the rice is well coated with the onion and turmeric mixture, and the chicken starts to brown slightly.
5. Pour in the chicken or vegetable broth and bring the mixture to a simmer. Reduce the heat to medium-low and let it simmer for about 15-20 minutes, or until the rice is almost cooked through and most of the liquid is absorbed.
6. Gently add the fresh mussels, shrimp, squid rings/strips, and thawed green peas to the pan. Arrange them evenly over the rice and chicken mixture.
7. Cover the pan and let it simmer for an additional 5-7 minutes or until the seafood is cooked through, the mussels have opened, the shrimp turns pink, and the chicken is cooked.
8. Season the paella with salt and pepper to taste.
9. Garnish with lemon wedges and fresh parsley.
10. Serve hot, and enjoy your delicious and flavorful paella with shrimp, squid, and chicken, with turmeric for color and flavor, perfectly portioned for 2 people!

SHRIMP TACOS with CREAMY CITRUS SAUCE

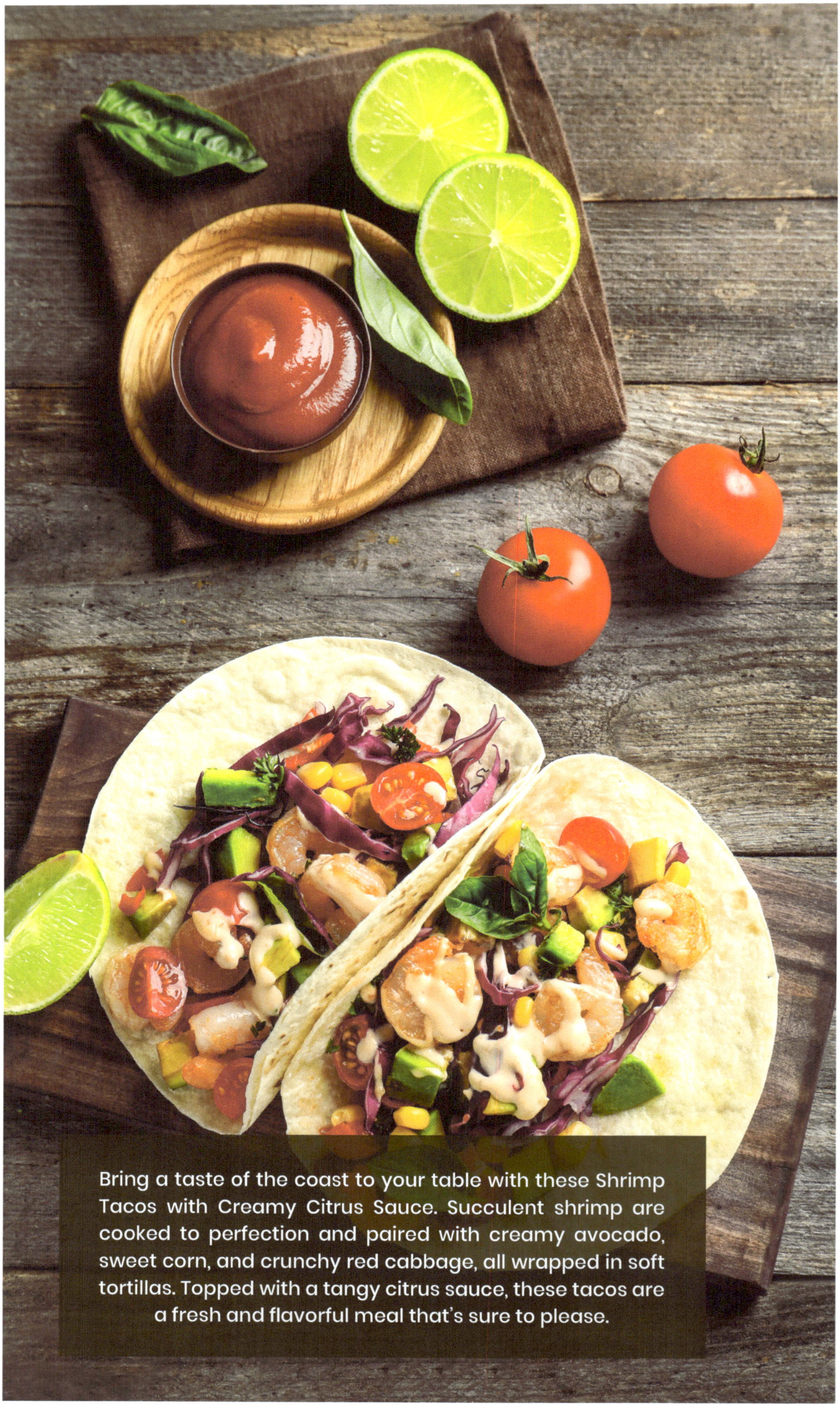

Bring a taste of the coast to your table with these Shrimp Tacos with Creamy Citrus Sauce. Succulent shrimp are cooked to perfection and paired with creamy avocado, sweet corn, and crunchy red cabbage, all wrapped in soft tortillas. Topped with a tangy citrus sauce, these tacos are a fresh and flavorful meal that's sure to please.

2 servings	25g P | 20g C 18g F	467 per serving	Prep Time: 10 minutes	Cooking Time: 10 minutes	Total Time: 20 minutes

INGREDIENTS

For the Tacos:

- 4 Mission Carb Balance Taco Size Soft Flour Tortillas (or use Almond Flour, Cassava Flour or White Corn)
- 24 large shrimp, peeled and deveined
- 1 ripe avocado, diced
- 1/4 cup yellow corn
- 12 grape tomatoes, halved
- 1 cup red cabbage, thinly shredded
- 4 lime wedges
- Fresh basil leaves and English parsley for garnish
- Optional: taco sauce

For Creamy Citrus Sauce:

- 1/4 cup Greek yogurt
- 1 tablespoon mayonnaise
- 1 tablespoon fresh lime juice
- 1 teaspoon honey
- 1/2 teaspoon paprika
- Salt and pepper to taste

DIRECTIONS

Prepare the Sauce:

1. In a small bowl, whisk together the Greek yogurt, mayonnaise, fresh lime juice, honey, paprika, salt, and pepper until smooth. Set aside.

Cook the Shrimp:

1. Heat a dry skillet over medium heat.
2. Add the shrimp and cook for 2-3 minutes on each side, until they are pink and opaque. Remove from heat and set aside.

Assemble the Tacos:

1. Heat a dry skillet over medium heat.
2. Warm each tortilla in the skillet for about 15-20 seconds on each side, or longer if you prefer them toasted.
3. On each tortilla, place 6 cooked shrimp.
4. Add diced avocado, yellow corn kernels, grape tomato halves, and shredded red cabbage on top of the shrimp.
5. Drizzle the creamy citrus sauce generously over the taco fillings.
6. Garnish the tacos with fresh basil leaves and English parsley.
7. Serve the tacos with lime wedges for squeezing and hot sauce for those who desire extra heat.

Breads & Toasts

- Artisanal Einkorn Bread Loaf
- Avocado Toast with Jammy Eggs
- Bagels & Lox Protein Deluxe
- Einkorn Flour and Greek Yogurt Everything Bagels
- Peanut Butter & Jelly Toast

Eggs & Savory Dishes

- Breakfast Tacos with Chorizo, Eggs, and Salsa
- Garden Fresh Veggie Frittata
- Hearty Cinnamon Spiced Sweet Potato Hash
- Sensational Shakshuka
- Spinach and Veggie Egg Bites

Smoothies & Bowls

- Blueberry Bliss Protein Smoothie
- Granola Breakfast Bowl
- Homemade Organic Granola
- Homemade Strawberry Chia Seed Jam
- High-Protein Sweet Banana Nut Overnight Oats
- Raspberry Chia Yogurt Cups
- Strawberry Chia Yogurt Parfait

Pancakes and Waffles

- Protein Blueberry Pancakes with Eggs & Bacon
- Protein Packed Belgian Waffle

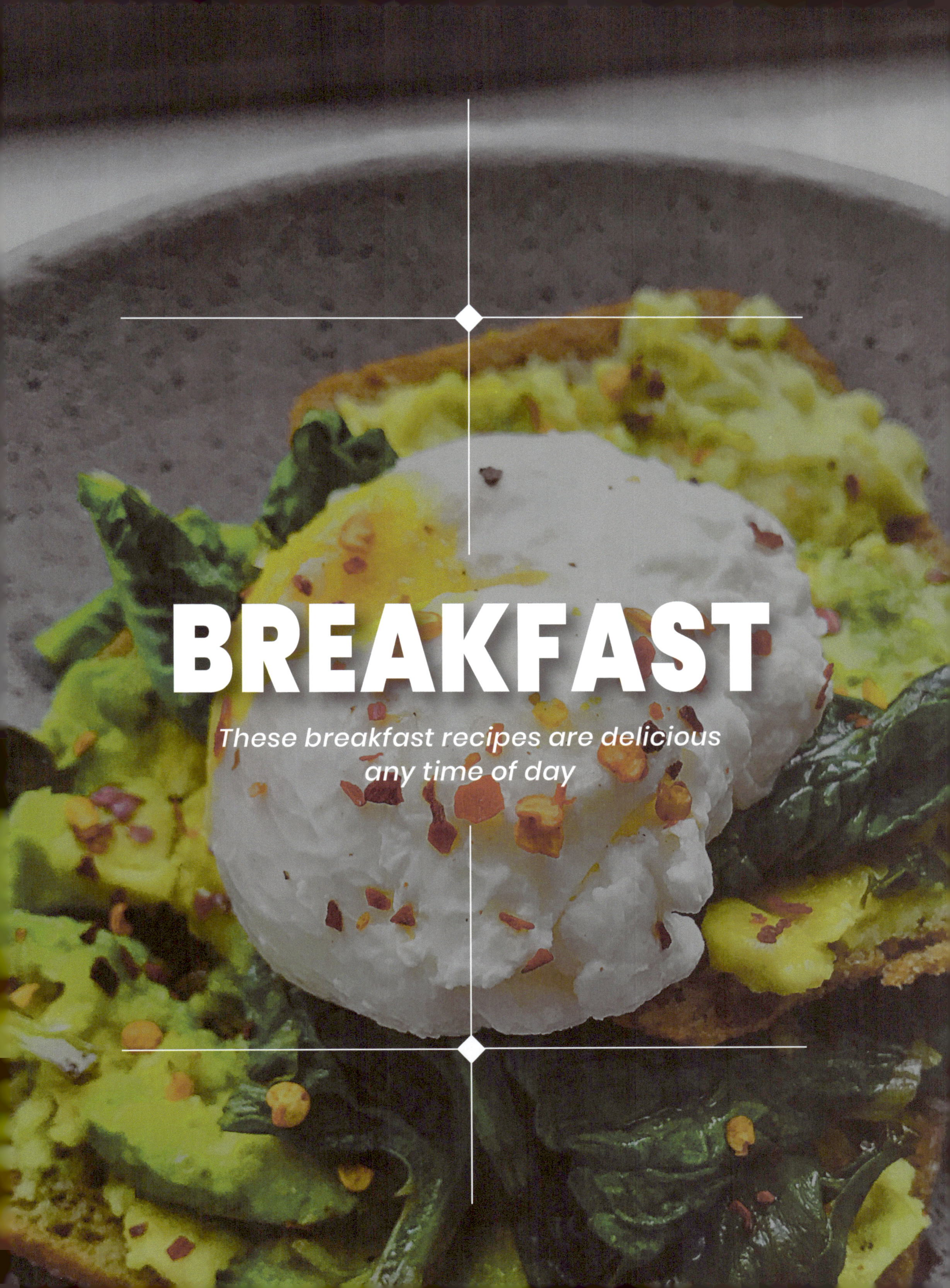

BREAKFAST

These breakfast recipes are delicious any time of day

Experience the rustic charm of homemade bread with this Artisanal Einkorn Bread Loaf. Made with nutrient-rich Einkorn flour and Greek yogurt, this loaf is soft inside with a crusty exterior. Einkorn flour, an ancient grain, is known for being easier to digest and causing fewer digestive issues compared to modern wheat flours. It is also rich in nutrients, making it a wholesome choice for your baking. Perfect for slicing and enjoying with butter, jam, or for making sandwiches, this bread brings a healthy and delicious touch to your meals.

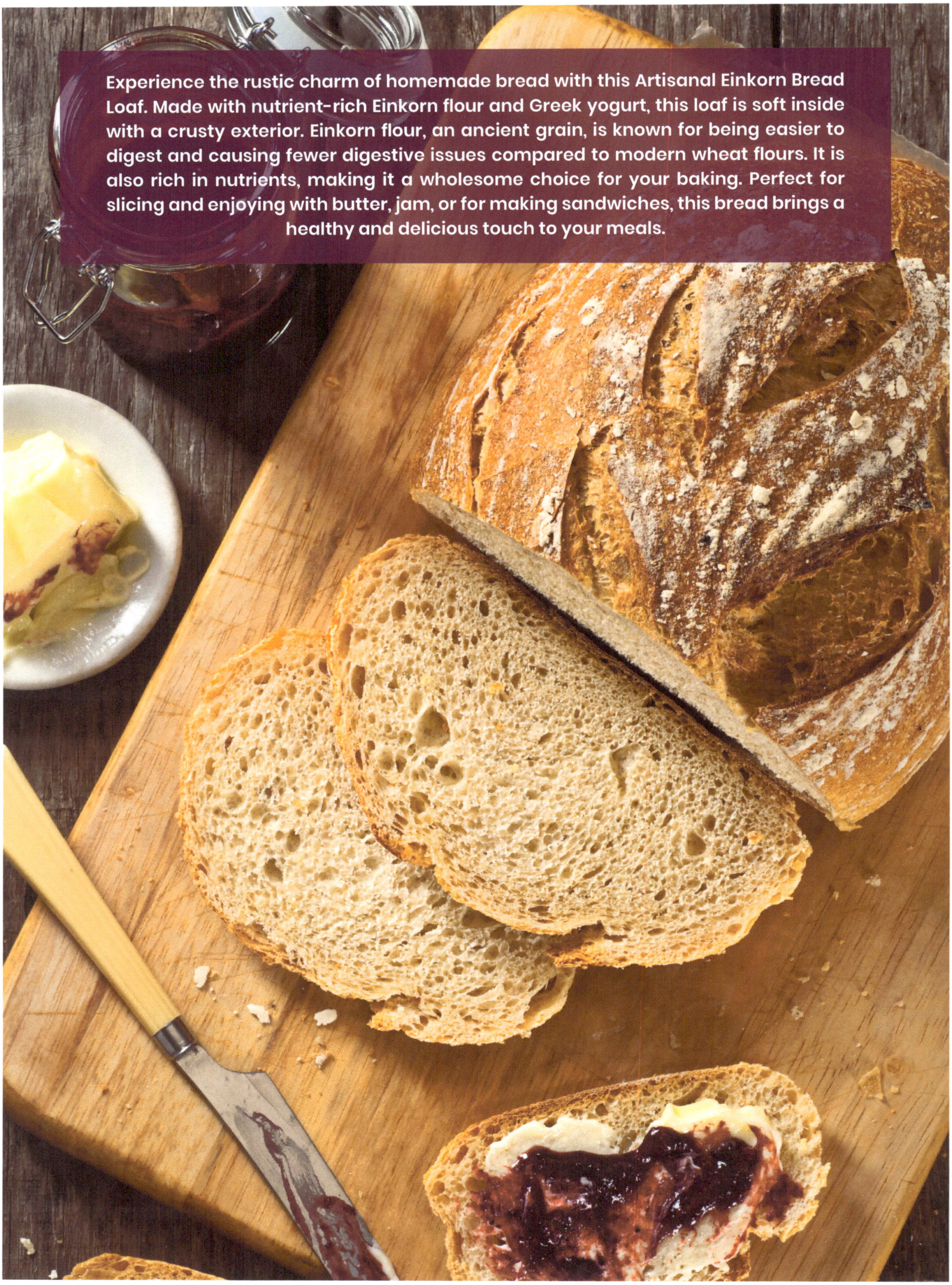

BREADS & TOASTS

ARTISANAL EINKORN BREAD LOAF

12 servings	5g P | 25g C 6g F	170 per serving	Prep Time: 15 minutes	Cooking Time: 30 minutes	Total Time: 45 minutes

INGREDIENTS

- 2 cups Einkorn flour
- 1 1/2 cups Greek yogurt
- 1 1/2 teaspoons baking powder
- 1/2 teaspoon salt
- 1 tablespoon honey (optional, for a touch of sweetness)
- 1/4 cup olive oil (or any preferred cooking oil)
- 2 large eggs

DIRECTIONS

1. Preheat your oven to 350°F (175°C). Line a baking sheet with parchment paper or lightly grease it.
2. Mix the dry ingredients. In a large mixing bowl, combine the Einkorn flour, baking powder, and salt. Stir until well mixed.
3. Mix the wet ingredients in a separate bowl. Whisk together the Greek yogurt, olive oil, eggs, and honey (if using). Mix until the wet ingredients are well combined.
4. Pour the wet ingredient mixture into the bowl with the dry ingredients. Stir everything together until you have a smooth batter.
5. After mixing the batter, transfer it to the prepared baking sheet. Shape it into a rectangular or oval shape for a rustic look. You can also score the top with a sharp knife to create a decorative pattern.
6. Place the baking sheet in the preheated oven and bake for about 30-35 minutes, or until the bread is golden brown on top and sounds hollow when tapped on the bottom. This will give the bread a crusty exterior.
7. Allow the bread to cool on a wire rack. Once cooled, slice it into rustic artisanal slices that can be used for your PB&J Toast recipe or other dishes where an artisanal appearance is desired.
8. Note: You can slice your loaf and freeze to use at a later time.

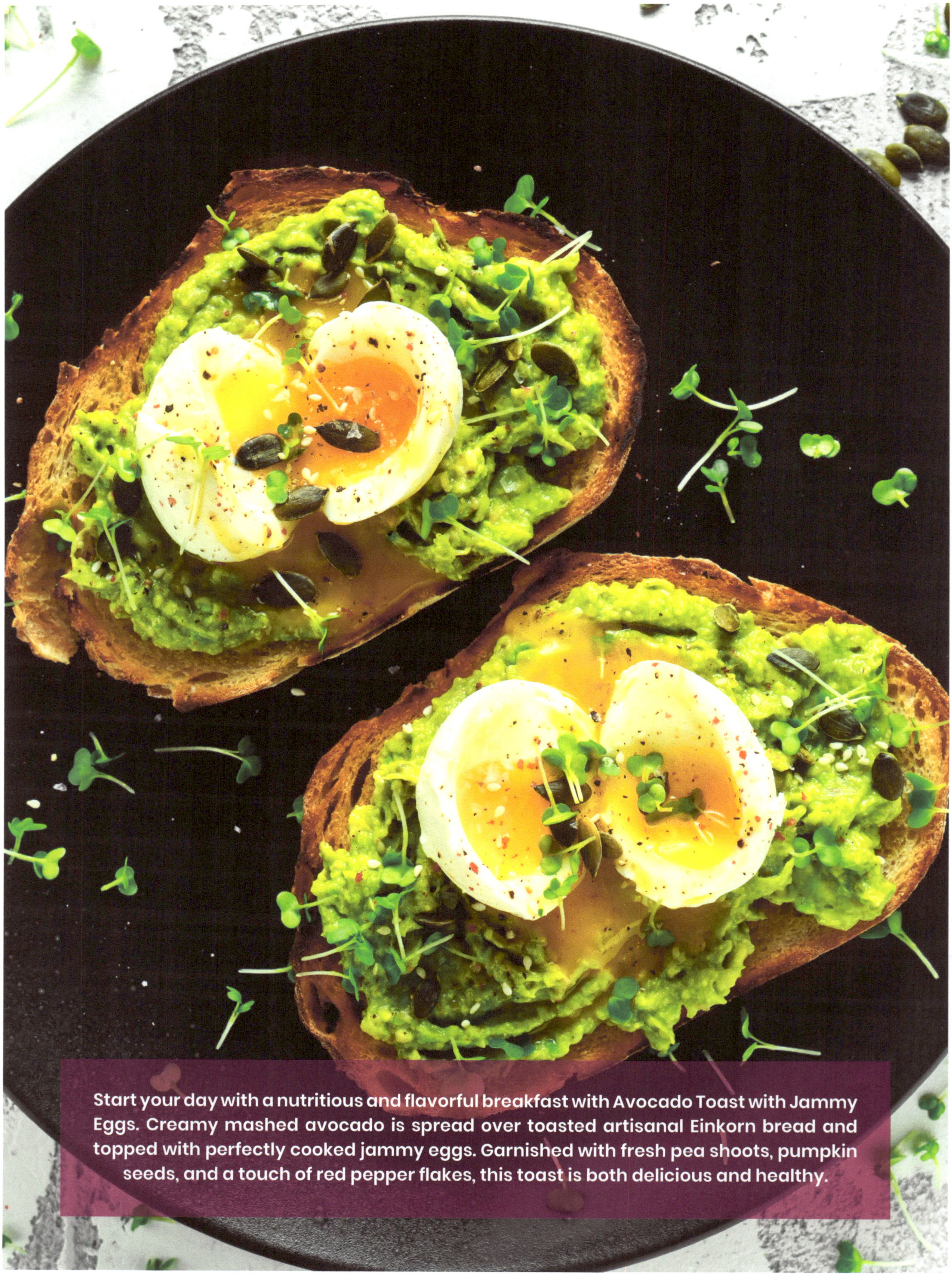

Start your day with a nutritious and flavorful breakfast with Avocado Toast with Jammy Eggs. Creamy mashed avocado is spread over toasted artisanal Einkorn bread and topped with perfectly cooked jammy eggs. Garnished with fresh pea shoots, pumpkin seeds, and a touch of red pepper flakes, this toast is both delicious and healthy.

AVOCADO TOAST with JAMMY EGGS

2 servings	24g P | 54g C 21g F	355 per serving	Prep Time: 8 minutes	Cooking Time: 7 minutes	Total Time: 15 minutes

INGREDIENTS

- 4 slices of Artisanal Einkorn Bread Loaf (see the recipe)
- 1 medium ripe avocado
- 4 large eggs
- Handful of pea shoots (for garnish)
- Salt and black pepper to taste
- Red pepper flakes (optional, for added spice)
- Pumpkin seeds (optional, for garnish)

DIRECTIONS

For Soft-Boiled Jammy Eggs:

1. Fill a medium saucepan with water and bring it to a boil. Add the eggs and simmer for 6-7 minutes for jammy yolks. Transfer eggs to ice water, peel, and set aside.
2. Toast the bread slices until golden brown and crisp.
3. Mash avocados, season with salt, pepper.
4. Spread mashed avocado onto toast slices and top with pea shoots.
5. Slice eggs in half and place one whole egg on each toast.
6. Season with salt, pepper, and optional red pepper flakes.
7. Garnish with pumpkin seeds.
8. Serve 2 slices per person as a delicious breakfast or brunch.

Alternative Options:

1. Grated Eggs: Hard boil and grate your eggs, distributing evenly over each slice.
2. Scrambled Eggs: Scramble your eggs, distributing evenly over each slice.
3. Poached Eggs: Gently poach your eggs in boiling water for 3-4 minutes until the whites are set but the yolks are still runny. Remove with a slotted spoon and enjoy over your toast!

BAGELS & LOX PROTEIN DELUXE

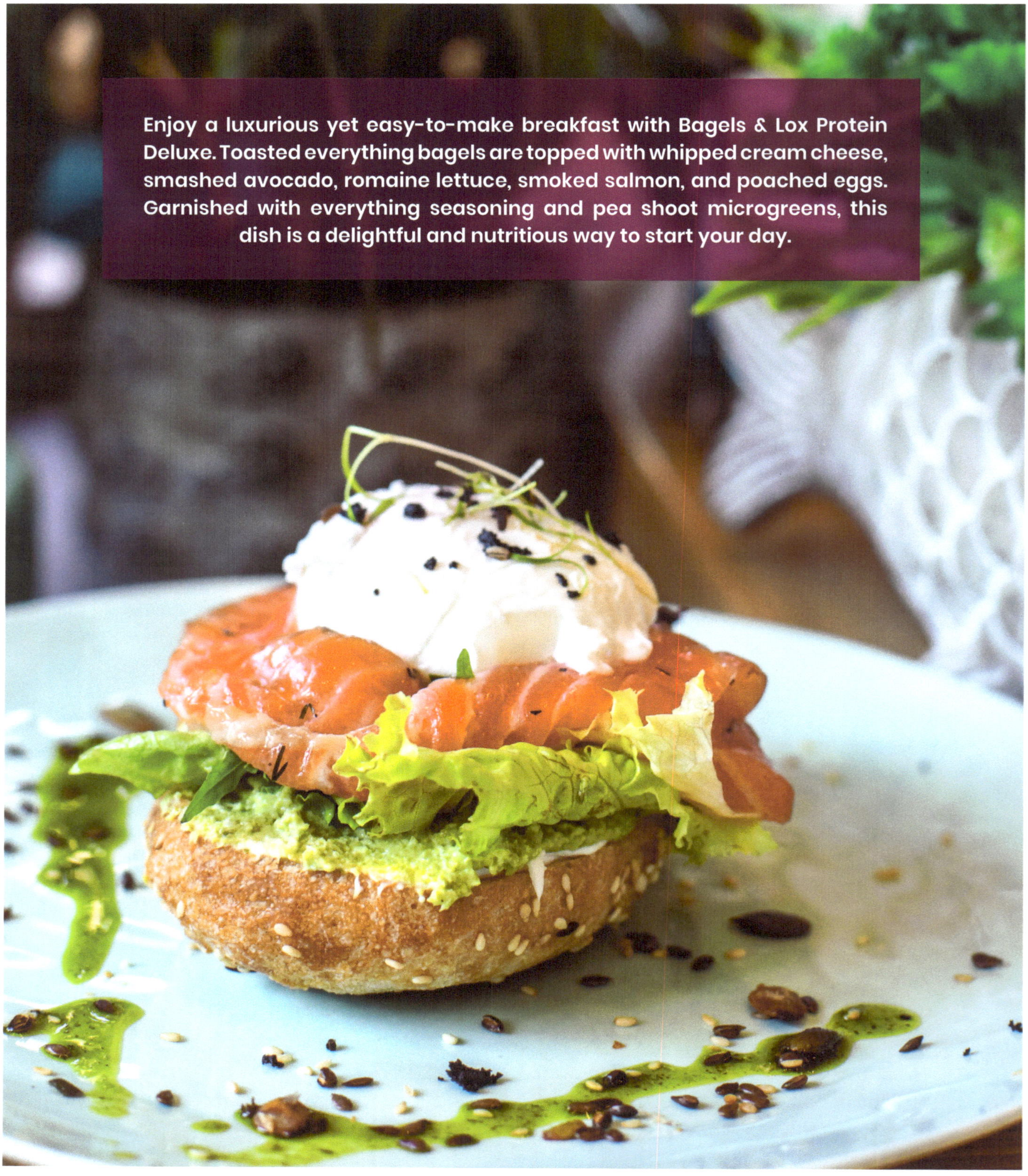

Enjoy a luxurious yet easy-to-make breakfast with Bagels & Lox Protein Deluxe. Toasted everything bagels are topped with whipped cream cheese, smashed avocado, romaine lettuce, smoked salmon, and poached eggs. Garnished with everything seasoning and pea shoot microgreens, this dish is a delightful and nutritious way to start your day.

2 servings	25g P | 41g C 27g F	490 per serving	Prep Time: 15 minutes	Cooking Time: 20 minutes	Total Time: 35 minutes

INGREDIENTS

- 2 Einkorn Flour and Greek Yogurt Everything Bagels (see the recipe)
- 2 tablespoons whipped cream cheese
- 1 medium avocado, smashed and divided (half for each bagel)
- 2 Romaine lettuce leaves, for layering
- 4 slices of smoked salmon
- 4 poached eggs
- Everything seasoning (to taste, for garnish)
- Pea shoots microgreens (for garnish)

DIRECTIONS

1. Place the bagel halves in a toaster or under a broiler until they are nicely toasted to your liking.
2. Once the bagels are toasted, spread 1 tablespoon of whipped cream cheese on each bagel, evenly dividing it between the bagel halves.
3. Take the ripe avocado and mash it, dividing the mashed avocado equally between the bagel halves,
4. Cut each romaine lettuce leaves into pieces and equally divide them between the bagel halves.
5. Lay 1 slice of smoked salmon on top of each lettuce-covered bagel half.

Prepare 4 poached eggs:

1. Fill a pot with water and bring it to a gentle simmer.
2. Add a splash of vinegar to the simmering water.
3. Crack each egg into a small bowl or ramekin.
4. Create a gentle whirlpool in the water by stirring it with a spoon.
5. Carefully slide each egg into the swirling water.
6. Poach for about 3-4 minutes until the whites are set but the yolks are still runny.
7. Use a slotted spoon to remove the poached eggs and let excess water drain.
8. Gently place one poached egg on each bagel half with smoked salmon.
9. Sprinkle Everything seasoning on top of each poached egg. Then, garnish with fresh microgreens.
10. Serve immediately and enjoy!

EINKORN FLOUR AND GREEK YOGURT EVERYTHING BAGELS

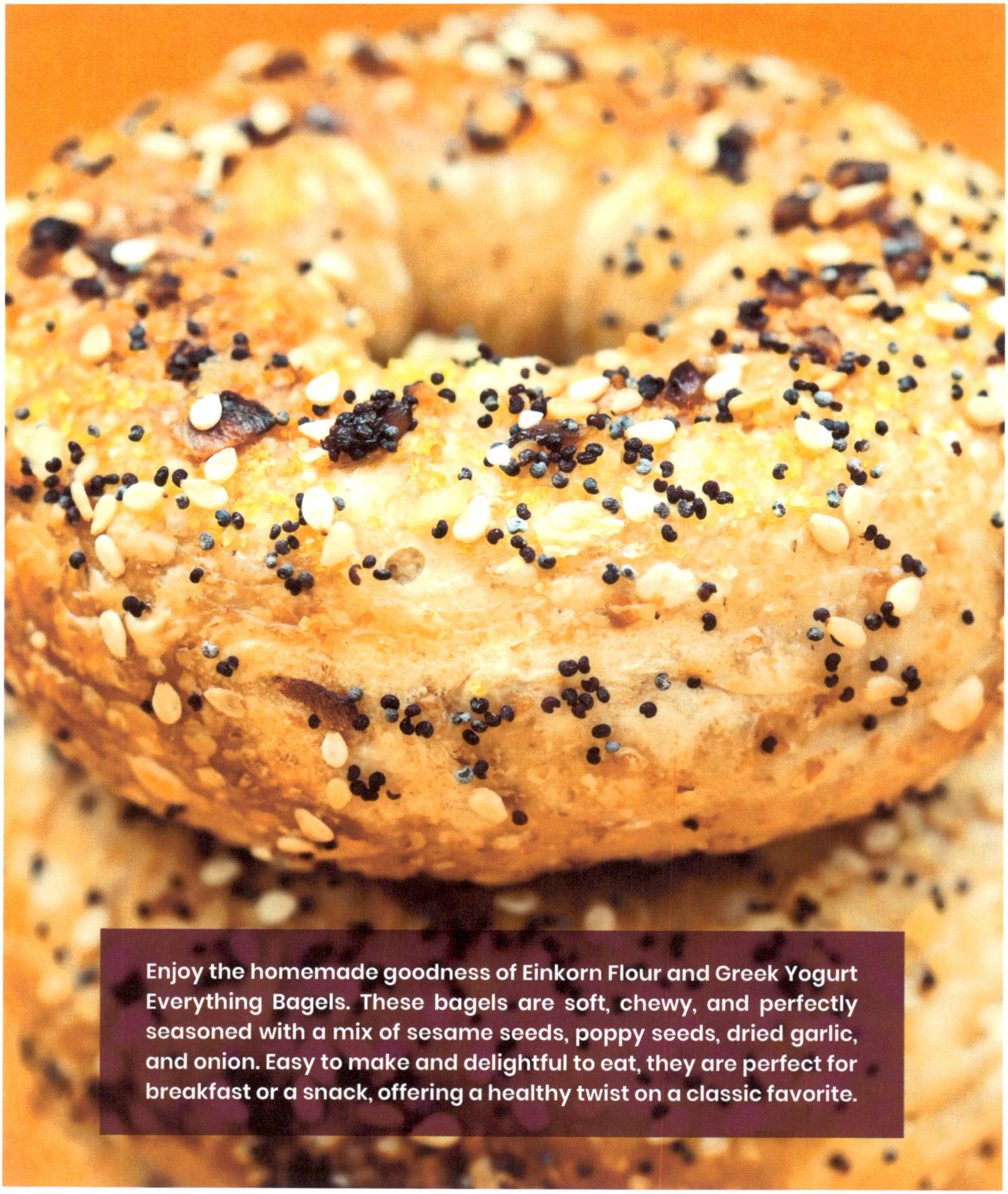

Enjoy the homemade goodness of Einkorn Flour and Greek Yogurt Everything Bagels. These bagels are soft, chewy, and perfectly seasoned with a mix of sesame seeds, poppy seeds, dried garlic, and onion. Easy to make and delightful to eat, they are perfect for breakfast or a snack, offering a healthy twist on a classic favorite.

4 servings	9g P | 33g C 6g F	380 per serving	Prep Time: 15 minutes	Cooking Time: 20 minutes	Total Time: 35 minutes

INGREDIENTS

For the Bagels:

- 1 cup Einkorn flour
- 1 cup Greek yogurt (full-fat or 2g for best results)
- 1 1/2 teaspoons baking powder
- 1/2 teaspoon salt
- 1 egg (for egg wash)

For the Everything Seasoning:

- 1 tablespoon sesame seeds
- 1 tablespoon poppy seeds
- 1 tablespoon dried minced garlic
- 1 tablespoon dried minced onion
- 1/2 teaspoon coarse sea salt

DIRECTIONS

1. Preheat your oven to 375°F (190°C). Line a baking sheet with parchment paper or lightly grease it.
2. In a mixing bowl, combine 1 cup of Einkorn flour, 1 1/2 teaspoons of baking powder, and 1/2 teaspoon of salt.
3. Add 1 cup of Greek yogurt (full-fat or 2g) to the dry ingredients and mix until a dough starts to form.
4. Turn the dough out onto a lightly floured surface and knead it for a few minutes until it becomes smooth and elastic. Add more flour if the dough is too sticky.
5. Divide the dough into 4 equal portions and roll each portion into a ball. Use your finger to poke a hole in the center, stretching it to form the classic bagel shape.
6. In a small bowl, beat an egg to create an egg wash.
7. Brush the tops of the bagels with the egg wash to give them a nice golden color when baked.
8. In a separate bowl, mix together 1 tablespoon sesame seeds, 1 tablespoon poppy seeds, 1 tablespoon dried minced garlic, 1 tablespoon dried minced onion, and 1/2 teaspoon coarse sea salt. Sprinkle this mixture generously over the egg-washed bagels.
9. Place the seasoned bagels on the prepared baking sheet and bake in the preheated oven for about 20-25 minutes, or until they are golden brown and cooked through. They should sound hollow when tapped on the bottom.
10. Allow the bagels to cool slightly on a wire rack before slicing and serving. Enjoy your homemade Einkorn flour everything bagels!

PEANUT BUTTER & JELLY TOAST

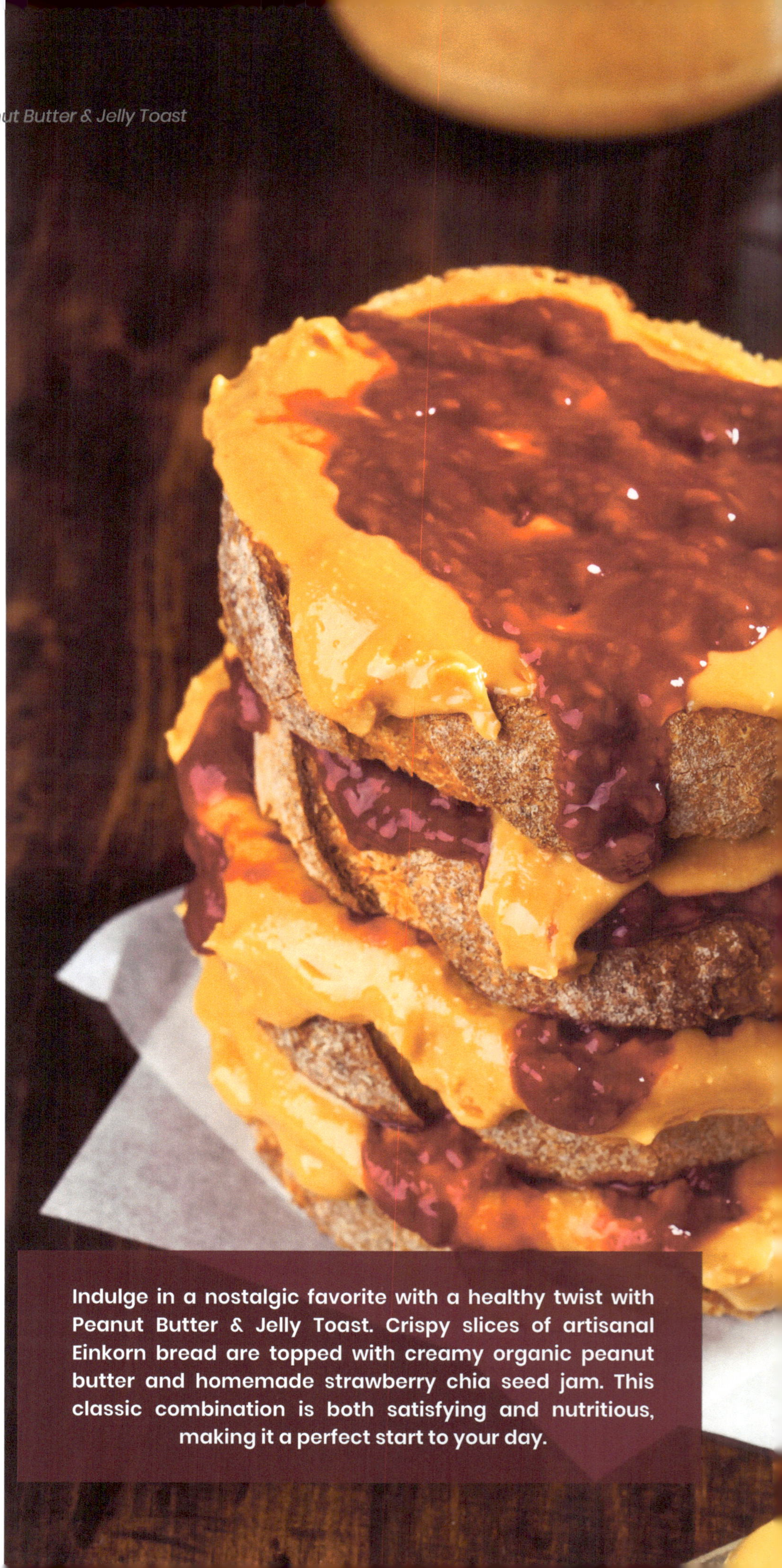

Indulge in a nostalgic favorite with a healthy twist with Peanut Butter & Jelly Toast. Crispy slices of artisanal Einkorn bread are topped with creamy organic peanut butter and homemade strawberry chia seed jam. This classic combination is both satisfying and nutritious, making it a perfect start to your day.

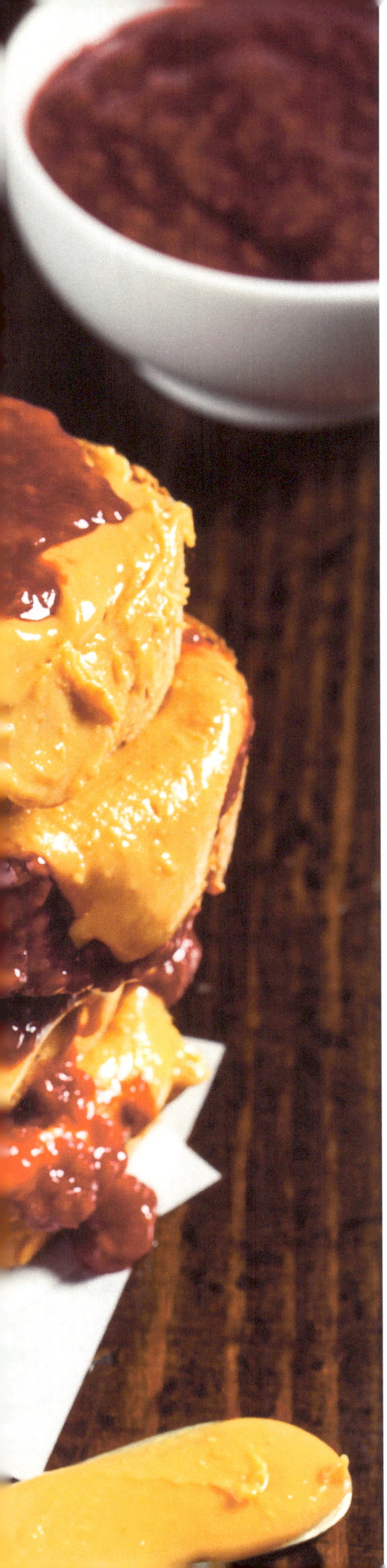

INGREDIENTS

- 4 slices of Artisanal Einkorn Bread Loaf (or 2 Einkorn Flour and Greek Yogurt Everything Bagels (see the recipe))
- 4 tablespoons creamy organic peanut butter
- 4 tablespoons Homemade Strawberry Chia Seed Jam (see the recipe)

4 servings

16g P | 58g C
26g F

490 per serving

Prep Time:
1 minutes

Cooking Time:
4 minutes

Total Time:
5 minutes

DIRECTIONS

1. Toast the bread slices until they are golden brown and have reached your desired level of crispiness.
2. Spread approximately 1 tablespoon of creamy organic peanut butter on one side of each toasted bread slice.
3. Once you've prepared the homemade Strawberry Chia Seed Jam according to the provided recipe, spread 1 tablespoon of jam on top of the peanut butter on each toasted bread slice.
4. Serve 2 toasted bread slices per person and enjoy!

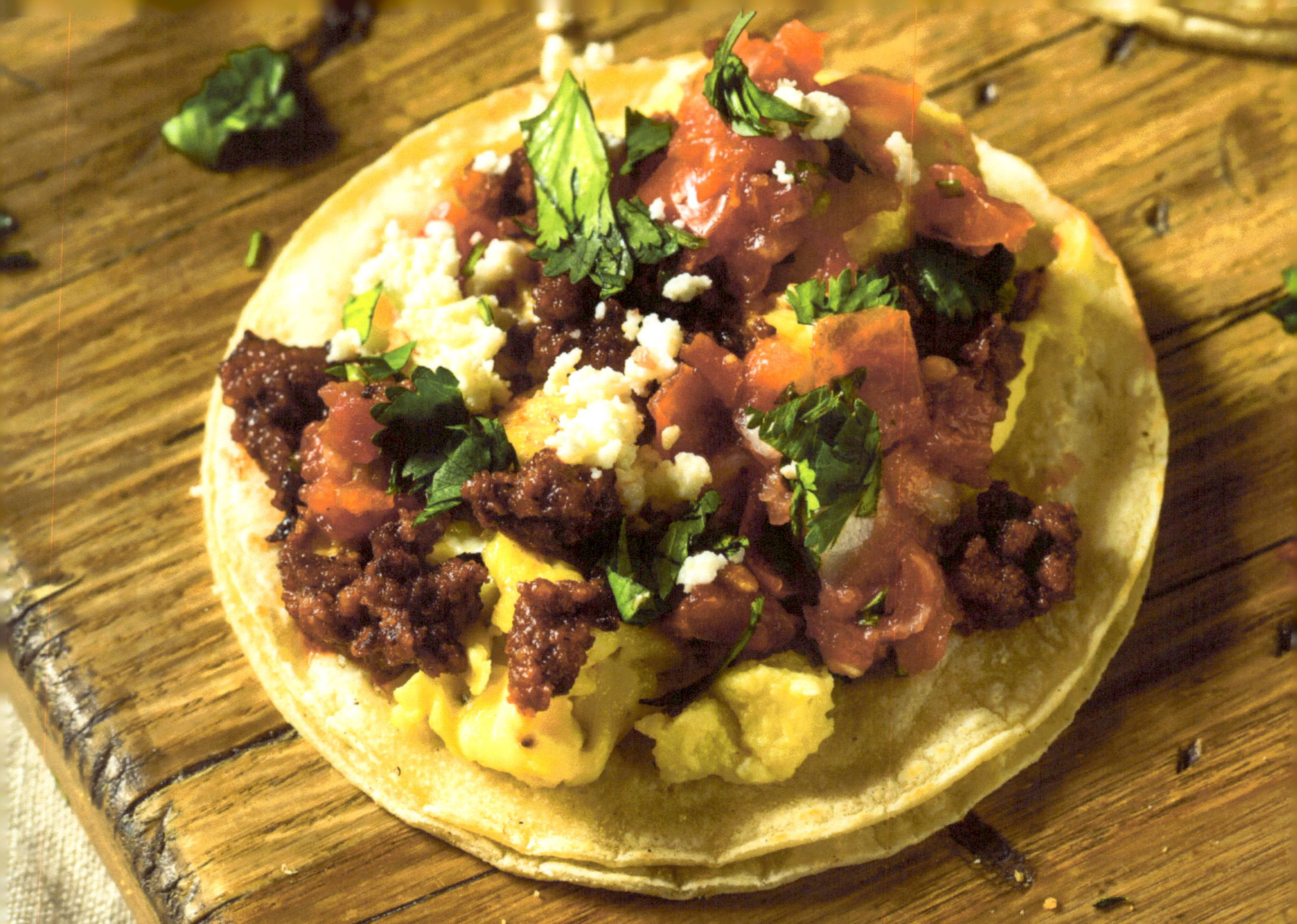

Start your day with the bold and vibrant flavors of these Breakfast Tacos with Chorizo, Eggs, and Salsa. Soft corn tortillas are filled with fluffy scrambled eggs and spicy chorizo, then topped with homemade chunky salsa, crumbled feta cheese, and fresh cilantro. These tacos bring together simple, authentic ingredients for a delicious and satisfying breakfast experience.

BREAKFAST TACOS WITH CHORIZO, EGGS AND SALSA

2 servings	25g P | 20g C 15g F	350 per serving	Prep Time: 10 minutes	Cooking Time: 15 minutes	Total Time: 25 minutes

EGGS & SAVORY DISHES

INGREDIENTS

For the Tacos:

- 4 small white corn tortillas
- 4 large eggs
- Salt and pepper to taste
- 1 tablespoon butter
- 4 oz Mexican chorizo, casing removed
- 1/4 cup crumbled feta cheese
- 1/4 cup fresh cilantro, chopped
- 1/2 cup chunky salsa (store-bought or homemade)

For Homemade Chunky Salsa:

- 1 can (14.5 oz) diced tomatoes, drained
- 1/4 cup finely chopped onion
- 1/2 jalapeño, seeded and finely chopped (optional for mild)
- 1 clove garlic, minced
- 1/4 cup fresh cilantro, chopped
- Juice of 1 lime
- 1/2 teaspoon ground cumin
- Salt and pepper to taste

DIRECTIONS

Make the Chunky Salsa (or use store-bought):

1. Combine drained diced tomatoes, onion, jalapeño (if using), garlic, cilantro, lime juice, cumin, salt, and pepper in a medium bowl. Mix well and set aside.

Cook the Chorizo:

1. Heat a skillet over medium heat. Add the chorizo (casing removed) and cook, breaking it up with a spoon, until fully cooked and browned, about 5-7 minutes. Remove from skillet and set aside before making the scrambled eggs.

Make the Scrambled Eggs:

1. In the same skillet, melt the butter over medium-low heat.
2. Crack the eggs into a bowl and season with salt, whisk the eggs until combined.
3. Pour the eggs into the skillet and gently stir with a spatula until soft curds form and the eggs are set but still slightly creamy.

Warm the Tortillas:

1. Heat the tortillas in a dry skillet over medium heat for about 30 seconds on each side, or until warm and pliable. Alternatively, you can warm them in the microwave wrapped in a damp paper towel for about 20 seconds.

Assemble the Tacos:

1. Divide the scrambled eggs evenly among the tortillas.
2. Top each taco with cooked chorizo, a spoonful of chunky salsa, crumbled feta cheese, and chopped cilantro.
3. Serve the breakfast tacos immediately while warm.

GARDEN FRESH VEGGIE FRITTATA

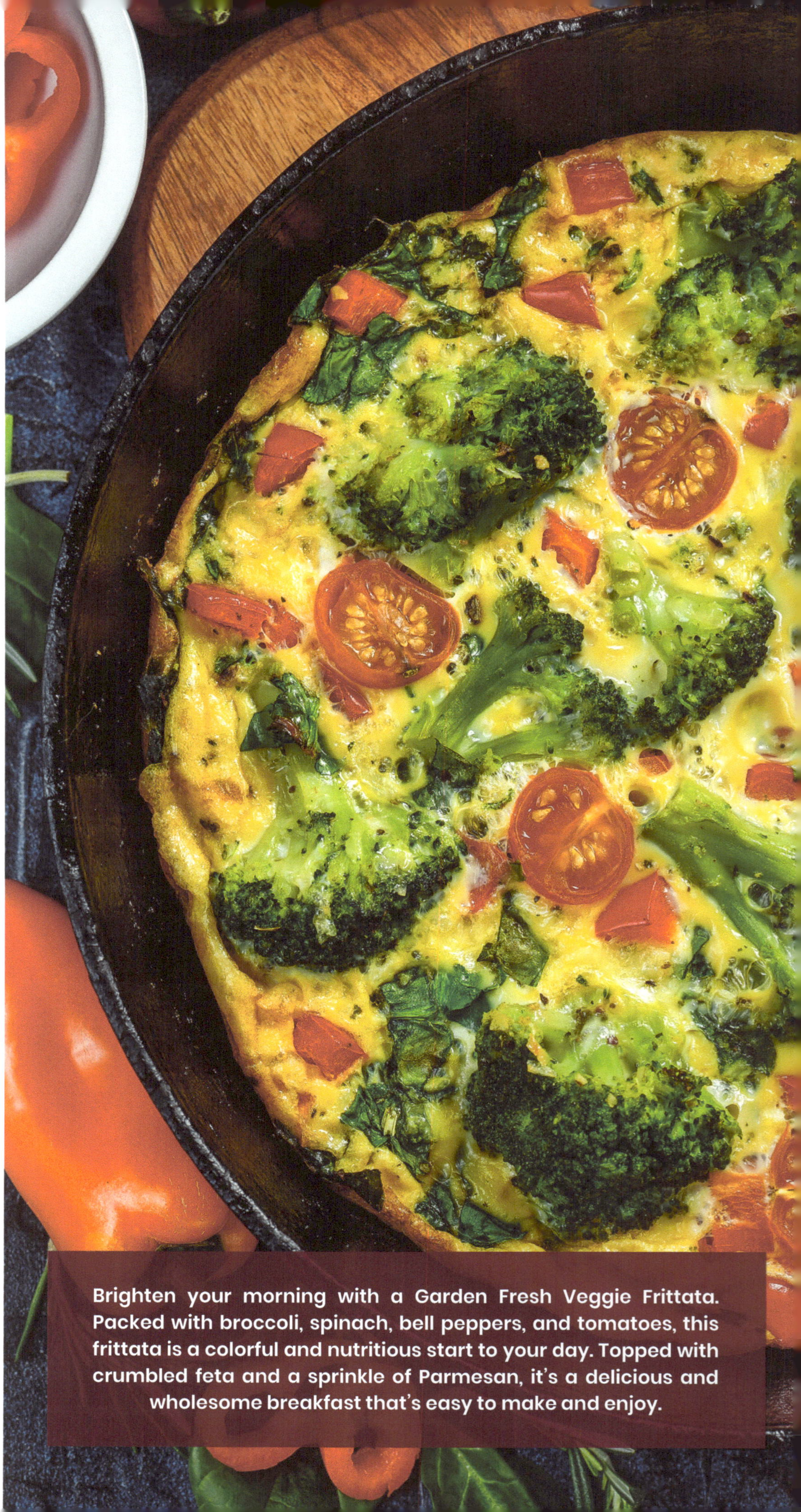

Brighten your morning with a Garden Fresh Veggie Frittata. Packed with broccoli, spinach, bell peppers, and tomatoes, this frittata is a colorful and nutritious start to your day. Topped with crumbled feta and a sprinkle of Parmesan, it's a delicious and wholesome breakfast that's easy to make and enjoy.

2 servings	14g P | 10g C 15g F	280 per serving	Prep Time: 10 minutes	Cooking Time: 20 minutes	Total Time: 30 minutes

INGREDIENTS

- 6 large eggs
- 1 cup broccoli florets, chopped
- 1 cup baby spinach leaves
- 1/2 red bell pepper, diced
- A handful of grape tomatoes, halved
- 1/4 cup crumbled feta cheese
- 1 clove garlic, minced
- 1/4 teaspoon dried basil
- 1/2 teaspoon salt
- Pepper to taste
- A pinch of red pepper flakes
- Grated Parmesan cheese for garnish
- Olive oil spray for cooking

DIRECTIONS

1. Preheat your oven to 350°F (175°C).
2. In an oven-safe skillet, heat a drizzle of olive oil over medium heat.
3. Sauté minced garlic for about 30 seconds until fragrant.
4. Add broccoli, red bell pepper, and grape tomatoes to the skillet. Sauté for 3 minutes until they begin to soften.
5. Stir in baby spinach and cook for an additional 1 minute until it starts to wilt.
6. Whisk eggs in a bowl, add dried basil, salt, pepper, and crumbled feta cheese. Mix well.
7. Pour the egg mixture evenly over the sautéed vegetables in the skillet.
8. Cook on the stove over medium heat for 3-4 minutes until edges set.
9. Transfer the skillet to the preheated oven and bake for 12-15 minutes until the frittata is set and slightly golden on top.
10. Remove from the oven, cool for a minute, sprinkle with grated Parmesan cheese, slice, and serve.

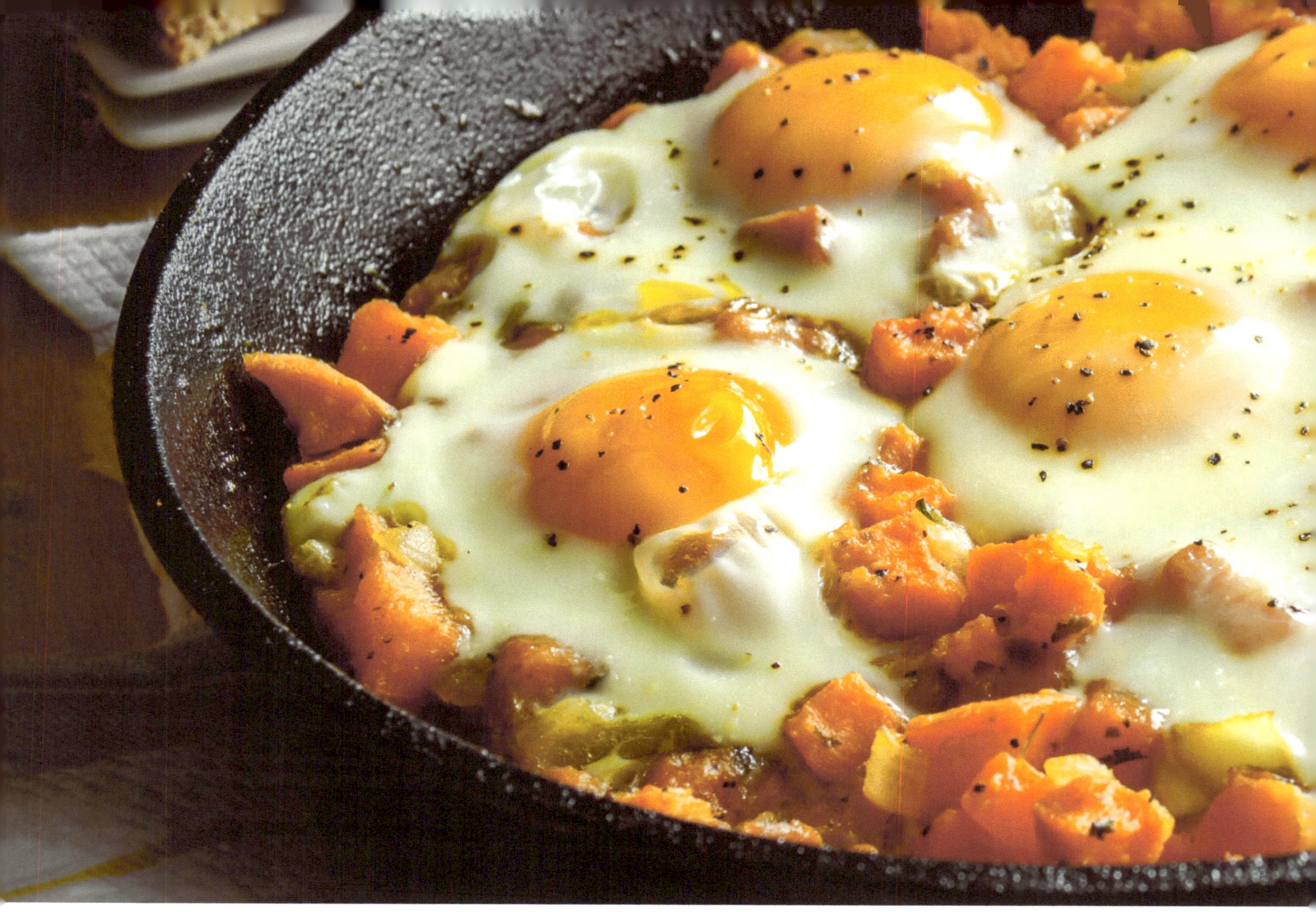

HEARTY CINNAMON SPICED SWEET POTATO HASH

INGREDIENTS

- 2 medium sweet potatoes, peeled and diced
- 1/2 medium white onion, finely chopped
- 1 small red bell pepper, diced
- 2 cloves garlic, minced
- 2 tablespoons olive oil
- 1/2 teaspoon paprika
- 1/2 teaspoon cinnamon
- Salt and black pepper to taste
- 4 large eggs
- 2 tablespoons Maple Syrup, for garnish (optional)

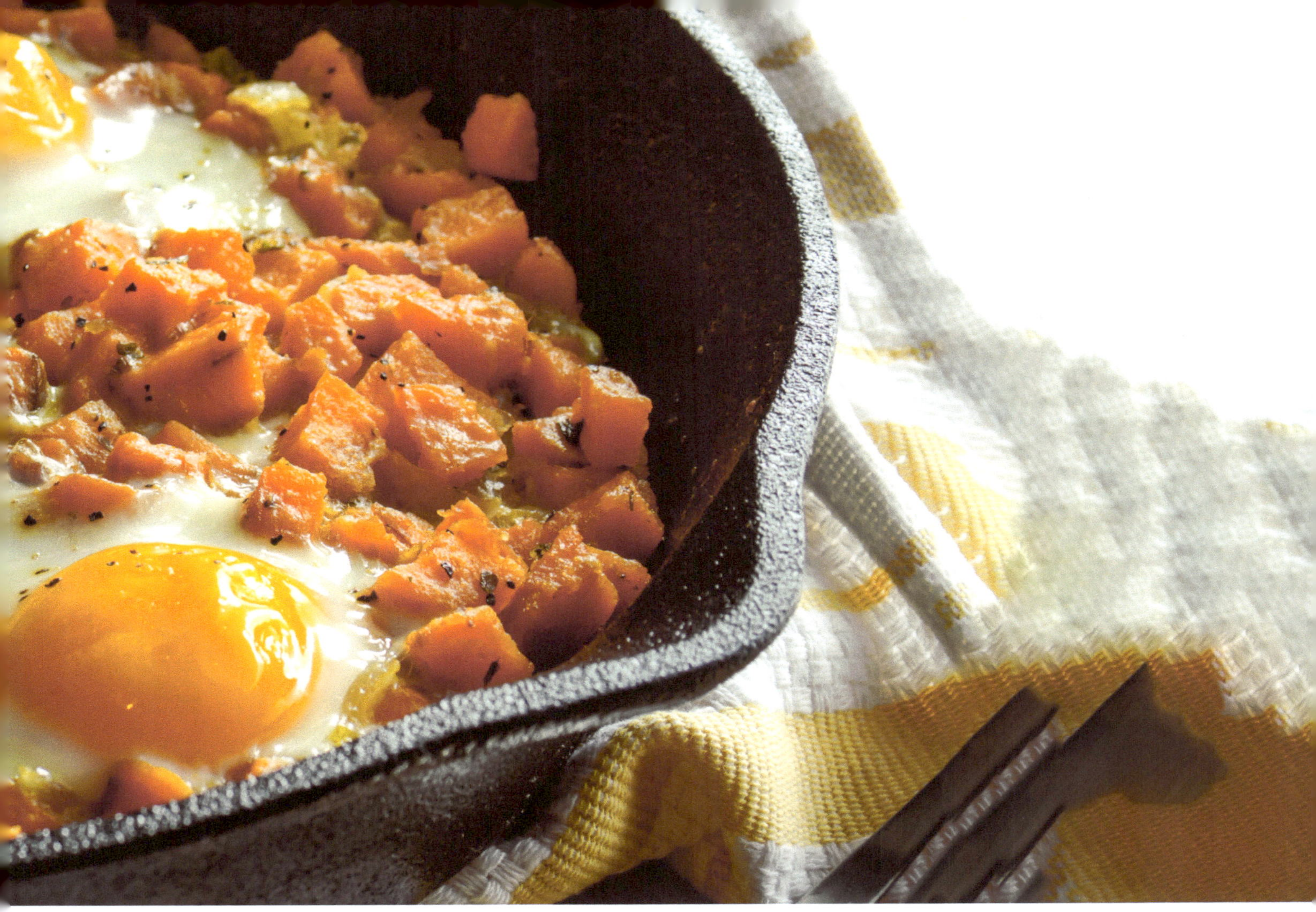

2 servings	11g P | 54g C 15g F	370 per serving	Prep Time: 15 minutes	Cooking Time: 20 minutes	Total Time: 35 minutes

DIRECTIONS

1. In a large skillet, heat olive oil over medium heat. Add the diced sweet potatoes and cook for about 10-12 minutes, or until they become tender and slightly crispy. Stir occasionally.
2. Add the chopped onion and red bell pepper to the skillet. Sauté for an additional 3-4 minutes, until the vegetables become soft and the onion is translucent.
3. Stir in the minced garlic, paprika, ground cinnamon, salt, and black pepper. Cook for another 1-2 minutes, allowing the flavors to meld.
4. Make four small wells in the sweet potato mixture with a spoon. Crack one egg into each well. Cover the skillet and cook for about 5-7 minutes, or until the egg whites are set but the yolks are still slightly runny. Adjust the cooking time if you prefer firmer yolks.
5. Once the eggs are cooked to your liking, garnish with salt and pepper to taste and maple syrup if desired.

SENSATIONAL SHAKSHUKA

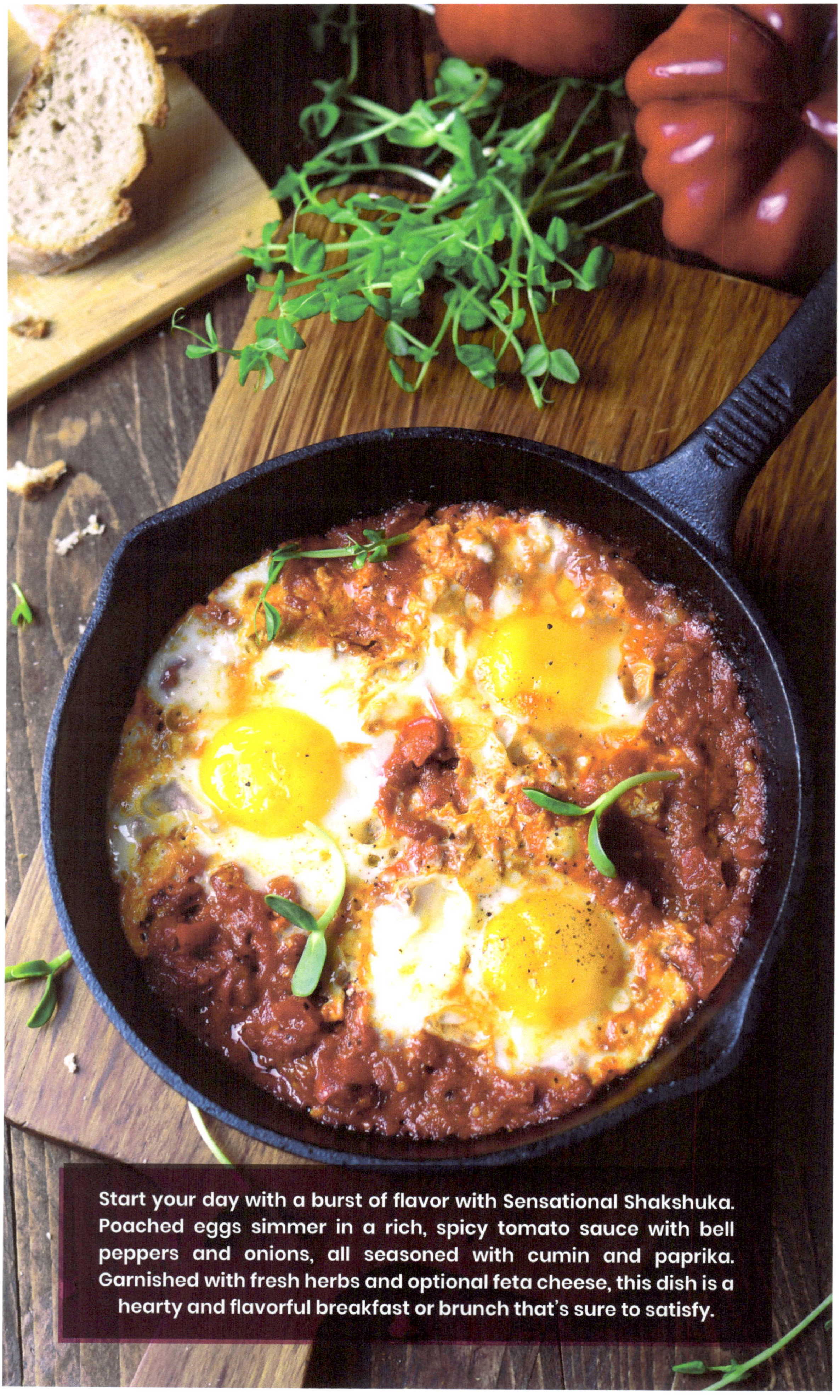

Start your day with a burst of flavor with Sensational Shakshuka. Poached eggs simmer in a rich, spicy tomato sauce with bell peppers and onions, all seasoned with cumin and paprika. Garnished with fresh herbs and optional feta cheese, this dish is a hearty and flavorful breakfast or brunch that's sure to satisfy.

2 servings	18g P | 17g C 15g F	260 per serving	Prep Time: 10 minutes	Cooking Time: 20 minutes	Total Time: 30 minutes

INGREDIENTS

- 2 tablespoons olive oil
- 1 onion, finely chopped
- 1 red bell pepper, diced
- 2 cloves garlic, minced
- 1 can (14 ounces) crushed tomatoes
- 1 teaspoon ground cumin
- 1/2 teaspoon paprika
- 1/4 teaspoon cayenne pepper (adjust to taste)
- Salt and pepper to taste
- 6 large organic, pasture raised, cage-free, eggs
- Fresh parsley or cilantro leaves for garnish
- Optional:
- Crumbled feta cheese for topping
- Artisanal Einkorn bread, slice (see the recipe)

DIRECTIONS

1. Heat the olive oil in a large skillet over medium heat. Add the finely chopped onion and diced red bell pepper. Sauté for 2-3 minutes or until the vegetables soften.
2. Stir in the minced garlic and cook for an additional minute until fragrant.
3. Add the crushed tomatoes, ground cumin, paprika, and cayenne pepper. Season with salt and pepper to taste. Simmer the sauce for 10 minutes, or until it thickens slightly.
4. Using a spoon, create small wells in the tomato sauce for the eggs. Crack each egg into a well.
5. Cover the skillet and let the eggs poach in the sauce for about 5-7 minutes or until the egg whites are set but the yolks are still runny. You can cook them longer if you prefer firmer yolks.
6. Garnish the Shakshuka with fresh parsley or cilantro leaves
7. Optional: Serve with crumbled feta cheese and toasted bread, if desired.

Enjoy a protein-packed breakfast with these Spinach and Veggie Egg Bites. Fresh spinach, tomatoes, bell peppers, and onions are combined with eggs and baked to perfection. These bites are convenient, nutritious, and perfect for a quick breakfast or snack on the go.

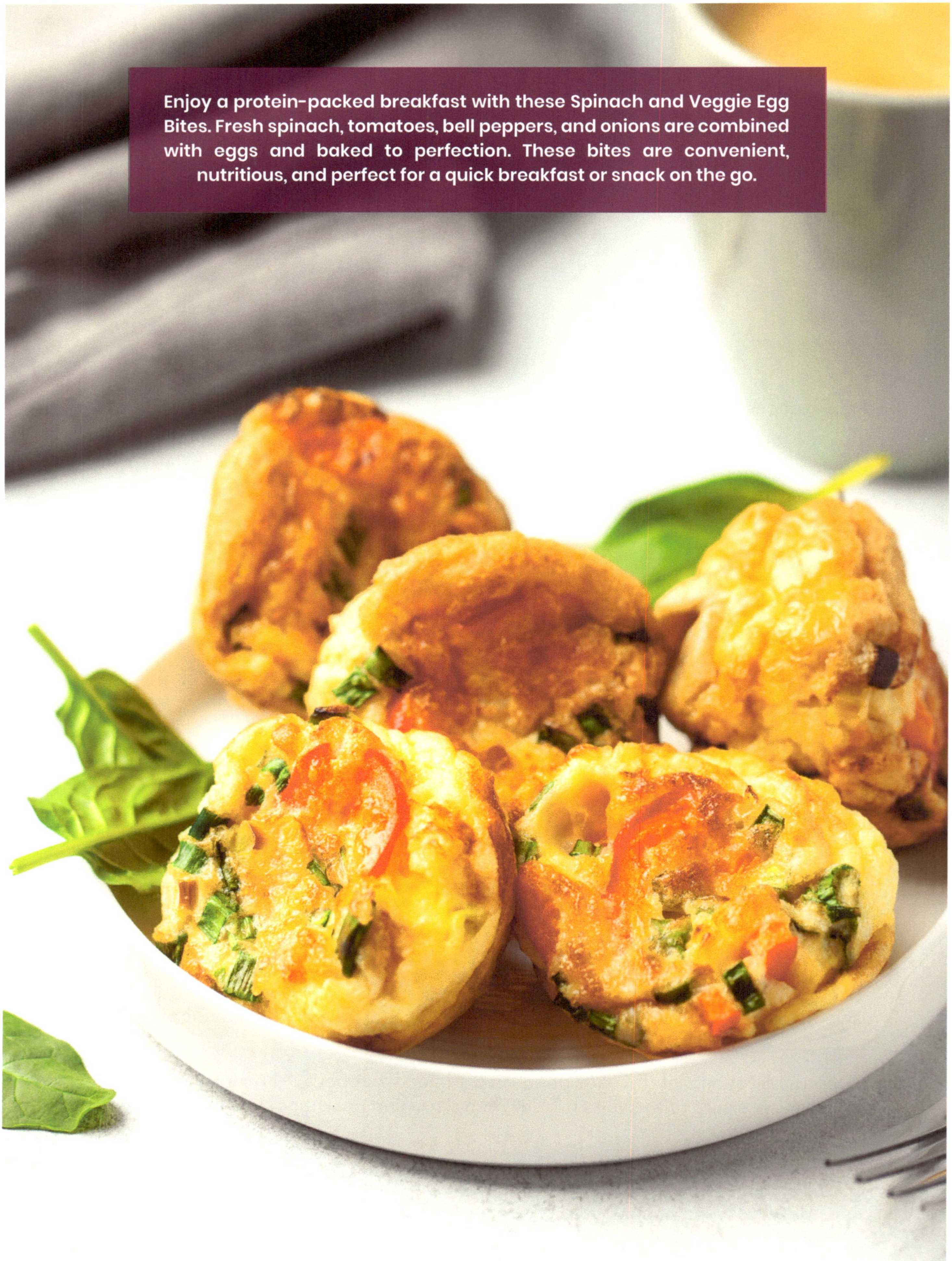

SPINACH AND VEGGIE EGG BITES

2 servings	18g P | 6g C 18g F	255 per serving	Prep Time: 10 minutes	Cooking Time: 10 minutes	Total Time: 30 minutes

INGREDIENTS

- 6 large eggs
- 1 cup fresh spinach, finely chopped
- 1/2 cup grape or cherry tomatoes, diced
- 1/4 cup diced red bell pepper
- 1/4 cup diced spring onion (green onion)
- 1/4 cup crumbled feta cheese (optional)
- Salt and black pepper to taste
- Cooking spray or butter for greasing the muffin tin

DIRECTIONS

1. Preheat your oven to 350°F (175°C). Grease a 6-cup muffin tin with cooking spray.
2. In a bowl, crack the eggs and whisk them until well beaten. Season with salt and black pepper to taste.
3. Divide the finely chopped spinach, quartered tomatoes, diced red bell pepper, diced spring onion, and crumbled feta cheese (if using) evenly among the 6 muffin cups.
4. Pour the beaten eggs over the veggies and cheese in each muffin cup, filling them about two-thirds full.
5. Use a fork or a small spatula to gently stir the mixture in each muffin cup, ensuring the eggs and veggies are evenly distributed.
6. Bake in the preheated oven for 20-25 minutes or until the egg bites are set and slightly puffed up. You can check for doneness by inserting a toothpick into the center of one; it should come out clean when they're done.
7. Remove the muffin tin from the oven and let the egg bites cool for a few minutes. They will deflate slightly as they cool.
8. Use a knife or spoon to carefully remove the egg bites from the muffin tin. Serve 3 bites per person while they are warm, creating a delicious and portable breakfast or snack.

SMOOTHIES & BOWLS

BLUEBERRY BLISS PROTEIN SMOOTHIE

1 servings	34g P | 28g C 3g F	255 per serving	Prep Time: 4 minutes	Blending Time: 1 minute	Total Time: 5 minutes

INGREDIENTS

- 1 cup blueberries (fresh or frozen)
- 1 scoop vanilla ice cream flavor protein powder by Maxpro Elite (or 1/2 cup Greek yogurt)
- 1/2 cup unsweetened nut milk (or water or dairy milk)

Optional:

- Blueberries for garnish
- 2 cubes of ice

DIRECTIONS

1. In a blender, combine the blueberries, vanilla protein powder (or Greek yogurt if using), unsweetened nut milk (or water or dairy milk) and ice cubes if using.
2. Blend until smooth and creamy.
3. Pour into a glass and garnish with extra blueberries if desired.
4. Serve immediately and enjoy!

Alternative Option:

1. Feel free to get creative with your smoothie combinations! If you'd like to switch things up while staying within a similar nutritional profile, consider using other fruits like strawberries, raspberries, blackberries or combine them all. These berries are also rich in antioxidants and can add a burst of flavor to your smoothie.

2. Enhance the flavor and nutrition of this smoothie by adding a tablespoon of unsweetened cacao powder. Cacao powder not only brings a rich chocolatey taste but also provides antioxidants and a natural boost of energy. Simply blend it in with the other ingredients to create a delicious blueberry-chocolate smoothie that's both satisfying and nutritious.

Kickstart your day with the refreshing and nutritious Blueberry Bliss Protein Smoothie. Packed with antioxidants from fresh blueberries and protein from vanilla ice cream flavor protein powder, this smoothie is creamy, delicious, and perfect for a quick breakfast or post-workout snack.

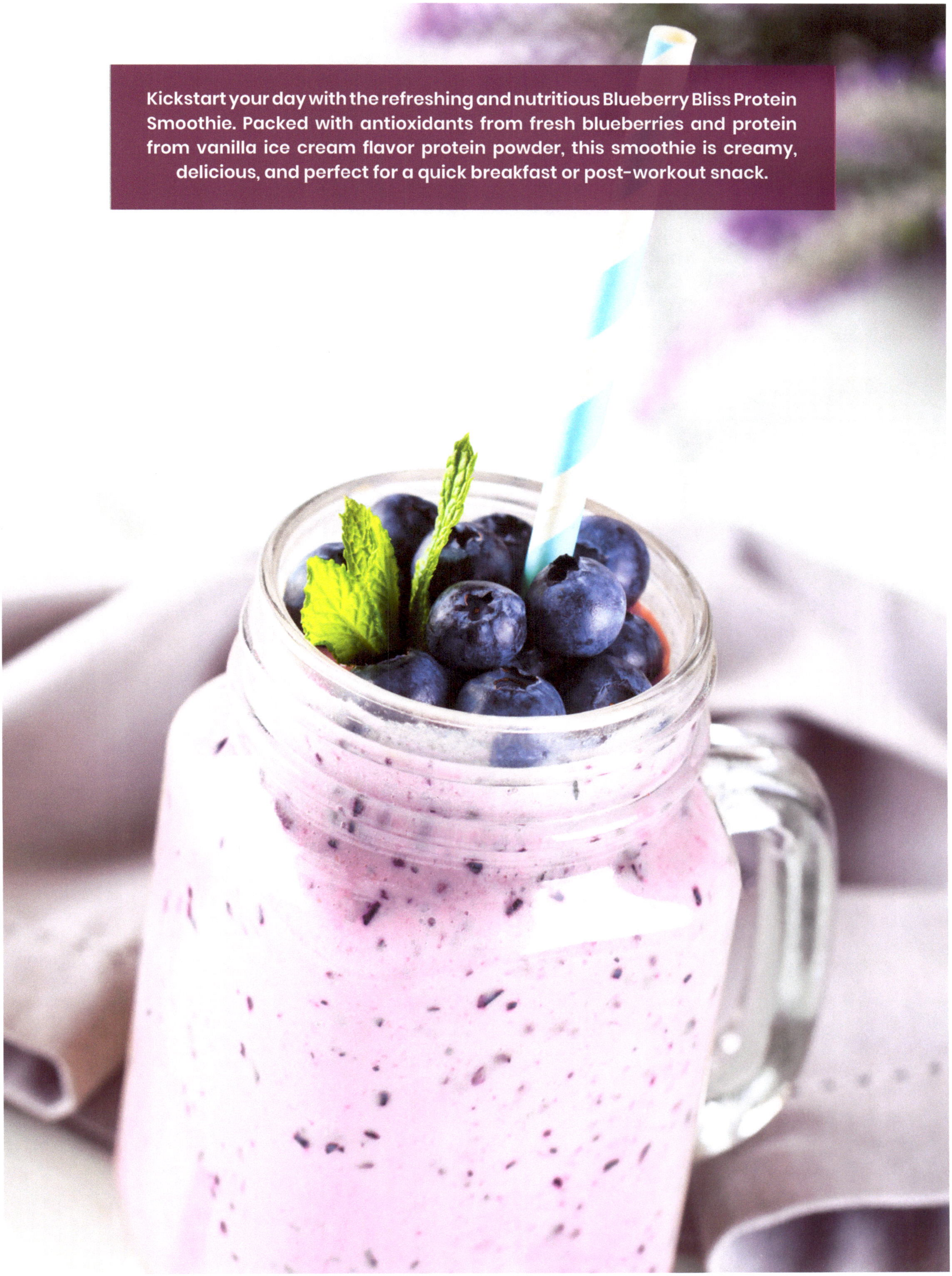

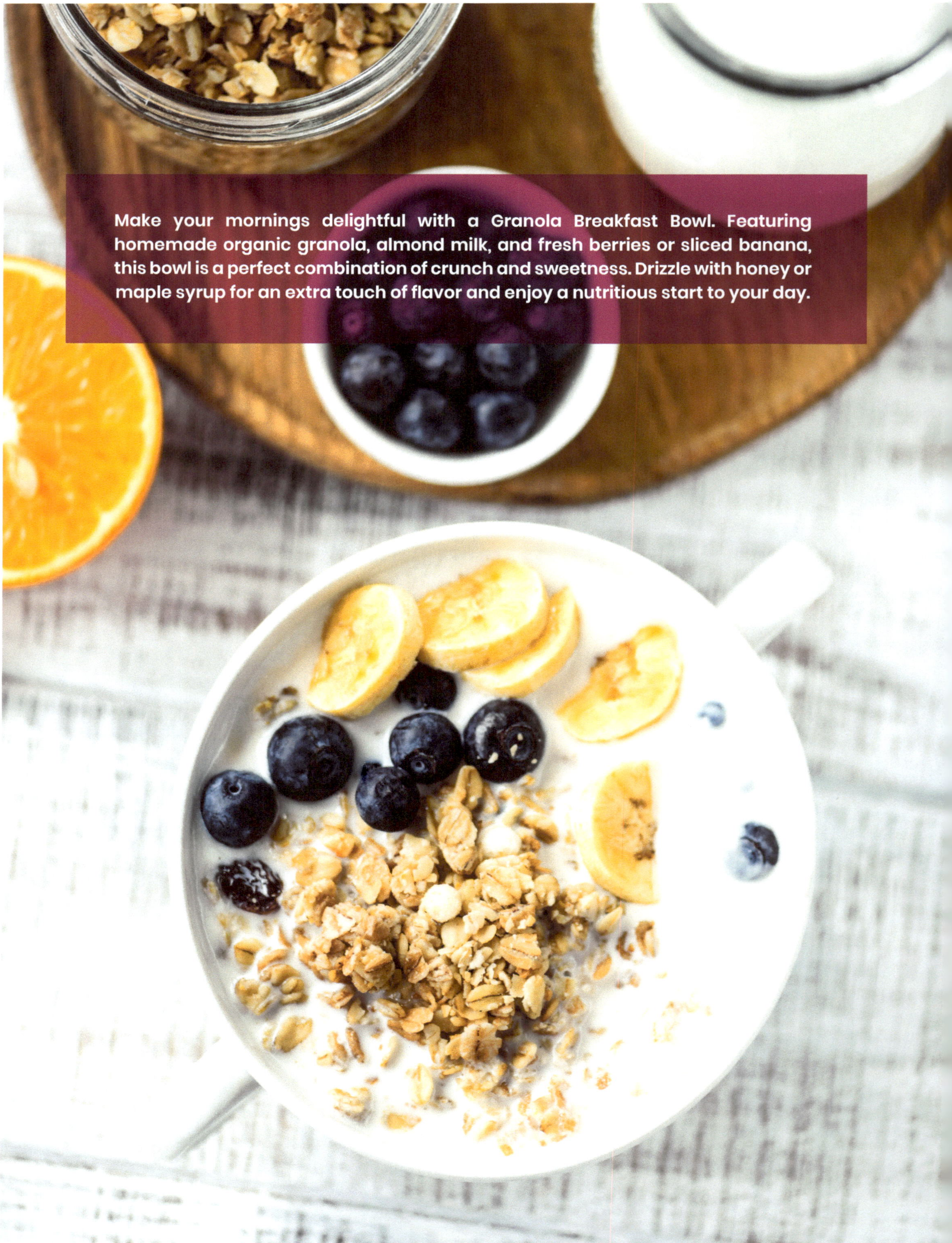

Make your mornings delightful with a Granola Breakfast Bowl. Featuring homemade organic granola, almond milk, and fresh berries or sliced banana, this bowl is a perfect combination of crunch and sweetness. Drizzle with honey or maple syrup for an extra touch of flavor and enjoy a nutritious start to your day.

GRANOLA BREAKFAST BOWL

1 servings	9g P | 38g C 20g F	372 per serving	Prep Time: 10 minutes	Cooking Time: 0 minutes	Total Time: Overnight

INGREDIENTS

- 1/2 cup Homemade Organic Granola (see the recipe)
- 1 cup almond milk (or your preferred milk of choice)

For the Topping (Optional):

- Fresh blueberries or sliced banana
- Honey or maple syrup for drizzling

DIRECTIONS

1. Start by preparing your homemade granola using the recipe you provided earlier.
2. Once the granola has cooled, take a serving bowl.
3. Add 1/2 cup of homemade granola to the bowl.
4. Pour 1 cup of organic almond milk (or your preferred milk of choice) over the granola.
5. Add fresh berries or sliced banana on top if desired.
6. Optionally, drizzle honey or maple syrup for sweetness, adjusting to your liking.

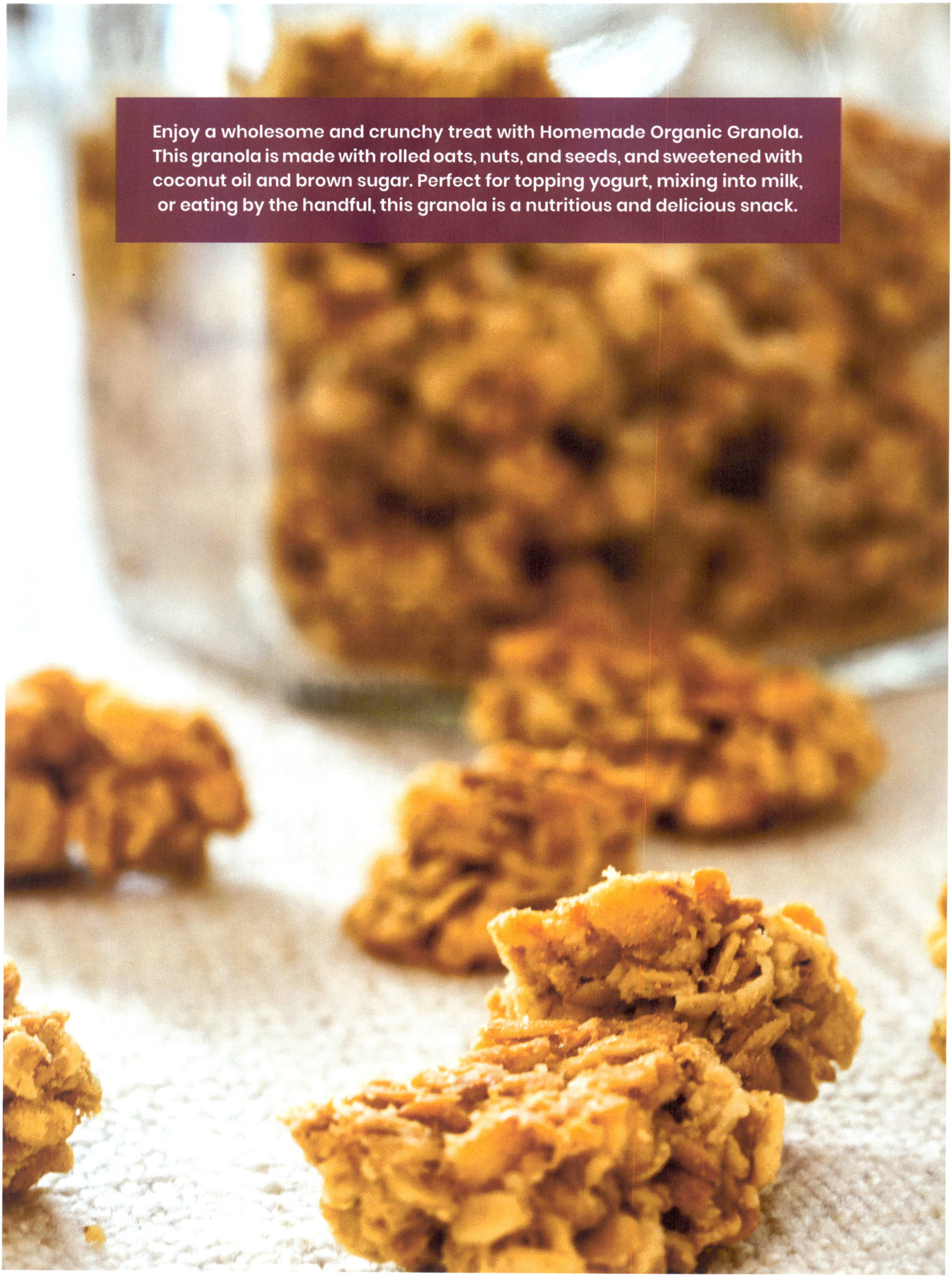

Enjoy a wholesome and crunchy treat with Homemade Organic Granola. This granola is made with rolled oats, nuts, and seeds, and sweetened with coconut oil and brown sugar. Perfect for topping yogurt, mixing into milk, or eating by the handful, this granola is a nutritious and delicious snack.

HOMEMADE ORGANIC GRANOLA

8 servings	8g P | 33g C 19g F	322 per serving	Prep Time: 10 minutes	Cooking Time: 20 minutes	Total Time: 30 minutes

INGREDIENTS

- 3 cups organic rolled oats
- 1 cup organic nuts (e.g., almonds, cashews, or walnuts), roughly chopped
- 1/2 cup organic seeds (e.g., pumpkin seeds or sunflower seeds)
- 1/4 cup organic brown sugar
- 1/4 cup organic coconut oil, melted
- 1 teaspoon organic vanilla extract
- 1/2 teaspoon organic ground cinnamon
- 1/4 teaspoon organic salt

DIRECTIONS

1. Preheat your oven to 325°F (163°C). Line a baking sheet with parchment paper or lightly grease it.
2. In a large mixing bowl, combine the organic rolled oats, chopped organic nuts, and organic seeds.
3. On the stovetop, combine the organic coconut oil, brown sugar, vanilla extract, ground cinnamon, and salt. Mix until everything is well combined and the sugar has dissolved into the mixture.
4. In a large mixing bowl, pour the liquid mixture over the oats, seeds, and nuts. Stir until the dry ingredients are evenly coated.
5. Spread the mixture evenly onto the prepared baking sheet.
6. Bake in the preheated oven for about 20-25 minutes or until the granola turns golden brown, stirring it gently every 10 minutes to ensure even cooking.
7. Remove the granola from the oven and let it cool completely on the baking sheet. It will take 30 minutes to completely cool and continue to crisp up as it cools.
8. Once cooled, store your homemade organic granola in an airtight container. It can be kept at room temperature for up to two weeks or in the refrigerator for longer freshness.

Enjoy the delightful taste of this Homemade Strawberry Chia Seed Jam any time of the year. Made with organic strawberries, chia seeds, and a hint of apple cider vinegar, this jam is naturally sweetened and packed with nutrients. Perfect for spreading on toast or mixing into yogurt, it's a healthy and delicious addition to your breakfast.

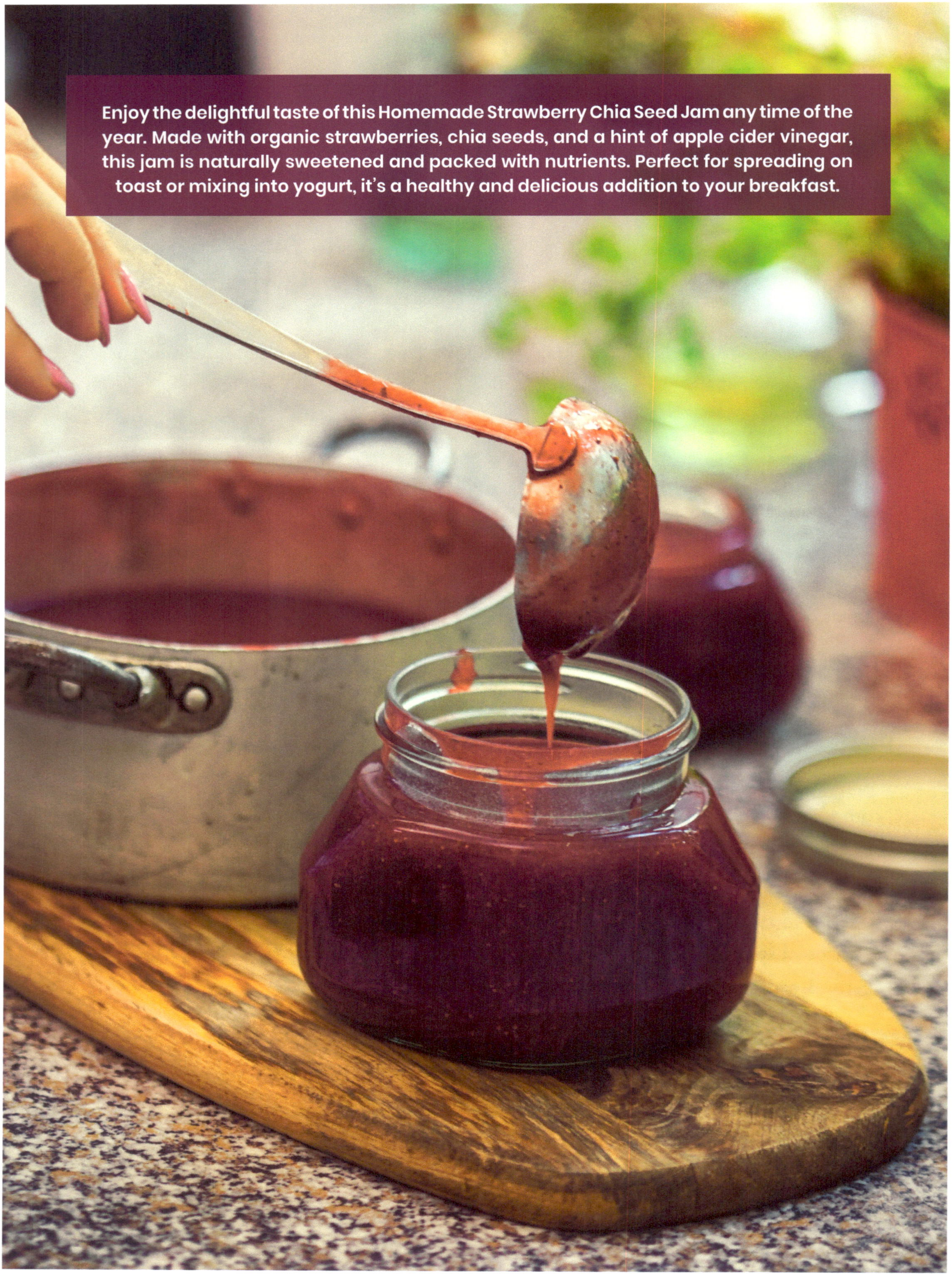

HOMEMADE STRAWBERRY CHIA SEED JAM

32 servings	0g P | 3g C 0g F	12 per serving	Prep Time: 5 minutes	Cooking Time: 20 minutes	Total Time: 25 minutes

INGREDIENTS

- 4 cups organic strawberries (fresh or frozen)
- 1/4 cup organic unprocessed cane sugar
- 1 tablespoon organic apple cider vinegar (or substitute with organic lemon juice)
- 3 tablespoons of chia seeds

DIRECTIONS

1. Prepare the strawberries. If using fresh strawberries, wash them thoroughly and remove the stems. If using frozen strawberries, you can start making the jam by placing them into the saucepan.
2. In a saucepan, add the strawberries and organic unprocessed sugar. Heat over medium heat, stirring occasionally until the strawberries release their juices and begin to break down. This should take about 5 minutes.
3. Stir in the organic apple cider vinegar (or substitute with organic lemon juice). This will add a pleasant tanginess to the jam and act as a natural preservative.
4. Continue to let the jam simmer on the stove for another 15 minutes, for a total cooking time of 20 minutes. The berries will naturally break down during the cooking process. Once the total cooking time has been reached, turn off the stove.
5. Stir in the chia seeds then let sit for 3 minutes, allowing the seeds to begin absorbing moisture and expanding. After 3 minutes, give the chia seed jam one more stir to ensure even distribution.
6. Carefully transfer the jam to a 16 oz glass jar or container with a lid. Place it in the refrigerator and allow it to cool and set overnight. This resting period will help the jam thicken to the perfect consistency. Your homemade strawberry chia jam can be stored in the refrigerator for up to two weeks.

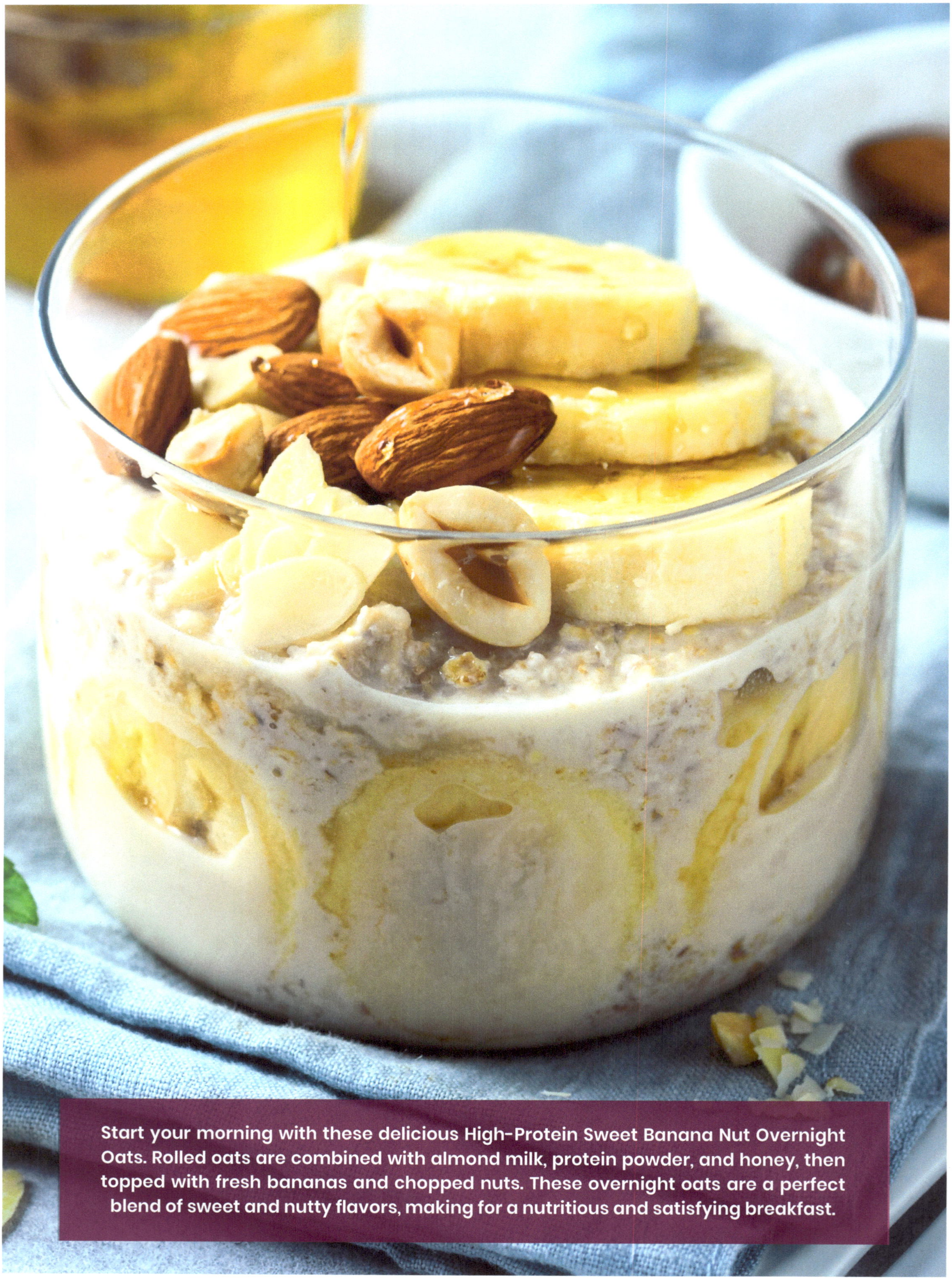

Start your morning with these delicious High-Protein Sweet Banana Nut Overnight Oats. Rolled oats are combined with almond milk, protein powder, and honey, then topped with fresh bananas and chopped nuts. These overnight oats are a perfect blend of sweet and nutty flavors, making for a nutritious and satisfying breakfast.

HIGH-PROTEIN SWEET BANANA NUT OVERNIGHT OATS

2 servings	10g P | 33g C 5g F	230 per serving	Prep Time: 5 minutes	Cooking Time: 0 minutes	Chilling Time: Overnight

INGREDIENTS

For the Banana Nut Overnight Oats:

- 1 cup rolled oats
- 1 1/2 cups unsweetened almond milk (or milk of choice)
- 1 scoop vanilla protein powder (plant-based or whey)
- 2 tablespoons honey or maple syrup
- 1/2 teaspoon ground cinnamon
- 1/2 teaspoon vanilla extract
- A pinch of salt

For Topping:

- 2 ripe bananas, sliced
- 1/4 cup chopped nuts (e.g., almonds or walnuts)
- Drizzle of honey

DIRECTIONS

1. In a 16 oz jar with lid or mixing bowl, combine the rolled oats, unsweetened almond milk, vanilla protein powder, chopped walnuts, honey, ground cinnamon, vanilla extract, and a pinch of salt.
2. Stir the mixture until all ingredients are well combined.
3. Seal the container and refrigerate it overnight to allow the oats to absorb the milk and flavors.

In the morning (or when serving):

1. Slice both bananas and distribute them evenly between two serving jars or bowls by placing a layer of banana slices at the bottom and/or sides of each dish, reserving some of the slices for garnish.
2. Pour the prepared overnight oat mixture over the banana slices in each jar.
3. Before serving, top each serving with the remaining banana slices, evenly distribute 1/4 cup of chopped nuts between the two servings, and drizzle with honey for extra nutrition and flavor.

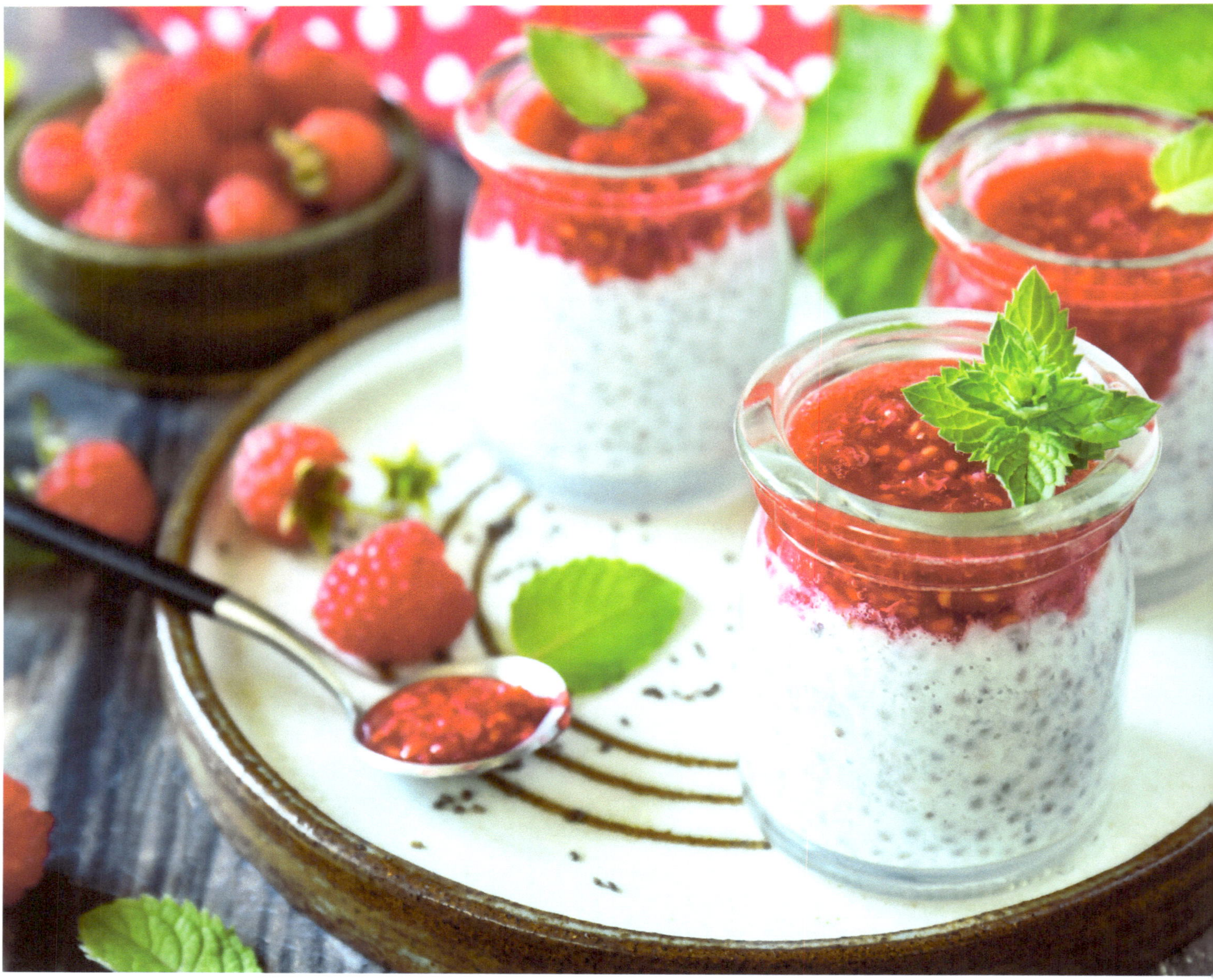

RASPBERRY CHIA YOGURT CUPS

- 2 servings
- 20g P | 18g C 5g F
- 200 per serving
- Prep Time: 10 minutes
- Chilling Time: Overnight
- Total Time: Overnight

INGREDIENTS

- 1 cup Greek yogurt
- 1/2 cup unsweetened almond milk (or milk of choice)
- 1 scoop vanilla protein powder
- 2 tablespoons chia seeds
- 1/2 cup fresh or frozen raspberries
- 2-3 tablespoons honey or maple syrup
- 1 teaspoon vanilla extract
- A pinch of salt

DIRECTIONS

Prepare the Yogurt Mix:

1. In a mixing bowl, combine the Greek yogurt, almond milk, 1-2 tablespoons of honey or maple syrup, and vanilla extract (if using plain yogurt). Mix until smooth.
2. Add the protein powder and mix well to ensure it's fully incorporated.
3. Stir in 1 tablespoon of chia seeds until evenly distributed.
4. Let the mixture sit for about 3 minutes to allow the chia seeds to start absorbing the liquid.

Prepare the Raspberry Reduction:

1. In a small saucepan, heat the raspberries over medium heat for about 5 minutes until they begin to break down and release their juices.
2. Stir in 1 tablespoon of honey or maple syrup and mix well.
3. Remove from heat and assemble the cups.

Assemble the Cups:

1. Spoon the yogurt and chia seed mixture into two serving cups or bowls.
2. Top with the raspberry reduction.
3. Cover and refrigerate overnight to let the chia seeds fully expand and the flavors meld.
4. *Note:* Allowing the chia yogurt cups to set overnight ensures that the chia seeds are fully bloomed, making them easier on digestion. If needed, you can let the mixture set for a minimum of 4 hours, but overnight is recommended for best results.

Treat yourself to these nutritious and delicious Raspberry Chia Yogurt Cups. Greek yogurt is combined with almond milk, protein powder, and chia seeds, then topped with a raspberry reduction. These cups are perfect for a make-ahead breakfast or snack, providing a balanced mix of protein, healthy fats, and carbohydrates.

STRAWBERRY CHIA YOGURT PARFAIT

INGREDIENTS

- 6 oz plain Greek yogurt
- 1 teaspoon organic lemon juice
- 1 teaspoon honey (or sweetener of choice, adjust to taste)
- 4 fresh strawberries (or raspberries) for layering
- 2 tablespoon Homemade Strawberry Chia Seed Jam (see the recipe)
- 1/2 cup homemade granola (see the recipe, or opt for store bought by Michele's Original Granola)

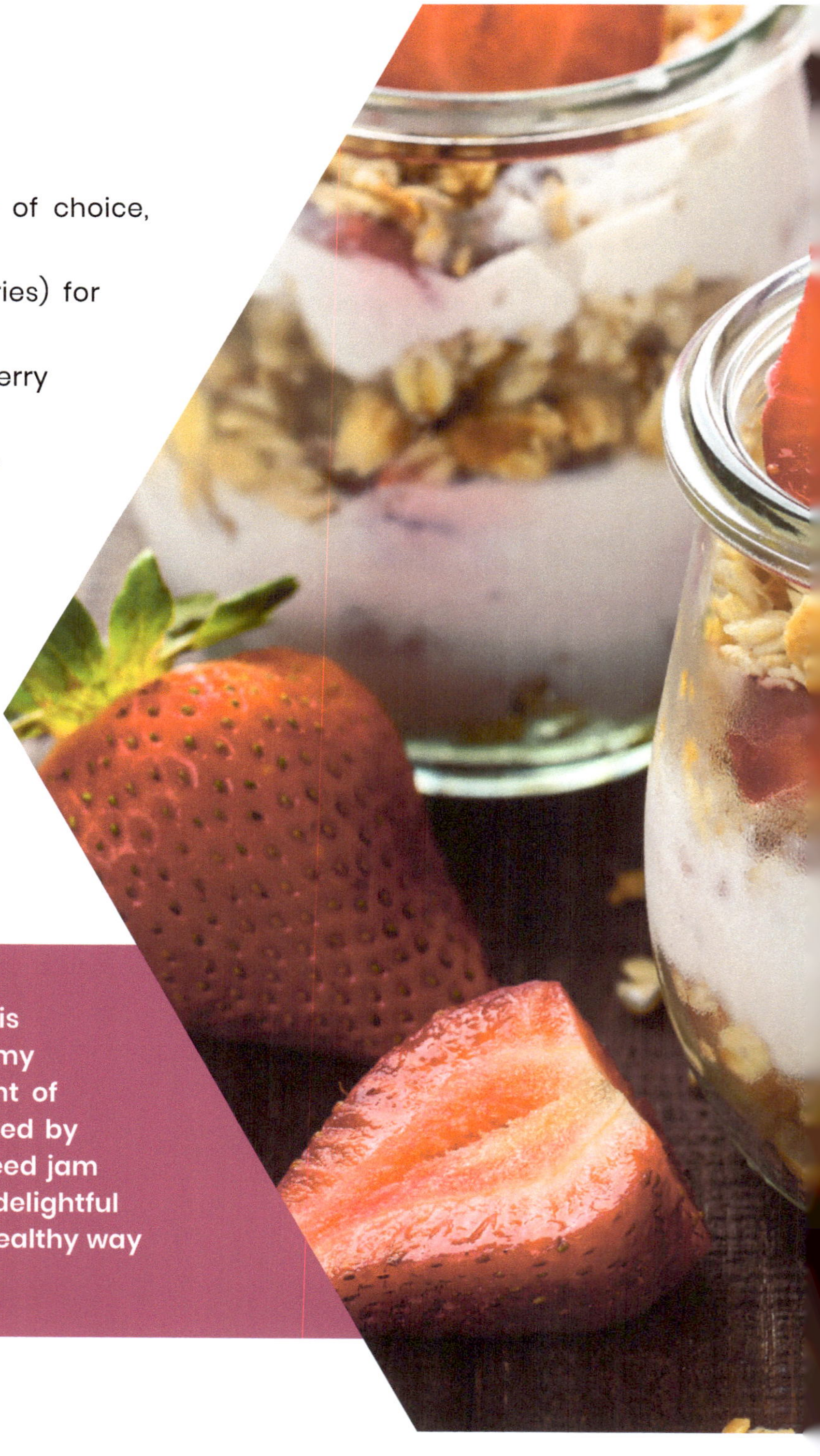

Indulge in the refreshing layers of this Strawberry Chia Yogurt Parfait. Creamy Greek yogurt is combined with a hint of lemon juice and honey, complemented by sweet homemade strawberry chia seed jam and crunchy granola. This parfait is a delightful blend of textures and flavors, and a healthy way to start your day or enjoy as a snack.

2 servings	7g P | 32g C 7g F	220 per serving	Prep Time: 10 minutes	Cooking Time: 0 minutes	Total Time: 10 minutes

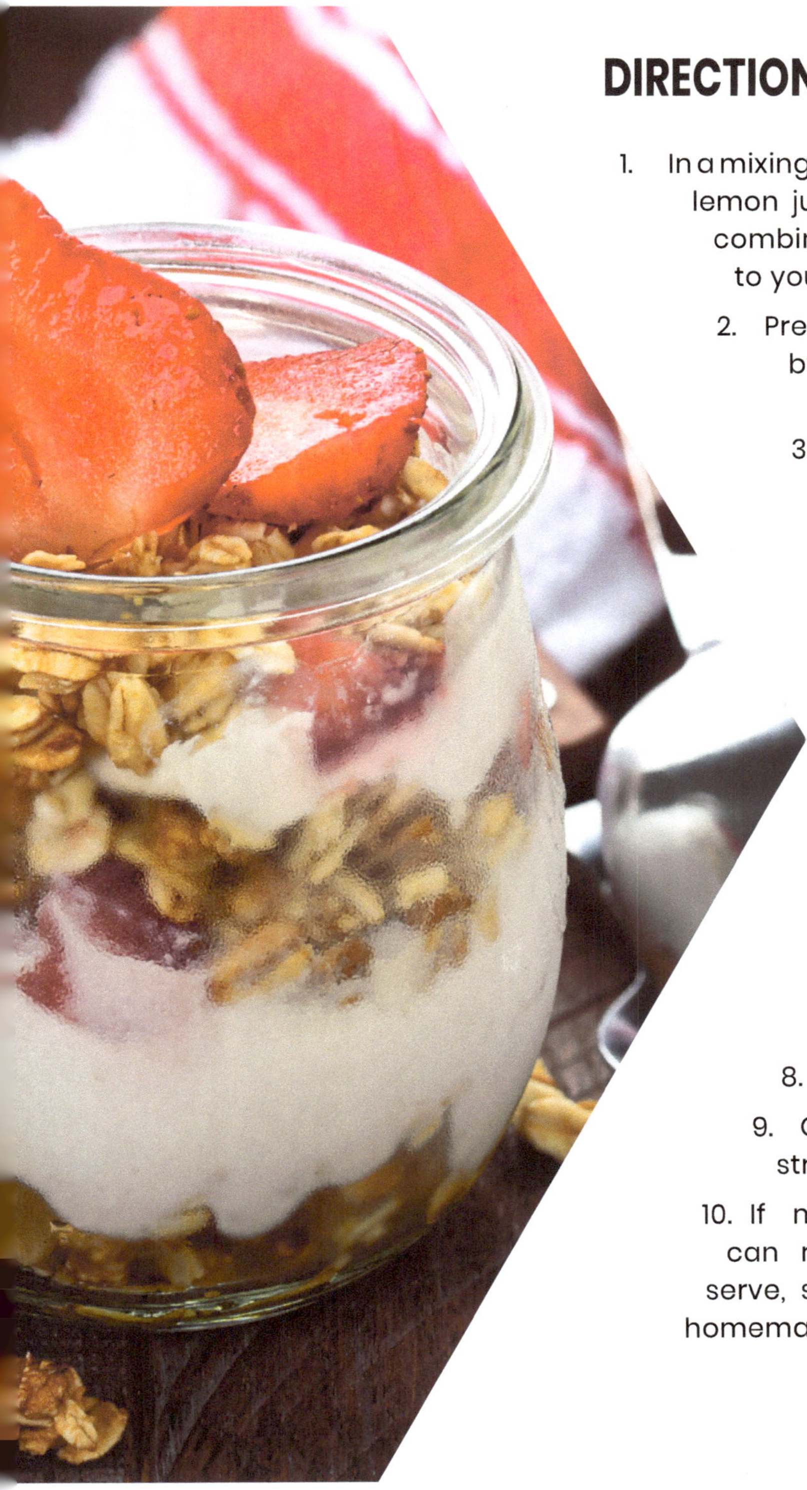

DIRECTIONS

1. In a mixing bowl, combine the Greek yogurt, organic lemon juice, and honey. Stir well to thoroughly combine all the ingredients. Adjust the honey to your desired level of sweetness.
2. Prepare for layering between 2 jars. Start by adding a small amount of homemade granola to the bottom of each jar.
3. Next, add a layer of the yogurt mixture over the granola in each jar.
4. Spoon 1 tablespoon of Homemade Strawberry Chia Seed Jam over the yogurt in each jar.
5. Add a layer of sliced strawberries on top of the jam in each jar.
6. Repeat the layering process by adding a small amount of homemade granola over the strawberries in each jar.
7. Add another layer of the yogurt mixture over the granola in each jar.
8. Finish with a final small layer of granola.
9. Garnish each parfait with a halved strawberry.
10. If making these the night before, you can refrigerate them and when ready to serve, simply top with fresh strawberries and homemade granola.

PROTEIN BLUEBERRY PANCAKES WITH EGGS & BACON

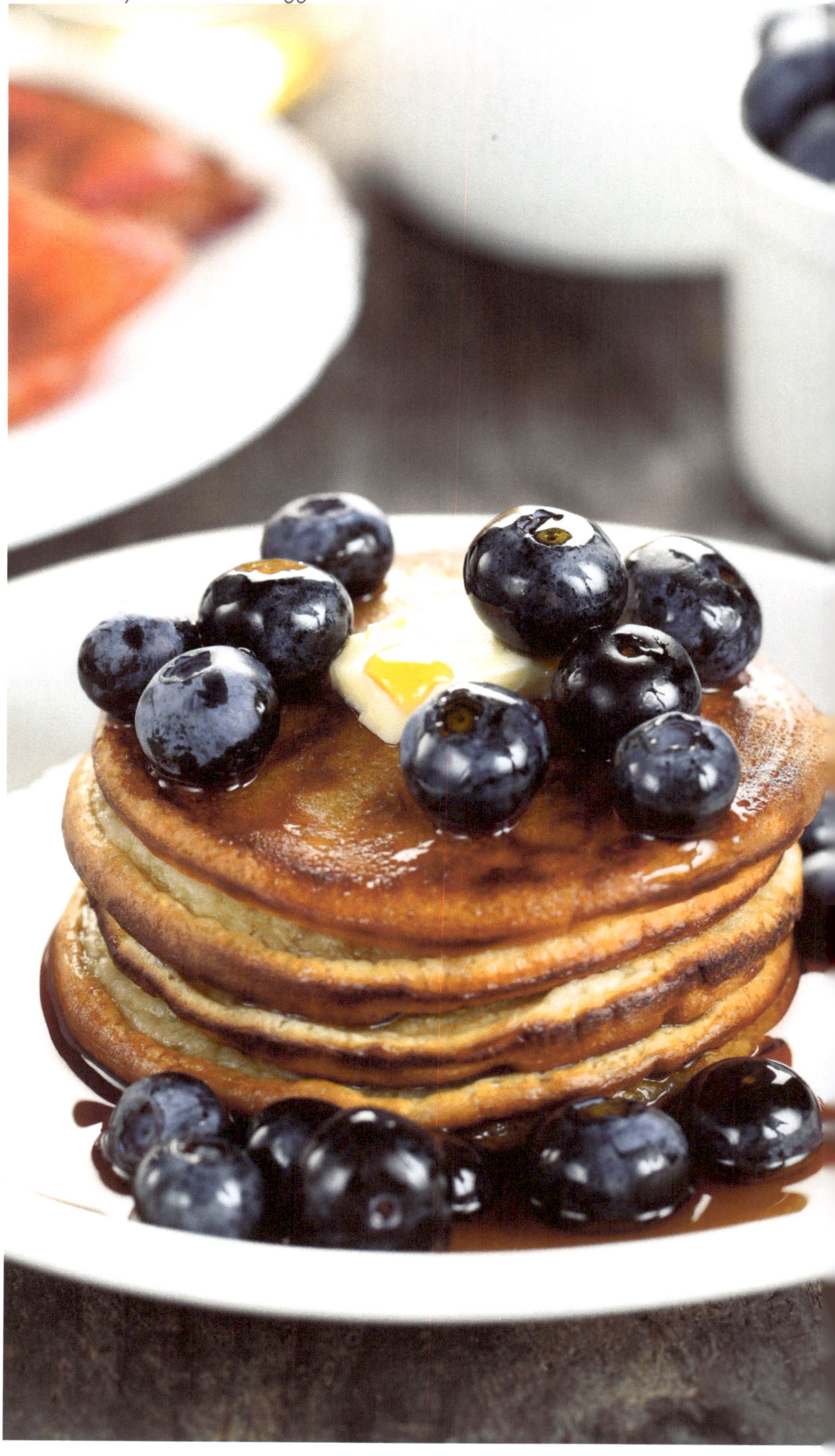

PANCAKES AND WAFFLES

2 servings	35g P | 40g C 20g F	450 per serving	Prep Time: 10 minutes	Cooking Time: 20 minutes	Total Time: 30 minutes

INGREDIENTS

For the Pancakes:

- 1 cup organic einkorn flour
- 1 scoop vanilla protein powder
- 1/2 teaspoon baking powder
- 1/4 teaspoon salt
- 1/2 teaspoon cinnamon
- 1/2 cup unsweetened almond milk (or any milk of your choice)
- 2 large eggs
- 1 teaspoon vanilla extract
- 1 tablespoon honey or maple syrup
- 1/2 cup fresh or frozen blueberries (plus extra for topping)
- Cooking spray or a small amount of butter for the pan

For the Over-Easy Eggs and Bacon:

- 4 large eggs
- Salt and pepper to taste
- 1 tablespoon butter
- 4 slices of bacon

For Topping:

- Fresh blueberries
- Maple syrup

Indulge in a hearty and nutritious breakfast with Protein Blueberry Pancakes with Over-Easy Eggs and Bacon. These fluffy pancakes, made with ancient Einkorn flour and protein powder, are served alongside perfectly cooked over-easy eggs and crispy bacon. Topped with fresh blueberries and a drizzle of maple syrup, this breakfast combines delicious flavors and wholesome ingredients for a satisfying start to your day.

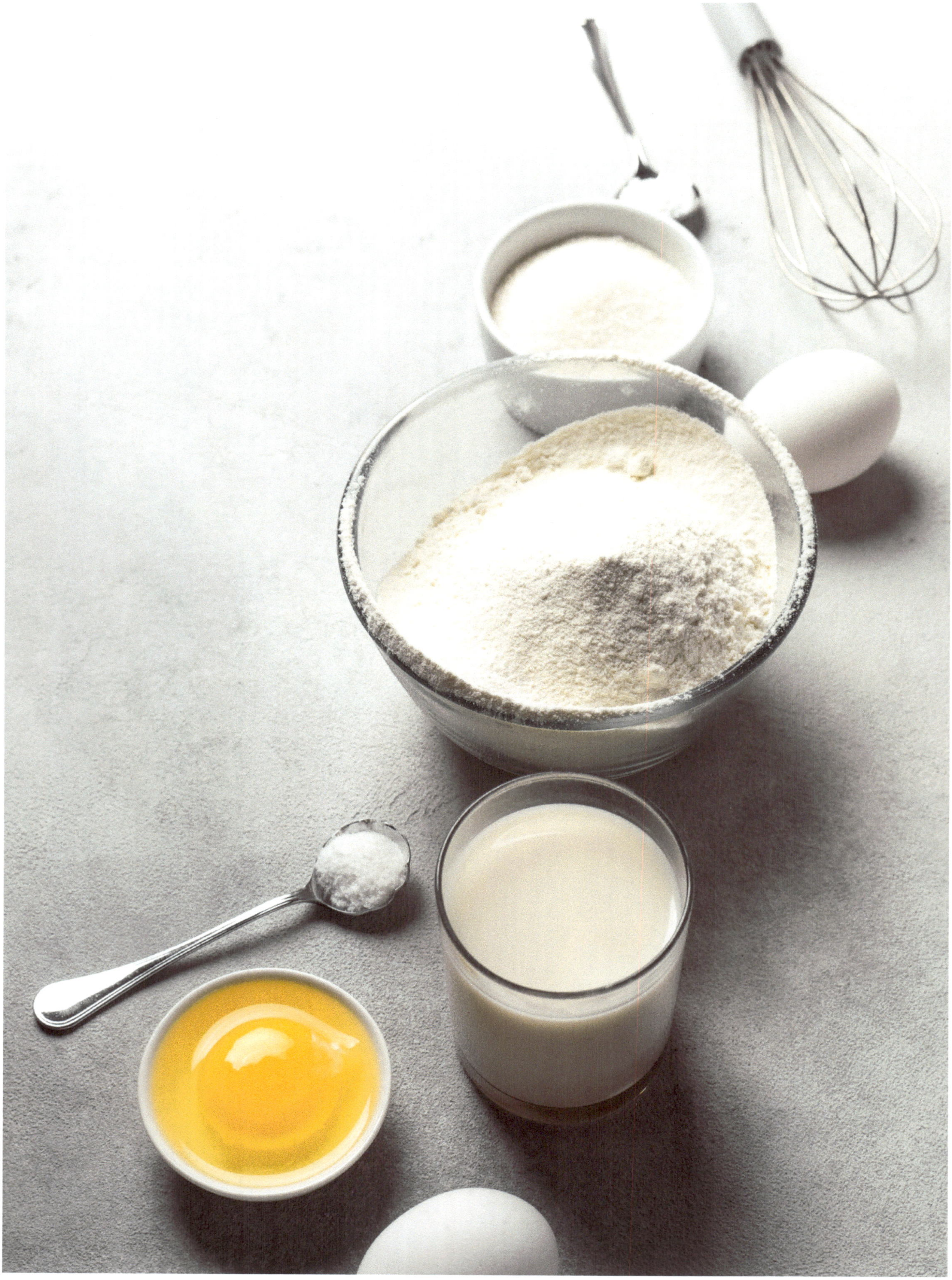

DIRECTIONS

Prepare the Pancake Batter:

1. In a large bowl, mix the einkorn flour, protein powder, baking powder, salt, and cinnamon.
2. In another bowl, whisk together the almond milk, eggs, vanilla extract, and honey or maple syrup.
3. Pour the wet ingredients into the dry ingredients and mix until just combined.
4. Gently fold in the blueberries.

Cook the Pancakes:

1. Heat a non-stick skillet or griddle over medium heat and lightly coat with cooking spray or butter.
2. Pour 1/4 cup of batter onto the skillet for each pancake.
3. Cook until bubbles form on the surface and the edges look set, about 2-3 minutes.
4. Flip and cook for another 1-2 minutes until golden brown.
5. Keep the pancakes warm.

Cook the Bacon:

1. Place a paper towel on a microwave-safe plate.
2. Lay the bacon slices on the paper towel in a single layer.
3. Cover the bacon with another paper towel.
4. Microwave on high for 3-4 minutes, or until crispy.
5. Remove and drain on paper towels.

Make the Over-Easy Eggs:

1. In a skillet, melt the butter over medium-low heat.
2. Crack the eggs into the skillet and cook until the whites are set, about 2-3 minutes.
3. Carefully flip the eggs and cook for another 1-2 minutes until the yolks are still runny but the whites are fully cooked.
4. Season with salt and pepper.

Serve:

1. Place two pancakes on each plate and top with fresh blueberries and a drizzle of maple syrup.
2. Add two over-easy eggs and two slices of bacon to each plate.

PROTEIN PACKED BELGIAN WAFFLE

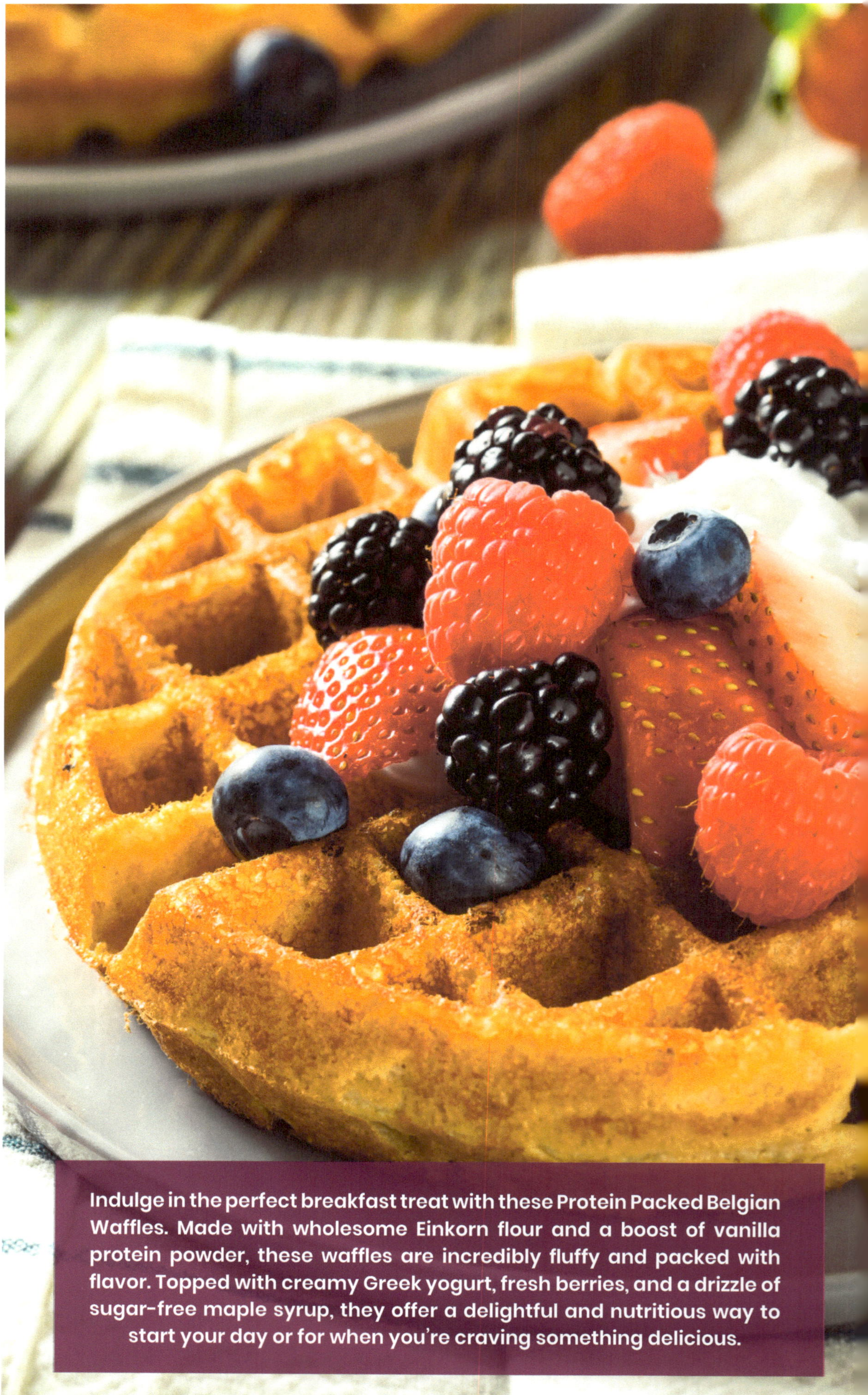

Indulge in the perfect breakfast treat with these Protein Packed Belgian Waffles. Made with wholesome Einkorn flour and a boost of vanilla protein powder, these waffles are incredibly fluffy and packed with flavor. Topped with creamy Greek yogurt, fresh berries, and a drizzle of sugar-free maple syrup, they offer a delightful and nutritious way to start your day or for when you're craving something delicious.

2 servings	38g P | 45g C 5g F	375 per serving	Prep Time: 15 minutes	Cooking Time: 10 minutes	Total Time: 25 minutes

INGREDIENTS

For the Belgian Waffles:

- 1 cup Einkorn flour by Jovial brand
- 1/2 cup vanilla protein powder by Maxpro Elite brand (2 scoops)
- 1 tablespoon maple syrup, sugar-free (or sweetener of your choice)
- 1 1/2 teaspoons baking powder
- 1/2 teaspoon baking soda
- 1/2 teaspoon cinnamon
- 1/4 teaspoon salt
- 2 large eggs
- 1 cup unsweetened almond milk (or milk of your choice)
- 2 tablespoons unsweetened applesauce
- Cooking spray (for waffle iron)

For Topping:

- 2 tablespoons Greek yogurt
- Fresh berries
- Sugar-free maple syrup for drizzling

DIRECTIONS

1. Preheat your waffle iron according to the manufacturer's instructions.
2. In a large mixing bowl, combine the Einkorn flour, vanilla protein powder, maple syrup, baking powder, baking soda, cinnamon, and salt. Mix well to ensure even distribution of dry ingredients.
3. In a separate bowl, whisk together the eggs, unsweetened almond milk, and unsweetened applesauce until well combined.
4. Pour the wet ingredients into the dry ingredients and stir until just combined. Be careful not to overmix; a few lumps are okay.
5. Lightly grease the waffle iron with cooking spray to prevent sticking.
6. Pour enough batter onto the preheated waffle iron to cover the waffle grid, following your waffle maker's instructions for the right amount.
7. Close the waffle iron and cook until the waffle is golden brown and crisp. Cooking times may vary depending on your waffle iron, but it usually takes 3-5 minutes.
8. Carefully remove the waffle and place it on a plate.
9. Top each waffle with 1 tablespoon of Greek yogurt, fresh berries, and a drizzle of sugar-free maple syrup.
10. Serve your waffles immediately while they're warm and enjoy!

Desserts

- Creamy Chocolate Protein Mousse with Cacao Powder
- Blueberry Cobbler
- Dark Chocolate Cacao Cookies
- Protein-Rich Dreamy Hot Chocolate

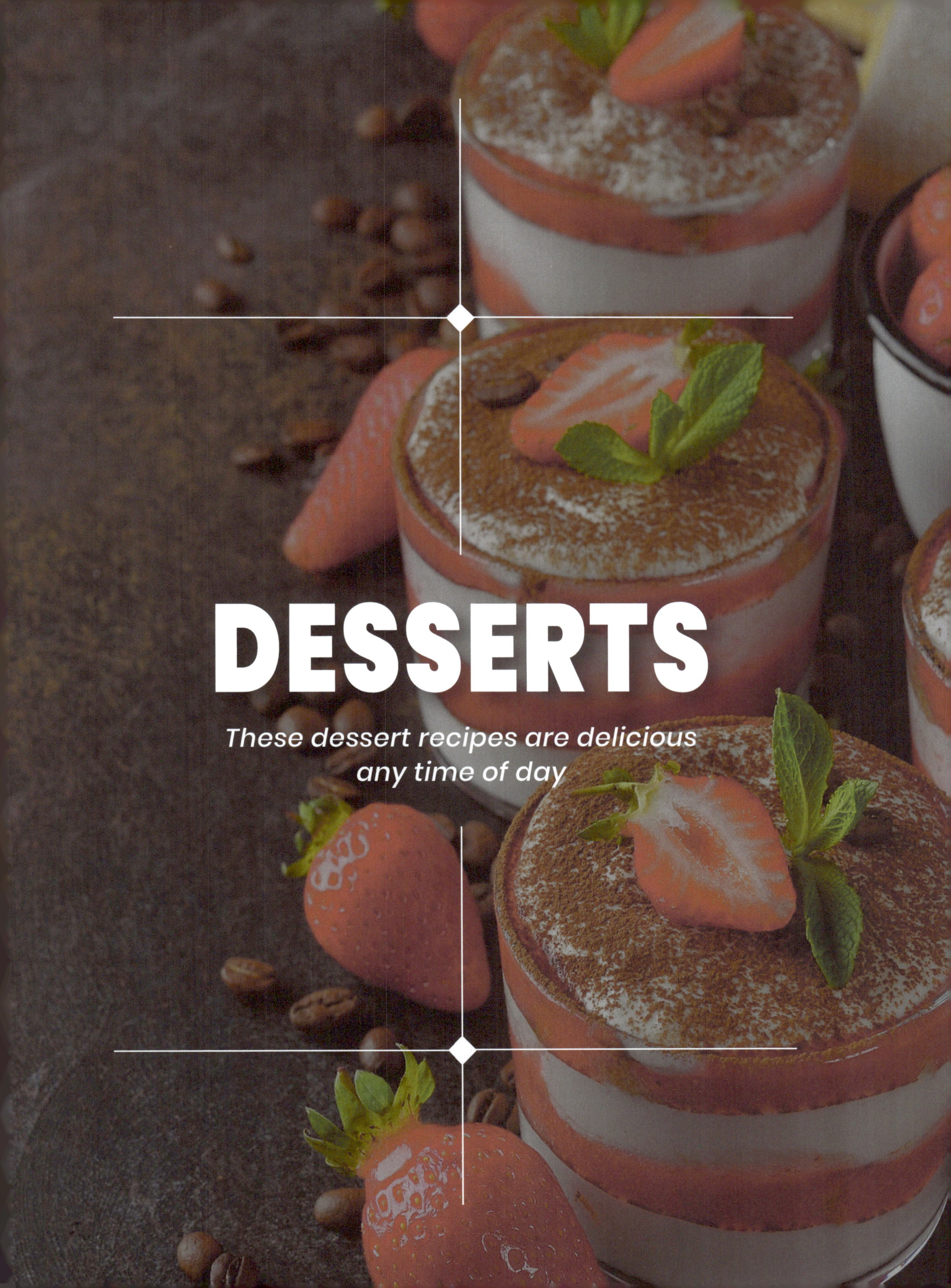

DESSERTS

These dessert recipes are delicious any time of day

CREAMY CHOCOLATE PROTEIN MOUSSE with CACAO POWDER

2 servings	12g P | 15g C 4g F	150 per serving	Prep Time: 5 minutes	Chilling Time: 1 hour

INGREDIENTS

- 1 cup cottage cheese
- 2 tablespoons cacao powder
- 2-3 tablespoons honey or maple syrup
- 1 teaspoon vanilla extract
- A pinch of salt
- Dark chocolate shavings or berries for topping (Optional):

DIRECTIONS

1. Blend the cottage cheese in a food processor or blender until smooth and creamy for about 30 seconds.
2. Add the cacao powder, sweetener, vanilla extract, and a pinch of salt. Blend again until well combined for another 30 seconds.
3. Taste and adjust sweetness if needed.
4. Transfer the mixture into serving bowls or glasses.
5. Chill in the refrigerator for at least an hour to set.
6. Before serving, top with dollop of whipped cream and dark chocolate shavings or berries if desired.

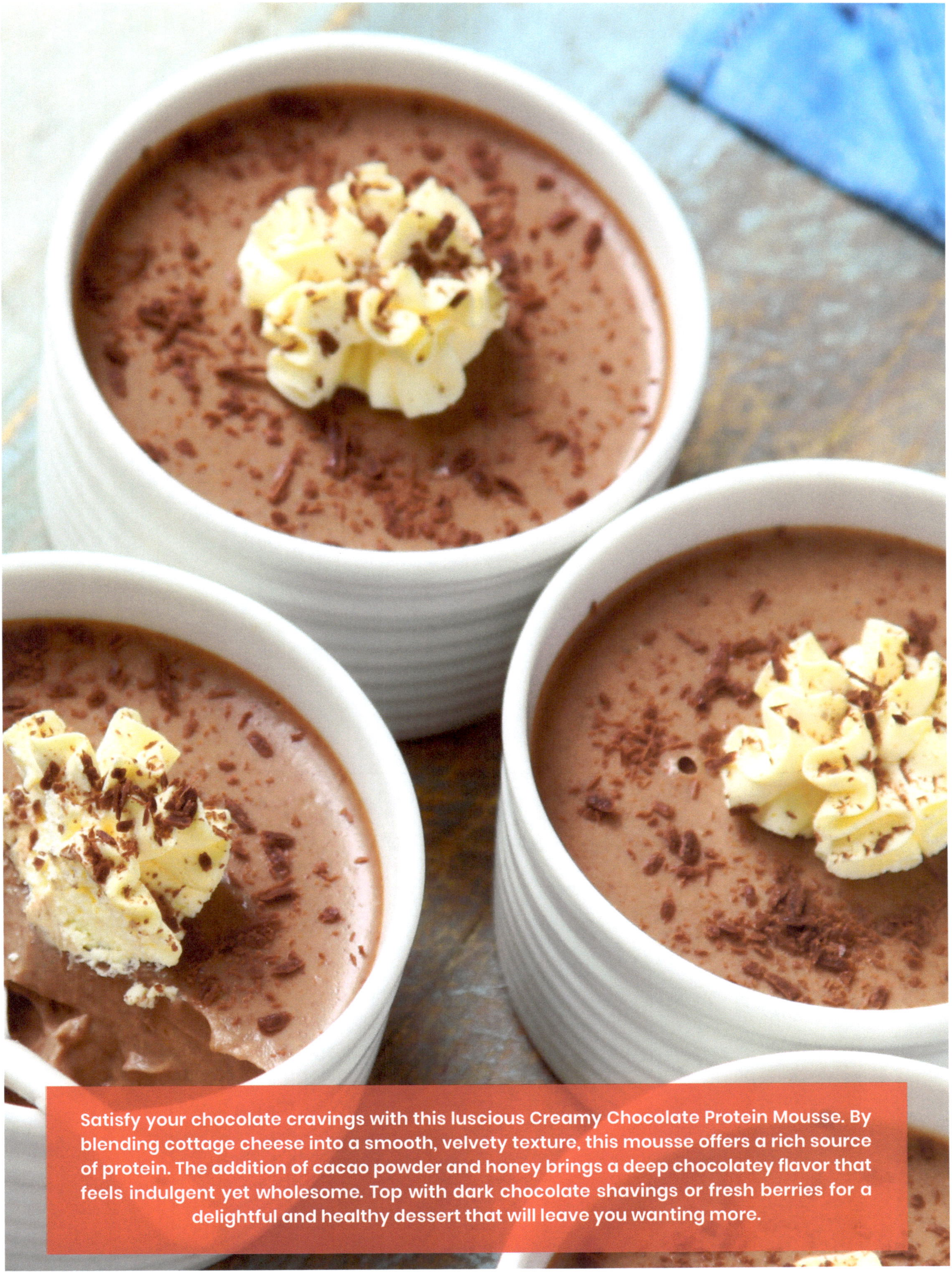

Satisfy your chocolate cravings with this luscious Creamy Chocolate Protein Mousse. By blending cottage cheese into a smooth, velvety texture, this mousse offers a rich source of protein. The addition of cacao powder and honey brings a deep chocolatey flavor that feels indulgent yet wholesome. Top with dark chocolate shavings or fresh berries for a delightful and healthy dessert that will leave you wanting more.

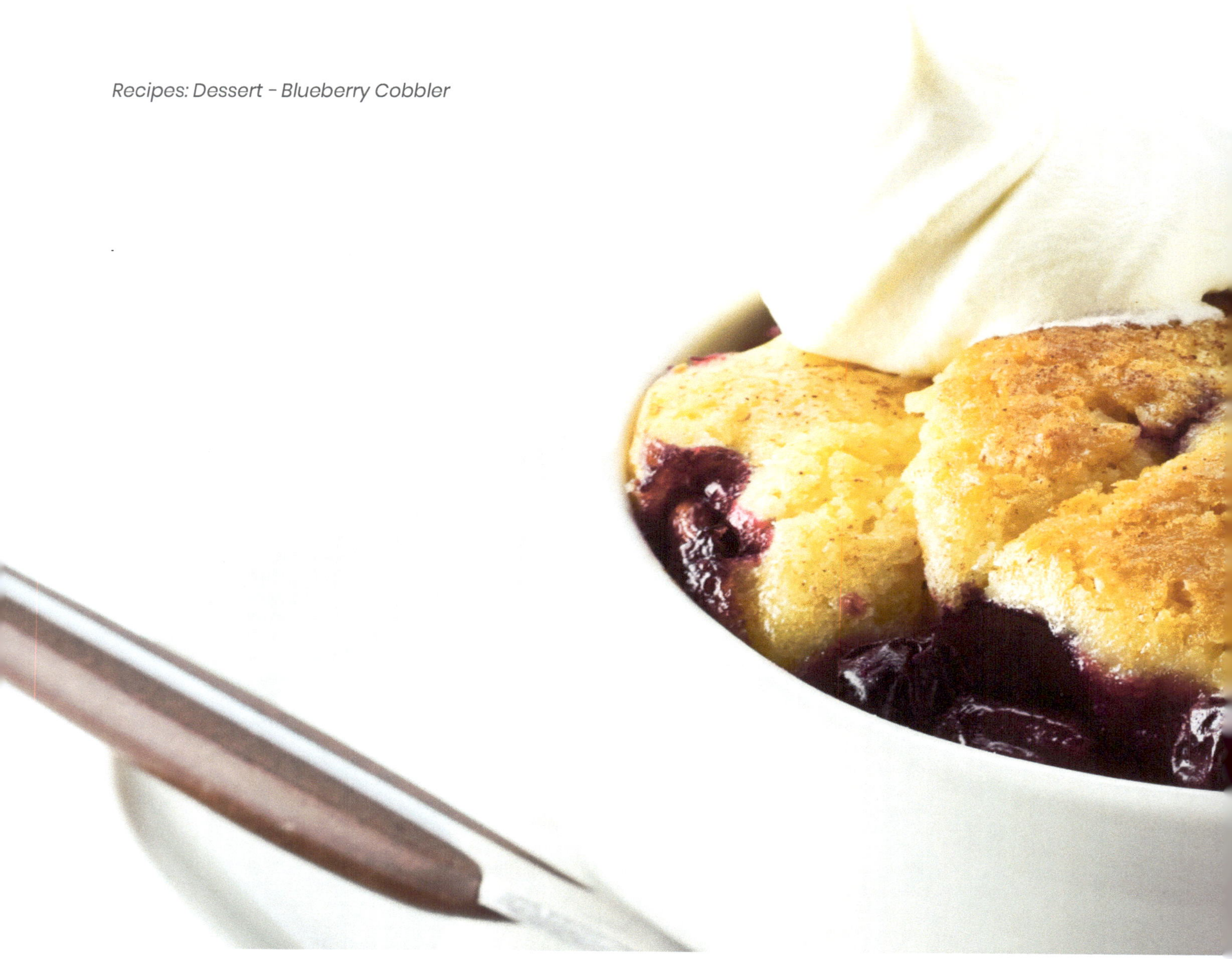

BLUEBERRY COBBLER

INGREDIENTS

For the Blueberry Filling:

- 4 cups fresh or frozen wild blueberries
- 2 tablespoons honey or maple syrup
- 1 teaspoon lemon juice
- 2 tablespoons chia seeds
- 1 teaspoon vanilla extract

For the Cobbler Topping:

- 1 cup organic einkorn flour
- 2 tablespoons coconut sugar or natural sweetener
- 1 teaspoon baking powder
- Pinch of salt
- 4 tablespoons unsalted butter, cold and cubed
- Whipped cream (optional)

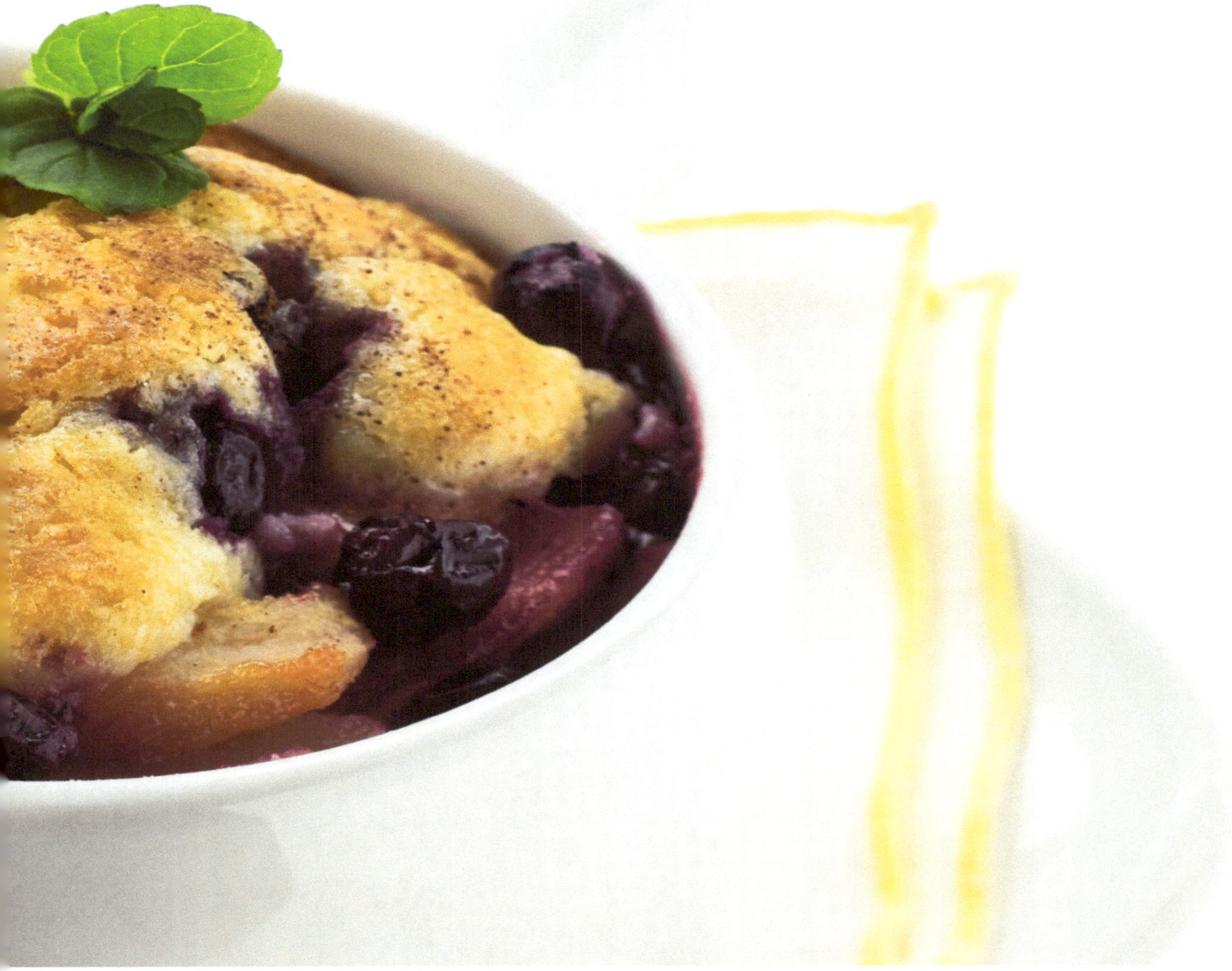

4 servings | 6g P | 35g C 7g F | 220 per serving | Prep Time: 25 minutes | Cooking Time: 30 minutes | Total Time: 55 minutes

DIRECTIONS

1. Combine blueberries, honey or maple syrup, lemon juice, chia seeds, and vanilla extract. Let sit for 15 minutes to thicken.
2. Preheat oven to 375°F (190°C). Grease an 8x8-inch baking dish.
3. Combine einkorn flour, coconut sugar, baking powder, and salt. Cut in cold butter until the mixture resembles coarse crumbs.
4. Pour thickened blueberry filling into the prepared baking dish. Sprinkle the crumb topping over the filling, leaving some gaps.
5. Bake for 30 minutes, or until the topping is golden brown and the filling is bubbly.
6. Let cool for a few minutes. Serve with a dollop of whipped cream if desired.

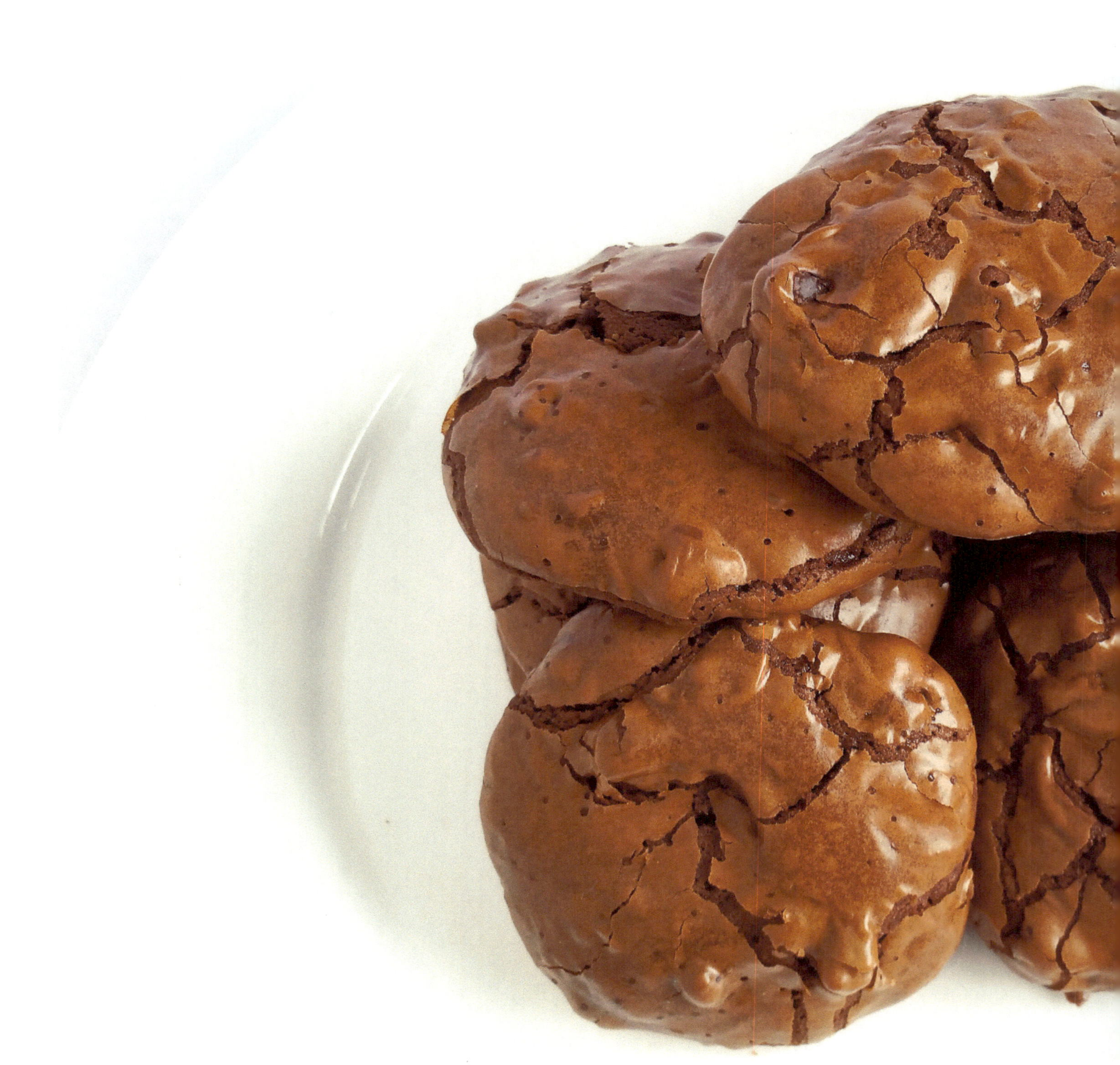

DARK CHOCOLATE CACAO COOKIES

Indulge in these rich and decadent Dark Chocolate Cacao Cookies. Made with ancient Einkorn flour and cacao powder, these eggless cookies are soft, chewy, and packed with deep chocolate flavor. Perfect for those with egg allergies or anyone seeking a simpler ingredient list, they offer a healthier twist on traditional chocolate cookies without compromising on taste.

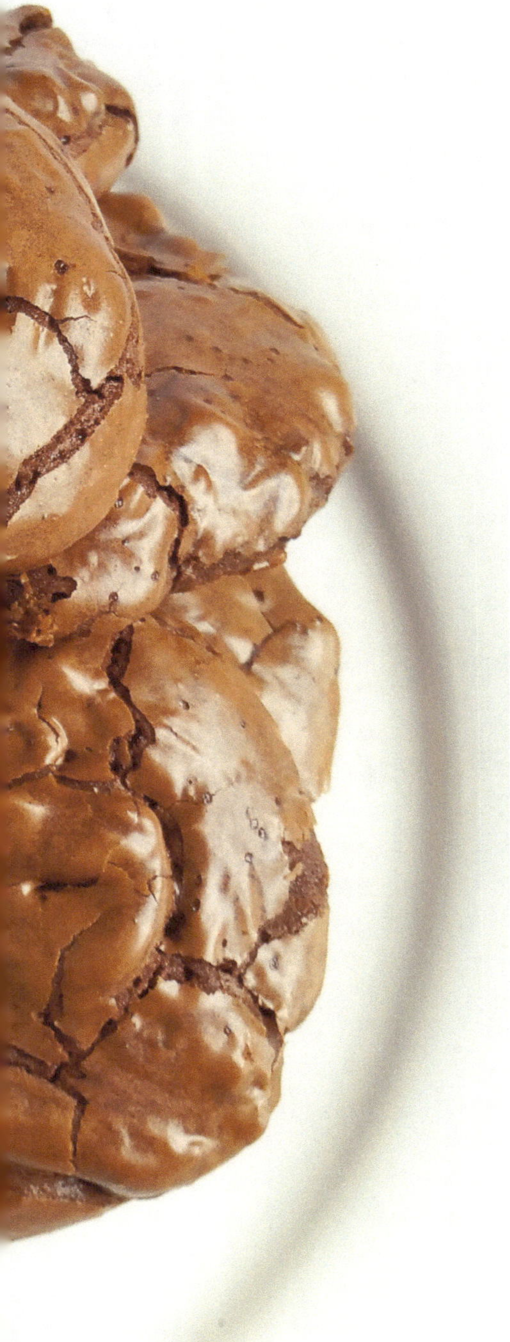

INGREDIENTS

- 1 cup einkorn flour
- 1/2 cup cacao powder
- 1/2 teaspoon baking soda
- 1/4 teaspoon salt
- 1/2 cup grapeseed oil
- 1 cup organic unprocessed sugar
- 1/4 cup unsweetened applesauce
- 1 teaspoon vanilla extract

DIRECTIONS

1. Preheat your oven to 350°F (175°C) and line a baking sheet with parchment paper.
2. In a medium bowl, whisk together the einkorn flour, cacao powder, baking soda, and salt.
3. In a large bowl, beat together the grapeseed oil and sugar until well combined.
4. Add the applesauce and vanilla extract to the wet mixture, and mix until smooth.
5. Gradually add the dry ingredients to the wet mixture, mixing until just combined.
6. Scoop small tablespoons of dough and roll them into balls.
7. Place the dough balls on the prepared baking sheet, about 2 inches apart.
8. Bake in the preheated oven for 8-10 minutes, or until the cookies are set and slightly cracked on top.
9. Let the cookies cool on the baking sheet for a few minutes before transferring them to a wire rack to cool completely. Enjoy your delicious, eggless dark chocolate cacao cookies!

24 servings	3g P | 15g C 7g F	130 per serving	Prep Time: 15 minutes	Cooking Time: 10 minutes	Total Time: 25 minutes

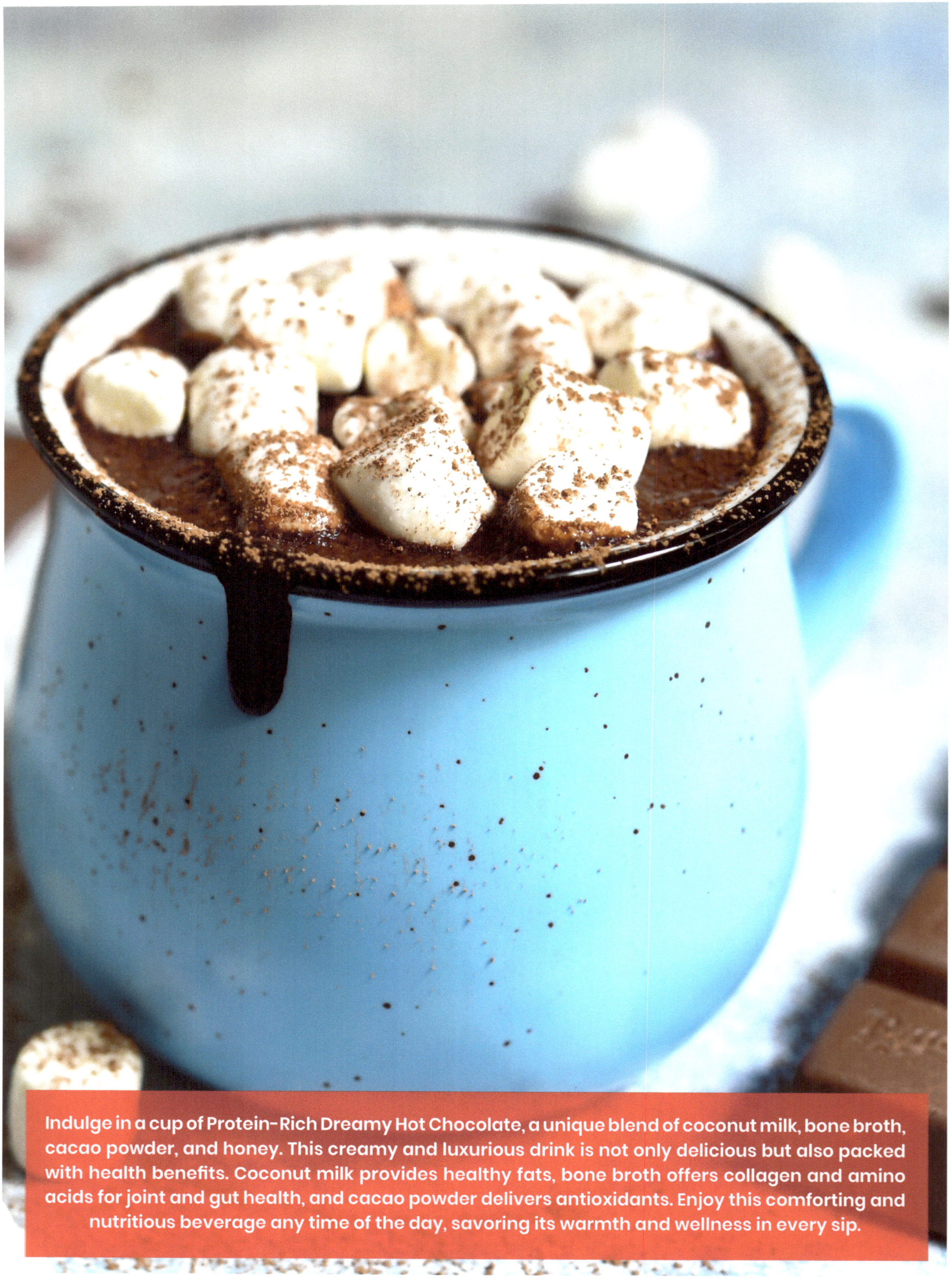

Indulge in a cup of Protein-Rich Dreamy Hot Chocolate, a unique blend of coconut milk, bone broth, cacao powder, and honey. This creamy and luxurious drink is not only delicious but also packed with health benefits. Coconut milk provides healthy fats, bone broth offers collagen and amino acids for joint and gut health, and cacao powder delivers antioxidants. Enjoy this comforting and nutritious beverage any time of the day, savoring its warmth and wellness in every sip.

PROTEIN-RICH DREAMY HOT CHOCOLATE

2 servings	10g P | 16g C 10g F	180 per serving	Prep Time: 5 minutes	Cooking Time: 5 minutes	Total Time: 10 minutes

INGREDIENTS

For the Hot Chocolate:

- 1 cup Native Forest Organic Coconut Milk (no guar)
- 1 cup Kettle & Fire Reduced Sodium Classic Chicken Bone Broth
- 3 tablespoons cacao powder
- 2-3 tablespoons honey or maple syrup (adjust to taste)
- 1 teaspoon vanilla extract
- A pinch of salt
- *Optional:* 1/4 teaspoon peppermint extract or 1 peppermint starlight mint, crushed

DIRECTIONS

1. In a small saucepan, heat the coconut milk and bone broth over medium heat until warm (do not boil).
2. Whisk in the cacao powder until fully dissolved.
3. Add the honey or maple syrup, vanilla extract, a pinch of salt, and if desired, the peppermint extract or crushed peppermint starlight mint.
4. Continue to whisk until all ingredients are well combined and the mixture is heated through.
5. Serve hot, and optionally top with a few marshmallows or a sprinkle of cacao powder.

"Wellness Insights: *Did You Know?*"

- ***Did you know...*** that incorporating turmeric into your recipes can help reduce inflammation, support joint health and cognitive function?
- ***Did you know...*** that adding chia seeds to your smoothies or oatmeal can boost your intake of omega-3 fatty acids, fiber, and protein?

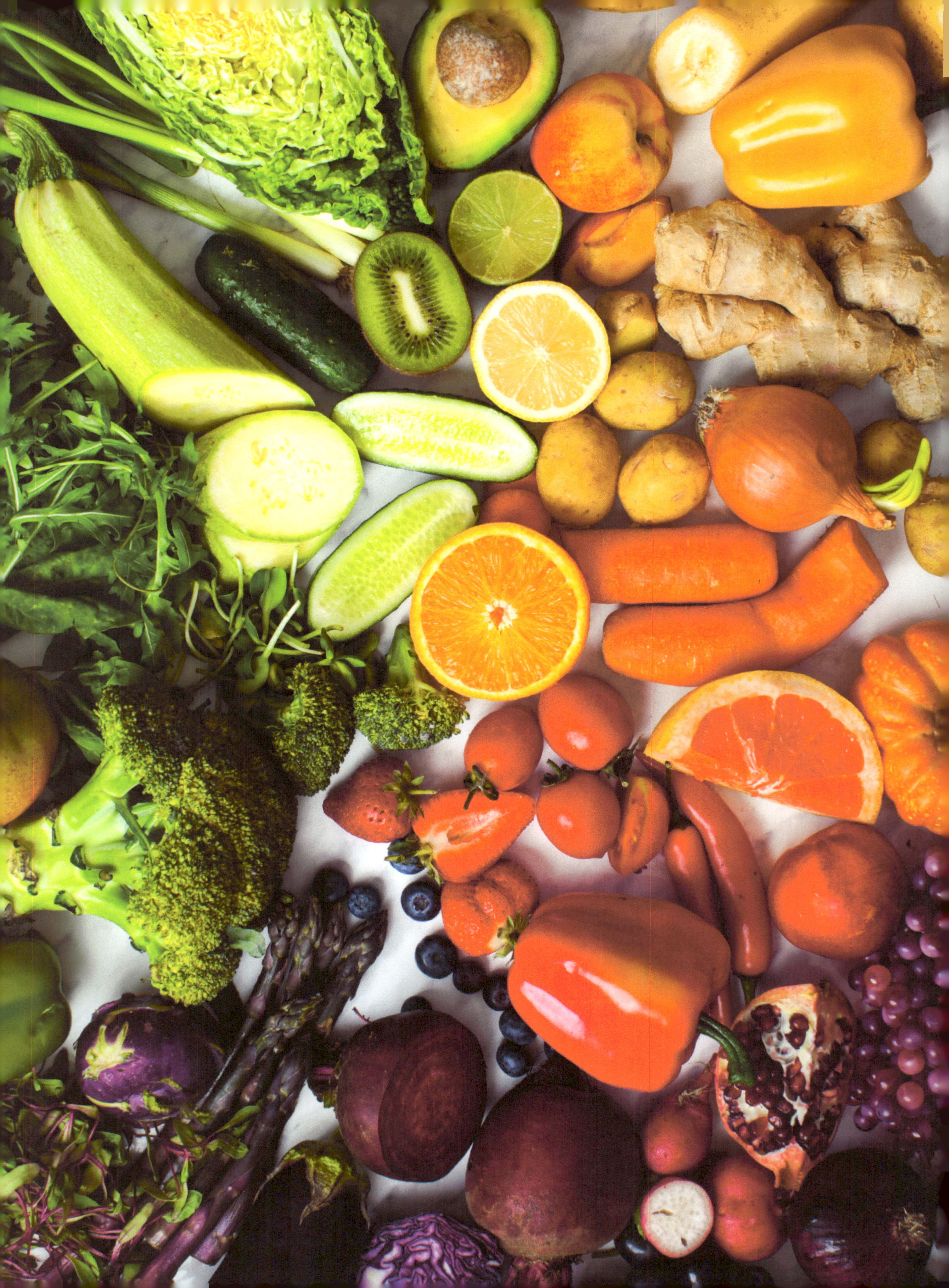

SECTION 5

SPECIAL RECIPE Collections

Welcome to the Special Recipe Collections section of "The Evolutionary Plate: From Taste to Transformation." In this section, you'll find an array of specially curated recipes designed to enhance your meals and support your wellness journey. These collections are crafted to offer versatility, convenience, and flavor, ensuring that you have a variety of options to suit your tastes and dietary needs.

Meat Marinades
Marinating your meats not only infuses them with rich flavors but also helps to tenderize and enhance their overall taste. While planning ahead and marinating meats the night before can yield the best results, these marinades can also be used for quick, immediate meal preparations. Simply coat your meat with the marinade, allow it to sit for a minimum of 30 minutes, and then cook as desired. These marinades can be applied to a variety of meats, including poultry, beef, pork, and even fish, adding a delightful burst of flavor to your dishes.

Assorted Salad Dressings
Salad dressings are more than just a topping for greens; they can elevate the taste of your salads and vegetables. Whether you're drizzling them over a fresh garden salad, tossing them with roasted veggies, or using them as a dip, these dressings add a burst of flavor to any meal. Experiment with different combinations to find your favorite pairings and enjoy the enhanced taste and nutrition they bring to your dishes.

Seasoning Blends
Seasoning blends are versatile additions to your culinary essentials. These custom blends can be sprinkled on poultry, meats, salads, vegetables, and even some sweet indulgences to bring out the best in your food. Whether you're looking to add a savory touch to your main course or a hint of spice to your dessert, these blends provide a simple yet effective way to elevate your cooking.

Super Smoothies Collection
Super smoothies are a fantastic way to prioritize your health and boost your nutrient intake. Packed with fruits, vegetables, and other wholesome ingredients, these smoothies are perfect for breakfast, a post-workout snack, or a quick meal on the go. Each recipe is designed to provide a balanced mix of vitamins, minerals, antioxidants, and fiber, ensuring you stay energized and nourished throughout the day. Enjoy the convenience and health benefits of these delicious blends, tailored to support various aspects of your wellness journey.

Wellness Shots Collection
Wellness shots are concentrated doses of nutrients that can give your immune system a boost and support overall health. These shots are quick to prepare and consume, making them an easy addition to your daily routine. With ingredients like ginger, turmeric, and citrus, they offer a potent blend o+f antioxidants and anti-inflammatory properties. Incorporate these wellness shots into your diet to enhance your vitality and well-being.
Each of these collections is designed to help you make the most of your meals, adding flavor, nutrition, and variety to your diet. Explore the recipes, try new combinations, and enjoy the journey to a healthier, more flavorful life.

MEAT MARINADES

Marinating meat not only enhances its flavor but also tenderizes it, making it more enjoyable to eat. Our collection of meat marinades includes a variety of flavors inspired by global cuisines. These marinades are designed to infuse your meats with rich, aromatic spices and herbs, turning a simple meal into a culinary delight.

Highlights:

- Mediterranean Herb Marinade
- Spicy Citrus Marinade
- Asian Ginger-Soy Marinade
- Smoky BBQ Marinade
- Zesty Lemon Garlic Marinade

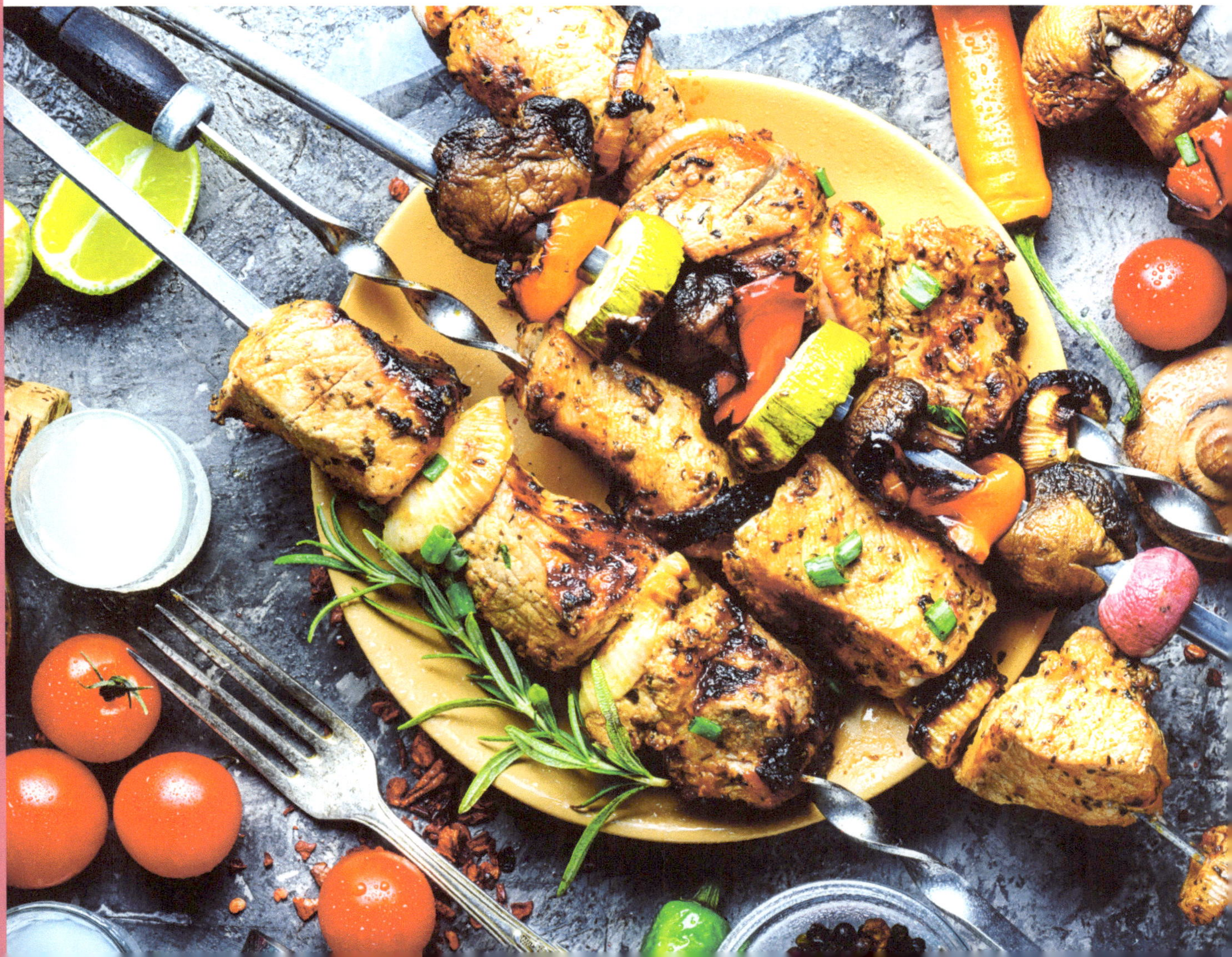

Mediterranean Herb Marinade

Ingredients:

- 1/4 cup olive oil
- 3 cloves garlic, minced
- 2 tablespoons fresh lemon juice
- 2 teaspoons dried oregano
- 1 teaspoon dried thyme
- 1 teaspoon dried rosemary
- 1 teaspoon sea salt
- ½ teaspoon black pepper

Note: Feel free to adjust the salt and pepper amounts to your taste preferences.

Instructions: Combine all ingredients in a bowl and whisk until well blended. Pour over meat (chicken, lamb, or beef) and marinate for at least 2 hours or overnight for best results. Grill, bake, or sauté as desired.

Spicy Citrus Marinade

Ingredients:

- 1/4 cup orange juice
- 1/4 cup lime juice
- 2 tablespoons olive oil
- 2 cloves garlic, minced
- 1 teaspoon ground cumin
- 1 teaspoon chili powder
- 1/2 teaspoon cayenne pepper
- 1 teaspoon sea salt
- ½ teaspoon black pepper

Note: Feel free to adjust the salt and pepper amounts to your taste preferences.

Instructions: Mix all ingredients in a bowl until well combined. Pour over meat (chicken or pork) and marinate for at least 1 hour. Cook using your preferred method.

Asian Ginger-Soy Marinade

Ingredients:

- 1/4 cup soy sauce
- 2 tablespoons rice vinegar
- 2 tablespoons honey
- 2 tablespoons sesame oil
- 2 cloves garlic, minced
- 1 tablespoon fresh ginger, grated
- 1 tablespoon sesame seeds
- 1 teaspoon sea salt
- ½ teaspoon black pepper

Note: Feel free to adjust the salt and pepper amounts to your taste preferences.

Instructions: Whisk all ingredients together in a bowl. Pour over meat (chicken, beef, or pork) and marinate for at least 1 hour. Grill, bake, or stir-fry as desired.

Smoky BBQ Marinade

Ingredients:

- 1/4 cup apple cider vinegar
- 1/4 cup ketchup
- 2 tablespoons molasses
- 2 tablespoons Worcestershire sauce
- 2 cloves garlic, minced
- 1 teaspoon smoked paprika
- 1/2 teaspoon ground mustard
- 1 teaspoon sea salt
- ½ teaspoon black pepper

Note: Feel free to adjust the salt and pepper amounts to your taste preferences.

Instructions: Combine all ingredients in a bowl and whisk until smooth. Pour over meat (beef, chicken, or ribs) and marinate for at least 2 hours or overnight. Cook on the grill or in the oven.

Zesty Lemon Garlic Marinade

Ingredients:

- 1/4 cup olive oil
- 1/4 cup fresh lemon juice
- 3 cloves garlic, minced
- 1 teaspoon dried oregano
- 1 teaspoon dried basil
- 1 teaspoon black pepper
- 1 teaspoon sea salt
- ½ teaspoon black pepper

Note: Feel free to adjust the salt and pepper amounts to your taste preferences.

Instructions: Mix all ingredients in a bowl until well combined. Pour over meat (chicken, fish, or shrimp) and marinate for at least 30 minutes. Grill, bake, or sauté as desired.

"Wellness Insights: *Did You Know?*"

» ***Did you know...*** that marinating meats in a mixture of olive oil, lemon juice, and garlic not only enhances flavor but also helps tenderize the meat and preserve its nutrients?

ASSORTMENT OF SALAD DRESSINGS

A great salad is only as good as its dressing. Our assortment of salad dressings is designed to elevate your salads with bold, delicious flavors. From creamy to tangy to sweet, these dressings are perfect for any type of salad, adding a burst of flavor while keeping your meals healthy and balanced.

Highlights:

- Classic Balsamic Vinaigrette
- Creamy Avocado Lime Dressing
- Honey Mustard Dressing
- Tahini Lemon Dressing
- Herbed Yogurt Dressing

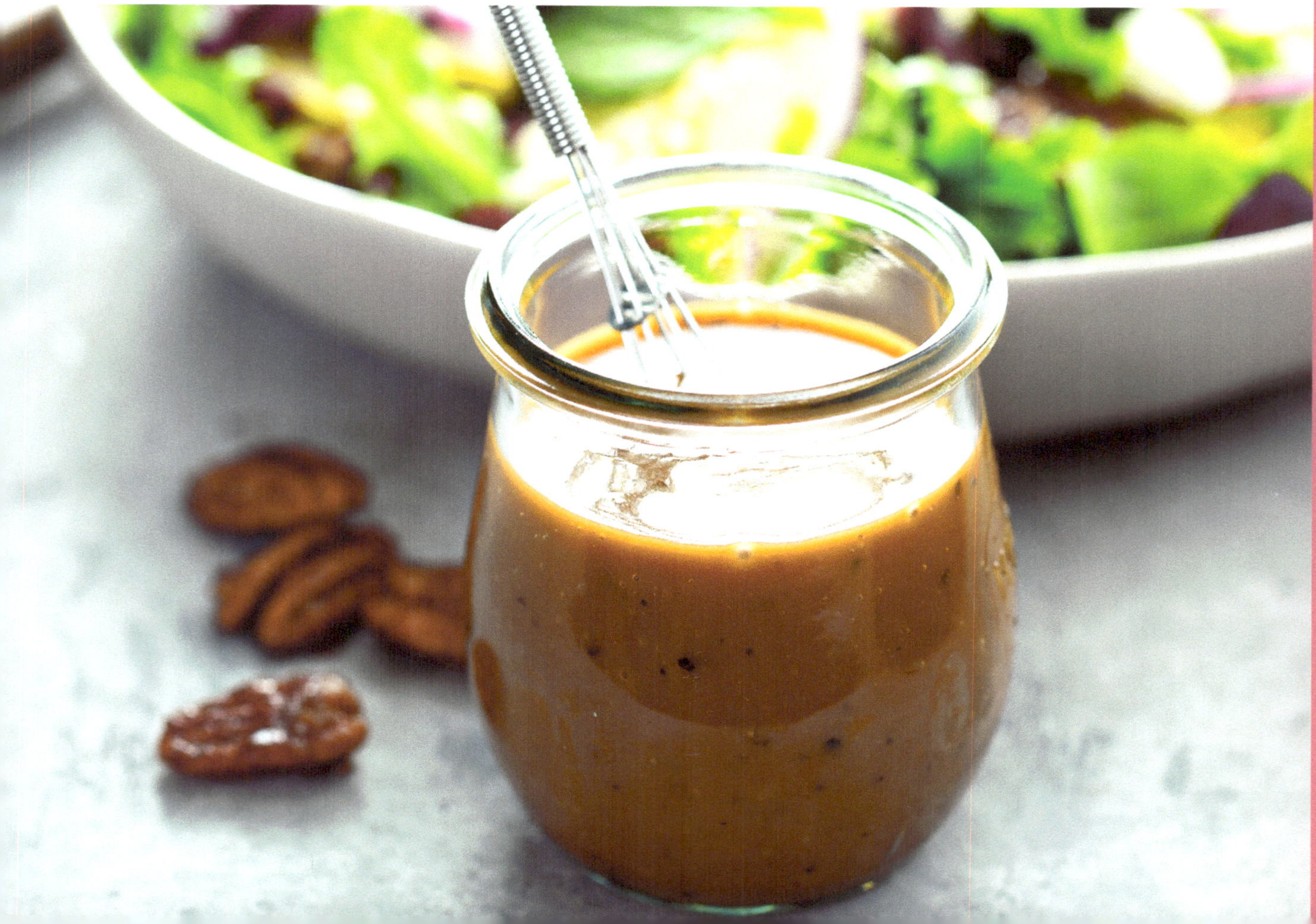

Classic Balsamic Vinaigrette

Ingredients:

- 1/4 cup balsamic vinegar
- 3/4 cup olive oil
- 1 tablespoon Dijon mustard
- 1 clove garlic, minced
- 1 teaspoon sea salt
- ½ teaspoon black pepper

Note: Feel free to adjust the salt and pepper amounts to your taste preferences.

Instructions: Combine all ingredients in a jar with a tight-fitting lid. Shake well until emulsified. Drizzle over your favorite salad and enjoy.

Creamy Avocado Lime Dressing

Ingredients:

- 1 ripe avocado
- 1/4 cup Greek yogurt
- Juice of 1 lime
- 2 tablespoons olive oil
- 1 clove garlic, minced
- 1 teaspoon sea salt
- ½ teaspoon black pepper

Note: Feel free to adjust the salt and pepper amounts to your taste preferences.

Instructions: Blend all ingredients in a food processor or blender until smooth. Adjust seasoning as needed. Serve over salads or as a dip.

Honey Mustard Dressing

Ingredients:

- 1/4 cup Dijon mustard
- 1/4 cup honey
- 1/4 cup apple cider vinegar
- 1/2 cup olive oil
- 1 teaspoon sea salt
- ½ teaspoon black pepper

Note: Feel free to adjust the salt and pepper amounts to your taste preferences.

Instructions: Whisk all ingredients together in a bowl. Taste and adjust seasoning if necessary. Drizzle over salads or use as a marinade.

Tahini Lemon Dressing

Ingredients:

- 1/4 cup tahini
- 1/4 cup water
- Juice of 1 lemon
- 1 tablespoon olive oil
- 1 clove garlic, minced
- 1 teaspoon sea salt
- ½ teaspoon black pepper

Note: Feel free to adjust the salt and pepper amounts to your taste preferences.

Instructions: Whisk all ingredients together until smooth. Add more water if needed to reach desired consistency. Serve over salads or as a dip.

Herbed Yogurt Dressing

Ingredients:

- 1 cup Greek yogurt
- 2 tablespoons fresh dill, chopped
- 2 tablespoons fresh parsley, chopped
- 1 clove garlic, minced
- Juice of 1 lemon
- 1 teaspoon sea salt
- ½ teaspoon black pepper

Note: Feel free to adjust the salt and pepper amounts to your taste preferences.

Instructions: Mix all ingredients in a bowl until well combined. Chill in the refrigerator for at least 30 minutes to let flavors meld. Serve over salads or as a dip.

"Wellness Insights: *Did You Know?*"

» ***Did you know...*** that homemade salad dressings with apple cider vinegar can help stabilize blood sugar levels and improve digestion due to its acetic acid content?

SEASONING BLENDS

Seasoning blends are a fantastic way to add depth and flavor to your dishes without the need for multiple spices and herbs. You may have many of these spices and herbs on hand in your pantry, putting them to good use to make a special blended seasoning. My unique blends are designed to enhance the flavor of poultry or meats, salads, and even ice cream or sorbets. Each blend combines carefully chosen ingredients to create a truly unique and delicious experience. These blends are versatile, flavorful, and easy to use, making them a staple in any kitchen.

Highlights:

- Heavenly Herb Blend
- Sunshine Salad Blend
- Sweet Serenade Blend
- Mediterranean Spice Blend
- Smoky BBQ Rub
- Zesty Citrus Blend

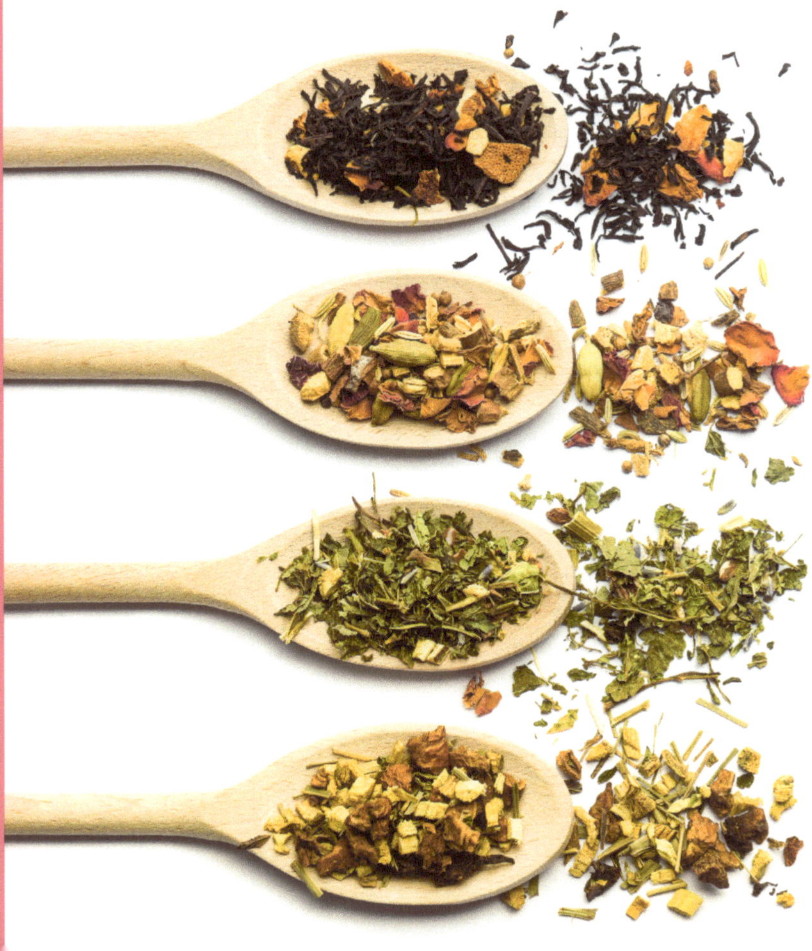

Heavenly Herb Blend

Purpose: Adds an aromatic and earthy flavor to poultry and meats.

Ingredients:

- 2 tbsp dried lavender
- 1 tbsp dried rosemary
- 1 tbsp dried thyme
- 1 tbsp dried sage
- 1 tbsp dried tarragon
- 2 tsp ground sumac
- 1 tsp black pepper
- 1 tsp salt

Instructions: Combine all ingredients in a small jar and shake well to blend. Store in an airtight container.

Usage: Rub onto poultry or meats before grilling, roasting, or pan-searing. Pairs well with chicken, turkey, pork, or lamb.

Sunshine Salad Seasoning

Purpose: Enhances the freshness and flavor of salads.

Ingredients:

- 3 tbsp dried orange zest
- 2 tbsp dried lemon zest
- 1 tbsp dried mint
- 1 tbsp dried basil
- 1 tbsp dried dill
- 1 tsp garlic powder
- 1 tsp onion powder
- 1 tsp salt

Instructions: Combine all ingredients in a small jar and shake well to blend. Store in an airtight container.

Usage: Sprinkle on salads or mix into salad dressings. Pairs well with leafy greens, cucumber, tomatoes, and avocado.

Sweet Serenade Spice

Purpose: Adds warmth and aromatic depth to sweet, frozen treats.

Ingredients:

- 2 tbsp ground cinnamon
- 1 tbsp ground ginger
- 1 tbsp ground cardamom
- 1 tbsp ground nutmeg
- 1 tbsp ground allspice
- 1 tbsp ground star anise
- 1 tsp ground cloves
- 1 tsp ground black pepper

Instructions: Combine all ingredients in a small jar and shake well to blend. Store in an airtight container.

Usage: Sprinkle over ice cream or sorbets, or mix into dessert bases before freezing. Pairs well with vanilla, chocolate, or caramel ice cream, as well as fruit-based sorbets like mango, peach, or raspberry.

Mediterranean Spice Blend

Purpose: Enhances the flavor of meats, vegetables, or grains with Mediterranean flavors.

Ingredients:

- 2 tbsp dried oregano
- 2 tbsp dried basil
- 1 tbsp dried rosemary
- 1 tbsp dried thyme
- 1 tbsp garlic powder
- 1 tbsp onion powder
- 1 tsp black pepper
- 1 tsp sea salt

Instructions: Combine all ingredients in a bowl and mix well. Store in an airtight container.

Usage: Use to season meats, vegetables, or grains.

Smoky BBQ Rub

Purpose: Adds a smoky, sweet, and spicy flavor to meats or roasted vegetables.

Ingredients:

- 2 tbsp smoked paprika
- 1 tbsp brown sugar
- 1 tbsp chili powder
- 1 tbsp garlic powder
- 1 tbsp onion powder
- 1 tsp black pepper
- 1 tsp sea salt
- 1/2 tsp cayenne pepper

Instructions: Mix all ingredients together in a bowl. Store in an airtight container.

Usage: Use as a dry rub for meats or to season roasted vegetables.

Zesty Citrus Blend

Purpose: Adds a bright, zesty flavor to fish, chicken, or vegetables.

Ingredients:

- 2 tbsp lemon zest (dried)
- 2 tbsp lime zest (dried)
- 1 tbsp dried thyme
- 1 tbsp dried basil
- 1 tbsp garlic powder
- 1 tsp sea salt
- 1 tsp black pepper

Instructions: Combine all ingredients in a bowl and mix well. Store in an airtight container.

Usage: Use to season fish, chicken, or vegetables.

"Wellness Insights: *Did You Know?*"

» ***Did you know...*** that using herbs and spices like cumin, coriander, and paprika in your seasoning blends can add not only flavor but also health benefits, such as improved digestion, reduced inflammation, and enhanced antioxidant levels?

SUPER SMOOTHIES

19 Nourishing Blends for Every Wellness Need

Smoothies are a quick and delicious way to pack a variety of nutrients into one convenient meal or snack. Whether you're looking to boost your energy, enhance your recovery, or simply enjoy a refreshing treat, my smoothie collection has something for everyone. Each recipe is designed to provide a balanced blend of vitamins, minerals, and macronutrients to support your wellness journey. From enhancing your energy and improving digestion to supporting weight loss and boosting overall health, these Super Smoothies have got you covered. Each drink is created with specific health benefits in mind, making it easy to find the perfect smoothie for your needs.

These smoothies range from creamy and refreshing to rich and filling, using natural ingredients to deliver vitamins, minerals, antioxidants, and fiber in every sip. Perfect for breakfast, post-workout recovery, or an afternoon snack, these nutritious blends are as versatile as they are beneficial.

Explore my top Super Smoothie recipes and discover how simple, wholesome ingredients can make a big impact on your health and well-being. Just blend and enjoy!

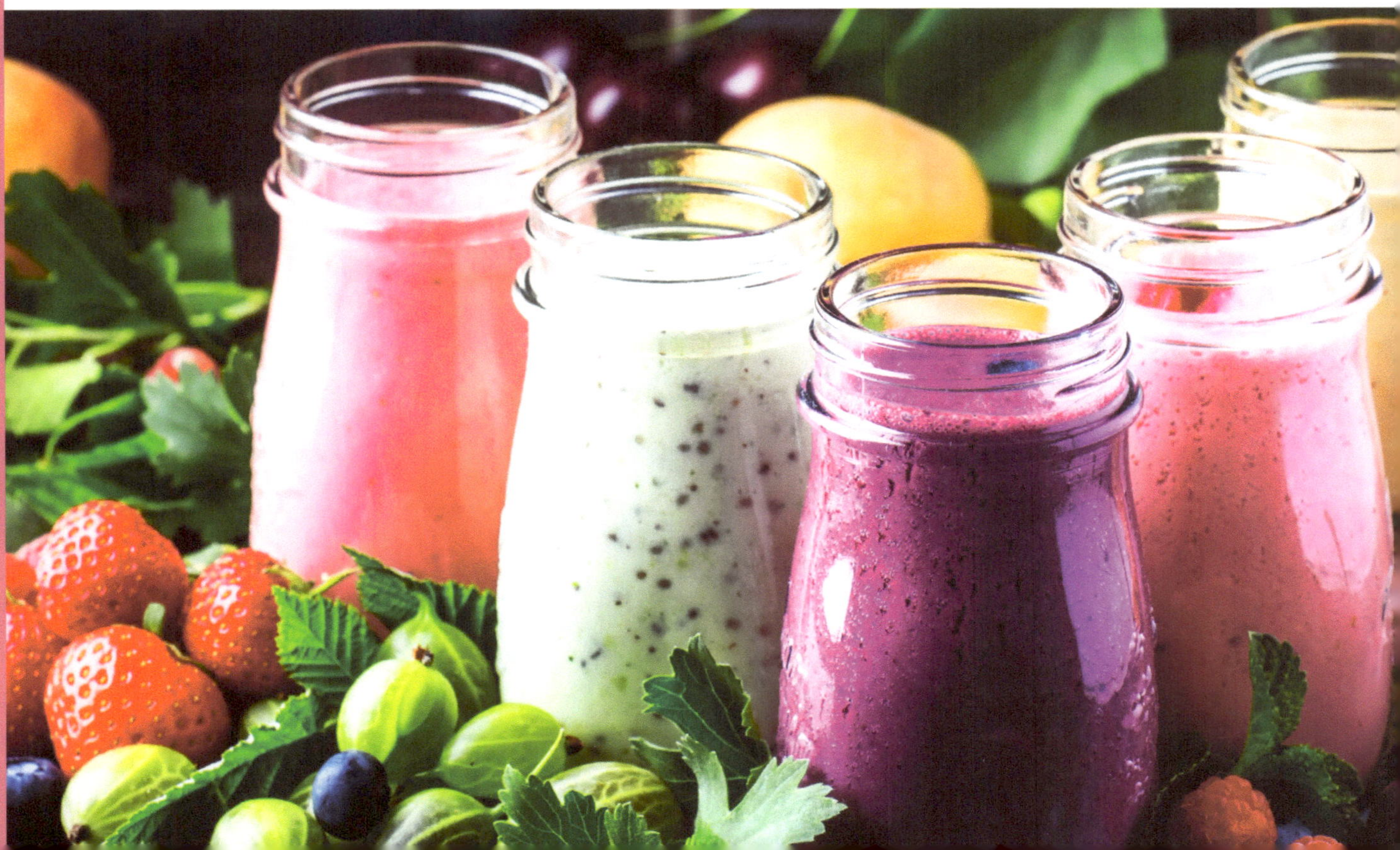

MEAL REPLACEMENT SMOOTHIES

These smoothies are more substantial and can keep you full for longer, making them ideal as meal replacements:

1. **Diabetes Management Smoothie** - Helps manage blood sugar levels with healthy fats and low carbs.
2. **Digestive Aid Smoothie** - Includes kefir or yogurt, which is filling and promotes gut health.
3. **Green Energy Smoothie** - Packed with spinach, avocado, and chia seeds for a hearty start.
4. **Protein Power Smoothie** - High in protein from the powder and peanut butter to support muscle recovery.
5. **Weight Loss Smoothie** - Contains ingredients that boost metabolism and keep you satiated.

SNACK SMOOTHIES

These smoothies are lighter and can be enjoyed as a snack between meals:

1. **Anti-Stress Cortisol Balancing Smoothie** - Calming adaptogens to help reduce stress.
2. **Berry Blast Smoothie** - Antioxidant-rich berries make for a refreshing snack.
3. **Breast Health Smoothie** - High in antioxidants to support breast health.
4. **Eye Health Smoothie** - High in beta-carotene to support vision and reduce inflammation.
5. **Heart Health Smoothie** - High in fiber and antioxidants, perfect for a heart-healthy snack.
6. **Hormonal Balance Smoothie** - Contains ingredients to support hormonal balance and boost energy.
7. **Immune Booster Smoothie** - A vitamin-packed option to boost your immune system.
8. **Kidney Health Smoothie** - Helps detoxify the body and support kidney function.
9. **Mental Health Smoothie** - Rich in nutrients that support mental health and mood.
10. **Mood Lifter Smoothie** - Nutrient-dense but light enough for a quick pick-me-up.
11. **Skin Glow Smoothie** - Hydrating and antioxidant-rich, great for a beauty boost.
12. **Thyroid Health Smoothie** - Supports thyroid function with nutrient-rich ingredients.
13. **Tropical Detox Smoothie** - Light and hydrating with pineapple and cucumber.
14. **Urinary Health Smoothie** - Contains ingredients that support urinary health and hydration.

21-DAY HEALTH GOAL
Smoothie Challenge

To maximize the benefits of these smoothies, consider doing a 21-Day Health Goal Smoothie Challenge. Here's how you can structure it to ensure you get a variety of health Benefits:

1. **Choose Your Health Goal:** (Select one health goal to focus on for 21 days)

Energy Boost
- Green Energy Smoothie
- Protein Power Smoothie
- Mood Lifter Smoothie

Digestive Health
- Digestive Aid Smoothie
- Tropical Detox Smoothie
- Urinary Health Smoothie

Immune Support
- Immune Booster Smoothie
- Berry Blast Smoothie
- Skin Glow Smoothie

Weight Loss
- Weight Loss Smoothie
- Green Energy Smoothie
- Diabetes Management Smoothie

Mental Health
- Mental Health Smoothie
- Mood Lifter Smoothie
- Heart Health Smoothie

Hormonal Balance
- Hormonal Balance Smoothie
- Anti-Stress Cortisol Balancing Smoothie
- Breast Health Smoothie

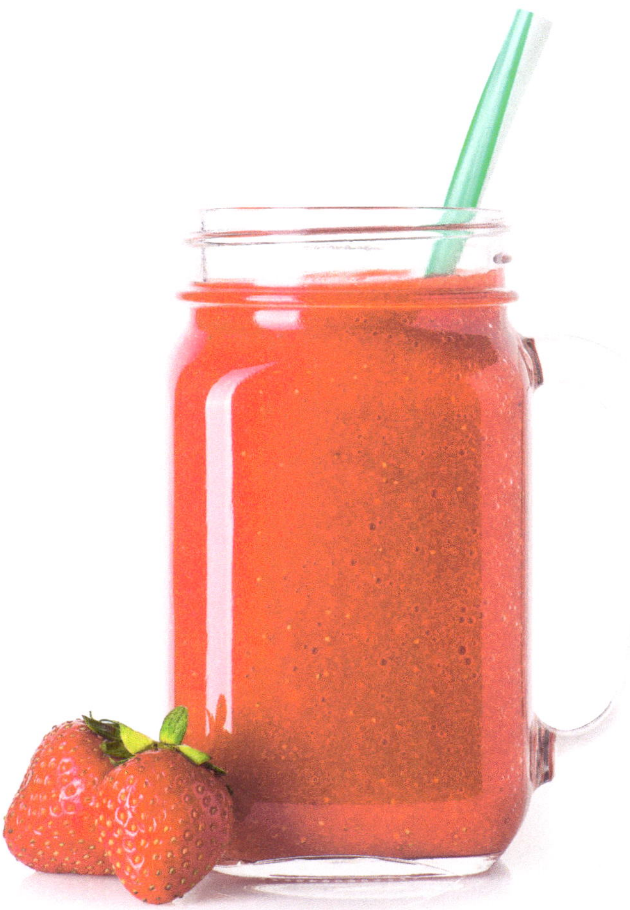

Skin and Beauty
- Skin Glow Smoothie
- Eye Health Smoothie
- Breast Health Smoothie

Organ Health

- Kidney Health Smoothie
- Urinary Smoothie
- Thyroid Smoothie

2. **Weekly Plan:** Replace your morning meal with a smoothie and rotate between the three smoothies corresponding to your chosen goal each week.

3. **Track Your Progress:** Keep a journal of how you feel each day.

Example Plan for Energy Boost:

- **Monday:** Green Energy Smoothie
- **Tuesday:** Protein Power Smoothie
- **Wednesday:** Mood Lifter Smoothie
- **Thursday:** Green Energy Smoothie
- **Friday:** Protein Power Smoothie
- **Saturday:** Mood Lifter Smoothie
- **Sunday:** Green Energy Smoothie

Repeat this plan for three weeks. After completing the 21-day cycle, choose another health goal and repeat the process for the next 21 days.

Not Interested in a Challenge? If you're not interested in a structured challenge, you can still enjoy the benefits of these smoothies:

- Pick any smoothie based on your current health needs or preferences and incorporate it into your daily routine.
- Enjoy one smoothie daily for three weeks, or mix and match any of these smoothies to replace your morning meal and boost your health.

Whether you need a quick energy boost, support for digestion, or an immune boost, there's a smoothie for every occasion.

"Wellness Insights: *Did You Know?*"

- ***Did you know...*** that 70% of your immune system resides in your gut? Adding probiotics to your smoothies can help boost your gut health and immunity.
- ***Did you know...*** that adding a handful of spinach to your smoothie can boost your intake of iron and vitamin K without altering the flavor significantly?

MEAL REPLACEMENT SMOOTHIES

Diabetes Management Smoothie - Manage Blood Sugar

1 serving
6g protein, 12g carbohydrates, 15g fat, 200 calories

Ingredients:
- 1 cup unsweetened almond milk
- 1/2 avocado
- 1/2 cucumber
- 1/4 cup frozen berries
- 1 tablespoon chia seeds

Benefits: Helps manage blood sugar levels, provides healthy fats, and supports overall health.

Digestive Aid Smoothie - Tummy Tamer

1 serving
8g protein, 40g carbohydrates, 7g fat, 250 calories

Ingredients:
- 1 cup kefir or yogurt
- 1/2 banana
- 1/2 cup papaya
- 1 tablespoon ground flaxseed
- 1 teaspoon ginger

Benefits: Promotes gut health, aids digestion, and reduces bloating.

Green Energy Smoothie - Fuel Your Day

1 serving
5g protein, 45g carbohydrates, 15g fat, 300 calories per serving

Ingredients:
- 1 cup spinach
- 1 banana
- 1/2 avocado
- 1 cup almond milk
- 1 tablespoon chia seeds
- 1 teaspoon honey

Benefits: Provides a natural energy boost, rich in antioxidants, and supports heart health.

Protein Power Smoothie - Strength and Recovery

1 serving
25g protein, 40g carbohydrates, 15g fat, 400 calories

Ingredients:
- 1 scoop protein powder (your choice)
- 1 banana
- 1 tablespoon peanut butter
- 1 cup almond milk
- 1 tablespoon oats

Benefits: Supports muscle recovery, provides sustained energy, and keeps you full longer.

Weight Loss Smoothie - Slim Down

1 serving
2g protein, 30g carbohydrates, 2g fat, 140 calories

Ingredients:
- 1/2 grapefruit, peeled
- 1/2 cucumber
- 1 cup green tea, cooled
- 1 tablespoon chia seeds
- 1 teaspoon honey

Benefits: Boosts metabolism, promotes fat burning, and keeps you full.

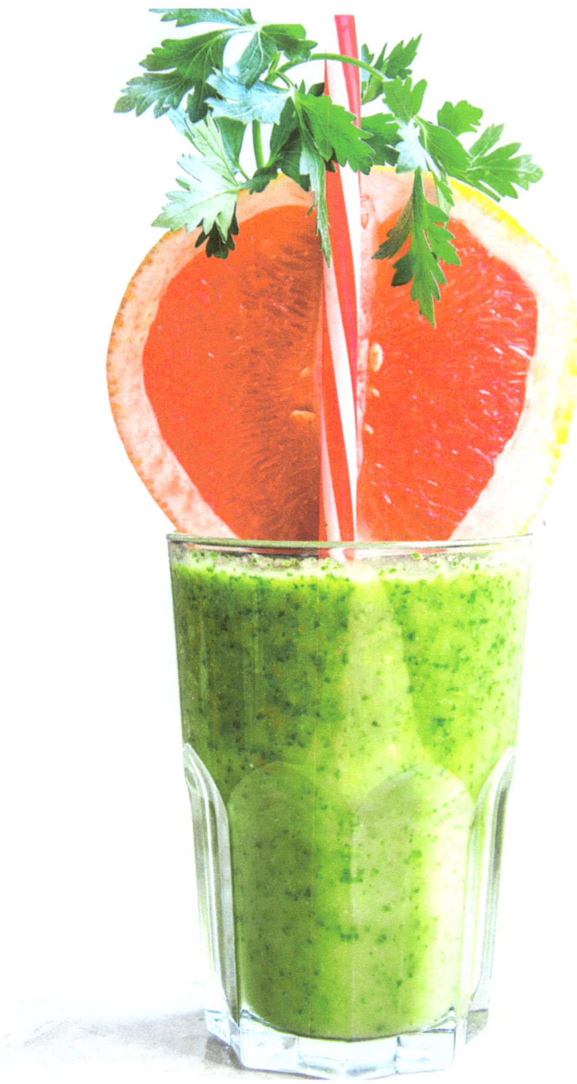

SNACK SMOOTHIES

Anti-Stress Cortisol Balancing Smoothie - Stress Relief and Hormonal Support

1 serving
8g protein, 30g carbohydrates, 10g fat, 275 calories

Ingredients:
- 1 cup unsweetened almond milk (or your preferred nut milk)
- 1/2 banana
- 1/2 cup spinach
- 1/2 cup blueberries
- 1 tablespoon almond butter
- 1 teaspoon ashwagandha powder
- 1 teaspoon honey or maple syrup (optional)
- 1/4 teaspoon cinnamon
- 1/2 teaspoon turmeric

Benefits: Helps reduce cortisol levels, rich in antioxidants, supports stress relief, and promotes hormonal balance.

Berry Blast Smoothie - Antioxidant Powerhouse

1 serving
8g protein, 35g carbohydrates, 5g fat, 220 calories

Ingredients:
- 1 cup mixed berries (blueberries, strawberries, raspberries)
- 1/2 cup Greek yogurt
- 1/2 cup orange juice
- 1 tablespoon flaxseed
- 1 teaspoon honey

Benefits: High in antioxidants, supports brain health, and boosts the immune system.

Breast Health Smoothie - Support Your Breast Health

1 serving
8g protein, 40g carbohydrates, 4g fat, 220 calories

Ingredients:
- 1 cup pomegranate juice
- 1/2 cup strawberries
- 1/2 cup Greek yogurt
- 1 tablespoon chia seeds

Benefits: High in antioxidants, supports breast health, and boosts the immune system.

Eye Health Smoothie - Protect Your Vision

1 serving
2g protein, 40g carbohydrates, 0g fat
150 calories

Ingredients:
- 1 cup carrot juice
- 1/2 mango
- 1 orange, peeled
- 1 teaspoon turmeric
- 1/4 teaspoon black pepper

Benefits: Supports eye health, high in beta-carotene, and reduces inflammation.

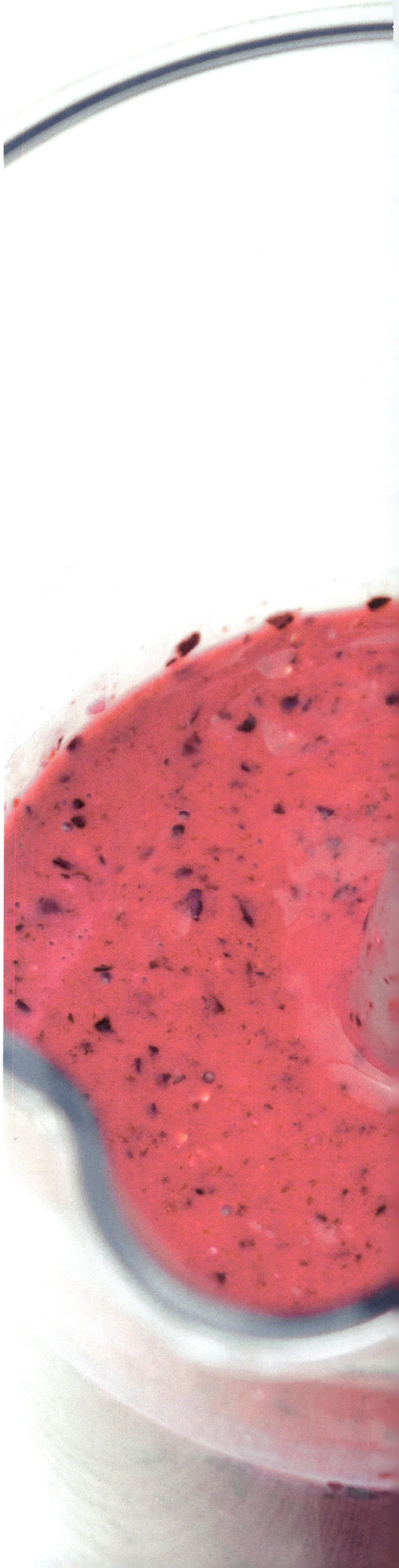

Heart Health Smoothie - Love Your Heart

1 serving
5g protein, 40g carbohydrates, 4g fat, 210 calories

Ingredients:
- 1 cup blueberries
- 1/2 banana
- 1 cup spinach
- 1 tablespoon ground flaxseed
- 1 cup almond milk

Benefits: Supports cardiovascular health, high in fiber and antioxidants, and reduces cholesterol.

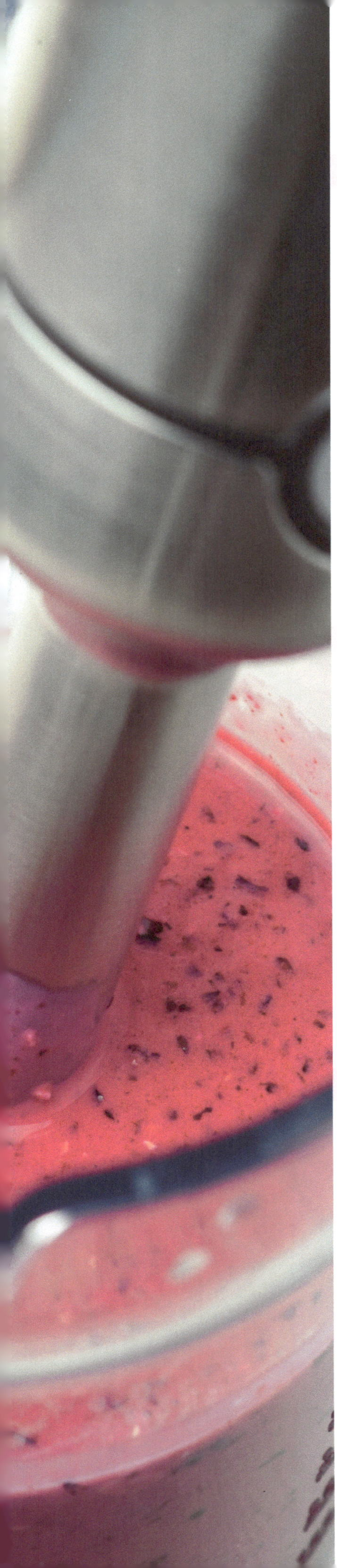

Hormonal Balance Smoothie - Balance Your Hormones

1 serving
8g protein, 30g carbohydrates, 7g fat, 200 calories per serving

Ingredients:
- 1 cup soy milk (contains phytoestrogens)
- 1 tablespoon ground flaxseed
- 1/2 banana
- 1/2 cup berries
- 1 teaspoon maca powder
- 1 serving

Benefits: Supports hormonal balance, provides essential nutrients, and boosts energy.

Immune Booster Smoothie - Stay Healthy

1 serving
2g protein, 45g carbohydrates, 0g fat, 180 calories

Ingredients:
- 1 orange, peeled
- 1/2 cup carrot juice
- 1/2 cup mango
- 1 tablespoon turmeric
- 1 teaspoon honey

Benefits: High in vitamin C, boosts the immune system, and reduces inflammation.

Kidney Health Smoothie - Support Your Kidneys

1 serving
3g protein, 20g carbohydrates, 0.5g fat, 90 calories

Ingredients:
- 1 cup kale
- 1/2 cucumber
- 1 apple, cored
- 1/2 lemon, juiced
- 1/4 cup parsley
- 1 cup water

Benefits: Supports kidney function, helps detoxify the body, and provides essential vitamins and minerals.

Mental Health Smoothie - Boost Your Mood

1 serving
6g protein, 35g carbohydrates, 8g fat, 230 calories

Ingredients:
- 1 banana
- 1/2 cup spinach
- 1 tablespoon almond butter
- 1 cup almond milk
- 1 teaspoon honey

Benefits: Supports mental health, rich in magnesium and potassium, and boosts mood.

Mood Lifter Smoothie - Feel Good

1 serving
5g protein, 40g carbohydrates, 10g fat, 270 calories

Ingredients:
- 1 banana
- 1/2 cup spinach
- 1/2 cup pineapple
- 1 cup almond milk
- 1 tablespoon almond butter

Benefits: Supports mental health, rich in magnesium and potassium, and boosts mood.

Skin Glow Smoothie - Radiate Beauty

1 serving
4g protein, 35g carbohydrates, 15g fat, 280 calories

Ingredients:
- 1/2 avocado
- 1 cup mixed berries
- 1 tablespoon chia seeds
- 1 cup coconut water
- 1 teaspoon honey

Benefits: Hydrates skin, rich in antioxidants, and promotes collagen production.

Thyroid Health Smoothie - Support Your Thyroid

5g protein, 30g carbohydrates, 7g fat, 180 calories

Ingredients:
- 1 cup coconut milk
- 1 tablespoon spirulina powder
- 1/2 banana
- 1 tablespoon ground flaxseed
- 1 teaspoon honey

Benefits: Supports thyroid function, rich in iodine, and provides essential nutrients.

Tropical Detox Smoothie - Cleanse and Refresh

1 serving
1g protein, 30g carbohydrates, 0g fat, 120 calories

Ingredients:
- 1 cup pineapple
- 1/2 cucumber
- 1/2 lime, juiced
- 1/2 cup coconut water
- 1 tablespoon mint leaves
- 1 teaspoon ginger

Benefits: Aids digestion, supports detoxification, and hydrates the body.

Urinary Health Smoothie - Maintain Urinary Health

1 serving
1g protein, 35g carbohydrates, 1g fat, 140 calories

Ingredients:
- 1 cup cranberry juice (unsweetened)
- 1/2 cucumber
- 1/2 cup watermelon
- 1 tablespoon chia seeds

Benefits: Supports urinary health, helps prevent UTIs, and hydrates the body.

WELLNESS SHOTS

10 Quick and Healthy Boosts for Every Need

Wellness shots are concentrated doses of nutrients designed to provide a quick and potent boost to your health. These small but powerful drinks are perfect for starting your day with a burst of energy, supporting your immune system, or aiding in digestion. My collection of wellness shots includes a variety of flavors and benefits, making it easy to incorporate these nutrient-packed drinks into your routine.

With busy schedules and endless to-do lists, keeping up with your health and energy levels can be a challenge. Whether you're looking to kickstart your morning, give your immune system a boost, or work towards specific health goals, my collection of wellness shots offers a quick and effective solution. These concentrated drinks provide targeted health benefits with each potent sip.

Each shot is packed with natural ingredients known for their powerful health-promoting properties. From enhancing digestion and reducing inflammation to improving skin health and supporting mental clarity, these wellness shots fit seamlessly into any routine. No juicer is needed to prepare them—they are easy to make and consume, delivering the nutrients your body craves without any artificial additives.

Discover how a simple, daily shot can transform your well-being with these recipes. Cheers to your health!

How to Take Wellness Shots: To incorporate wellness shots into your routine, consume one shot daily, ideally in the morning on an empty stomach. This helps your body absorb the nutrients more effectively and gives you a healthy start to your day.

Choose a Wellness Shot Based on Your Specific Needs:

1. **Anti-Anxiety Shot - Calm and Collected:** Reduce stress and foster relaxation.
2. **Anti-Inflammatory Shot - Soothe and Heal:** Alleviate inflammation and promote healing.
3. **Detox Shot - Cleanse and Renew:** Purify your system and refresh your body.
4. **Digestive Health Shot - Tummy Tamer:** Calm your digestive system and ease discomfort.
5. **Energy and Focus Shot - Sharp and Alert:** Enhance your concentration and stay sharp.
6. **Energy Boost Wellness Shot - Ignite Your Day:** Energize your morning with a natural boost.
7. **Heart Health Shot - Love Your Heart:** Support your cardiovascular health and function.
8. **Immune Boosting Shot - Shield Your System:** Strengthen your defenses during cold and flu season.
9. **Mood-Boosting Shot - Happiness in a Glass:** Elevate your mood and feel uplifted.
10. **Skin Health Shot - Glow from Within:** Hydrate your skin and enhance your complexion.

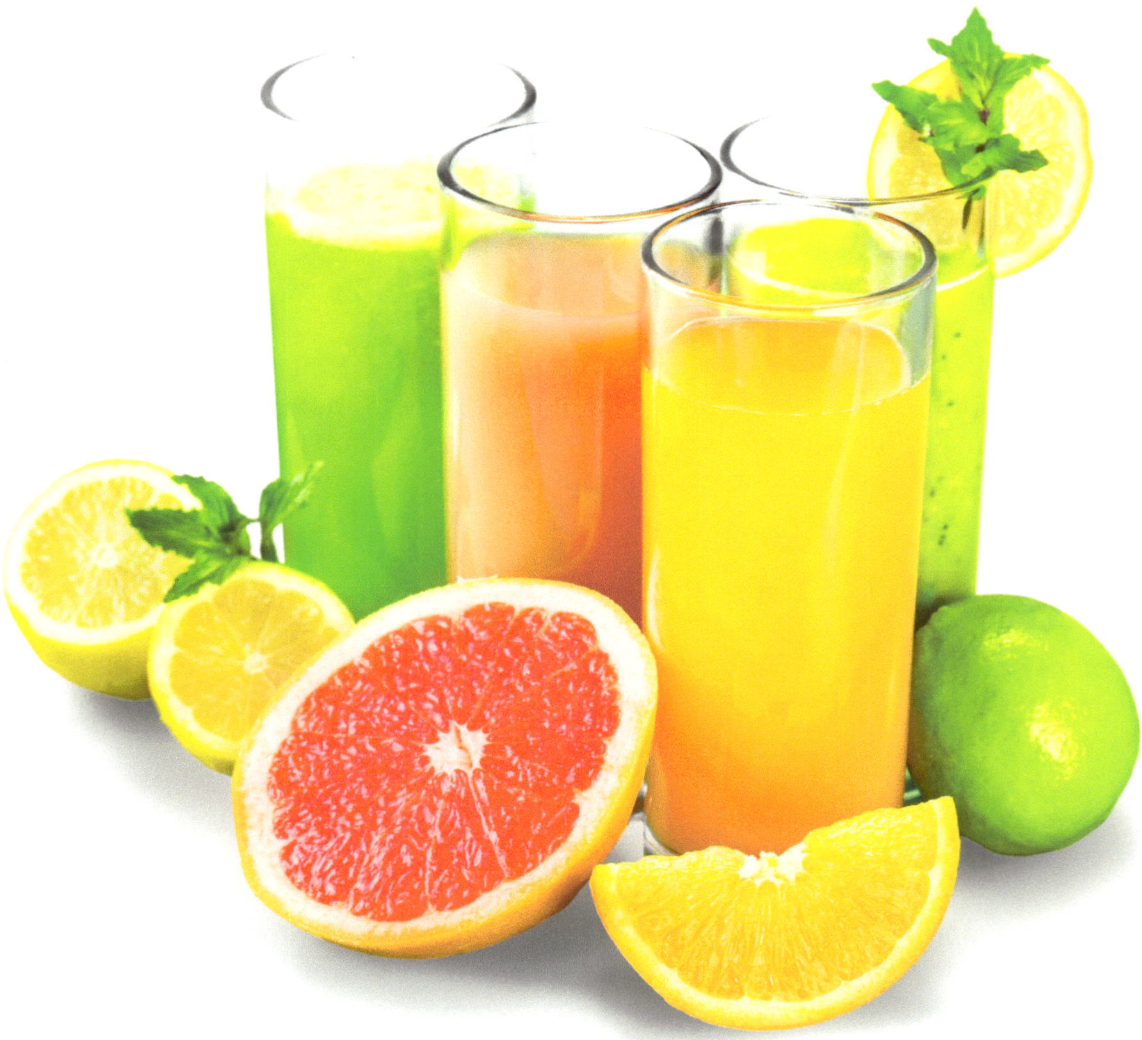

10 QUICK AND HEALTHY BOOSTS FOR EVERY NEED

Anti-Anxiety Shot – Calm and Collected

Ingredients:
- 1 teaspoon ashwagandha powder
- 1 tablespoon honey
- Juice of 1/2 lemon
- 1/4 cup chamomile tea (cooled)

Instructions: Blend or shake all ingredients together and drink immediately.
Benefits: Reduces anxiety, promotes relaxation, and supports overall mental health through a blend of ashwagandha and chamomile tea.

Anti-Inflammatory Shot – Soothe and Heal

Ingredients:
- 1-inch piece of turmeric root
- 1/4 teaspoon black pepper
- Juice of 1 orange
- 1 tablespoon apple cider vinegar
- 1/4 cup water

Instructions: Blend all the ingredients together. Alternatively, finely grate the turmeric root, shake all ingredients together, strain if desired, and drink immediately.
Benefits: Reduces inflammation, supports joint health, and boosts the immune system with the combination of turmeric and black pepper.

Detox Shot – Cleanse and Renew

Ingredients:
- Juice of 1 lemon
- 1 tablespoon apple cider vinegar
- 1/4 teaspoon cayenne pepper
- 1 teaspoon honey
- 1/4 cup water

Instructions: Blend or shake all ingredients together and drink immediately.
Benefits: Supports liver detoxification, boosts metabolism, and aids digestion with lemon juice and apple cider vinegar.

Digestive Health Shot – Tummy Tamer

Ingredients:

- 1-inch piece of ginger root
- 1 tablespoon apple cider vinegar
- Juice of 1/2 lemon
- 1 tablespoon aloe vera juice
- 1/4 cup water

Instructions: Blend all the ingredients together. Alternatively, finely grate the ginger root, shake all ingredients together and drink immediately.
Benefits: Aids digestion, soothes the stomach, and reduces bloating with ginger root and aloe vera juice.

Energy and Focus Shot – Sharp and Alert

Ingredients:

- 1 teaspoon matcha powder
- Juice of 1/2 lemon
- 1 tablespoon honey
- 1/4 cup coconut water

Instructions: Blend or shake all ingredients together and drink immediately.
Benefits: Provides a natural energy boost, enhances focus, and hydrates the body with matcha powder and coconut water.

Energy Boost Wellness Shot - Ignite Your Day

Ingredients:

- 1-inch piece of ginger root
- 1-inch piece of turmeric root
- 1/4 teaspoon cayenne pepper
- 1 teaspoon cinnamon (Cassia (regular store-bought))
- Pinch of black pepper
- 2 ounces lemon juice
- 1/4 cup water
- 1 teaspoon honey

Instructions:
Finely grate the ginger and turmeric roots, shake all ingredients together and drink immediately for a quick energy and digestion boost. Eat the honey separately.
Benefits: This shot provides a natural energy boost, aids digestion, and supports weight loss with ginger and turmeric, making it perfect for powering through workouts without the need for synthetic thermogenics.

Heart Health Shot – Love Your Heart

Ingredients:

- 1 small beet, juiced or finely grated
- Juice of 1/2 pomegranate
- 1 tablespoon flaxseed oil
- 1/4 teaspoon ground cinnamon
- 1/4 cup water

Instructions: Blend all the ingredients together. Alternatively, juice or finely grate the beet, then shake all ingredients together. Strain if desired, and drink immediately.
Benefits: Beets improve blood flow and lower blood pressure, pomegranate juice is rich in antioxidants, flaxseed oil provides omega-3 fatty acids, and cinnamon helps regulate blood sugar levels.

Immune Boosting Shot - Shield Your System

Ingredients:

- 1-inch piece of ginger root
- 1 clove garlic
- Juice of 1 lemon
- 1 tablespoon honey
- Pinch of cayenne pepper
- 1/4 cup water

Instructions: Blend all the ingredients together. Alternatively, finely grate the ginger root, shake all remaining ingredients together and drink immediately.
Benefits: Supports immune function, reduces inflammation, and fights infections with ginger root and lemon juice.

Mood-Boosting Shot – Happiness in a Glass

Ingredients:

- 1 teaspoon maca powder
- Juice of 1/2 orange
- 1 tablespoon honey
- 1/4 teaspoon turmeric powder
- 1/4 cup water

Instructions: Blend or shake all ingredients together and drink immediately.
Benefits: Maca powder is known to balance hormones and improve mood, while turmeric reduces inflammation. Orange juice provides vitamin C and antioxidants, and honey adds a touch of natural sweetness.

Skin Health Shot – Glow from Within

Ingredients:
- Juice of 1/2 grapefruit
- 1-inch piece of cucumber
- 1 tablespoon aloe vera juice
- 1/4 cup water

Instructions: Blend all the ingredients together. Alternatively, finely grate the cucumber, shake all remaining ingredients together, and drink immediately.
Benefits: Hydrates the skin, provides antioxidants, supports collagen production, and repairs skin with grapefruit juice and aloe vera juice.

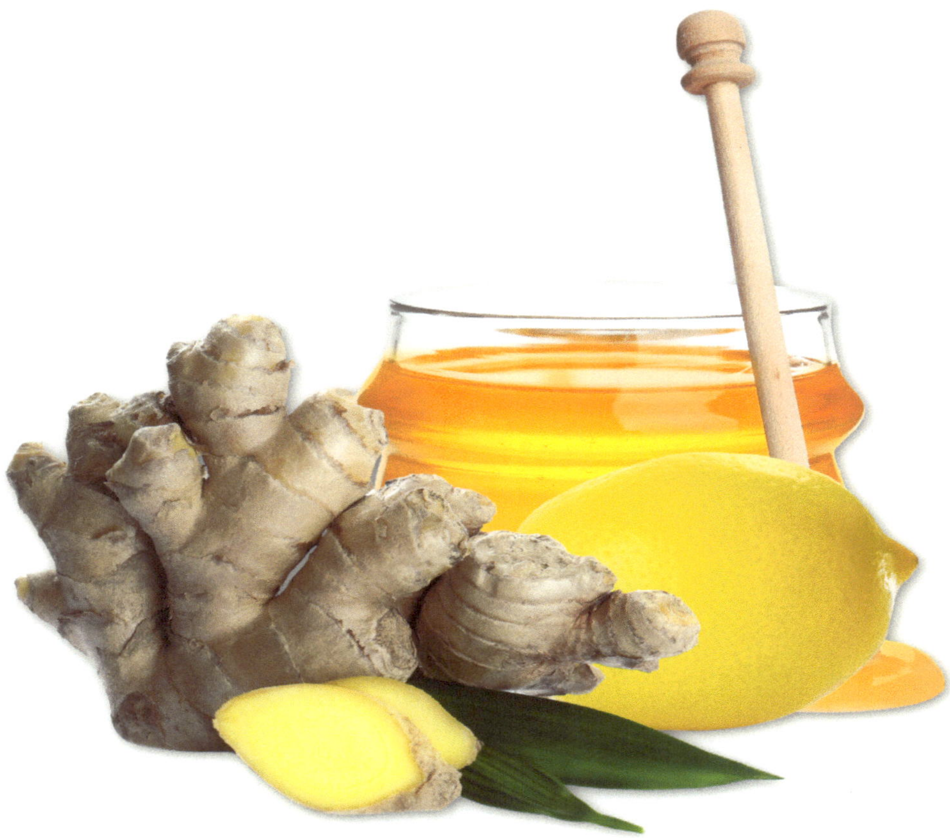

"Wellness Insights: *Did You Know?*"

» ***Did you know...*** that ginger shots can help boost your immune system and improve digestion due to their high levels of gingerol?

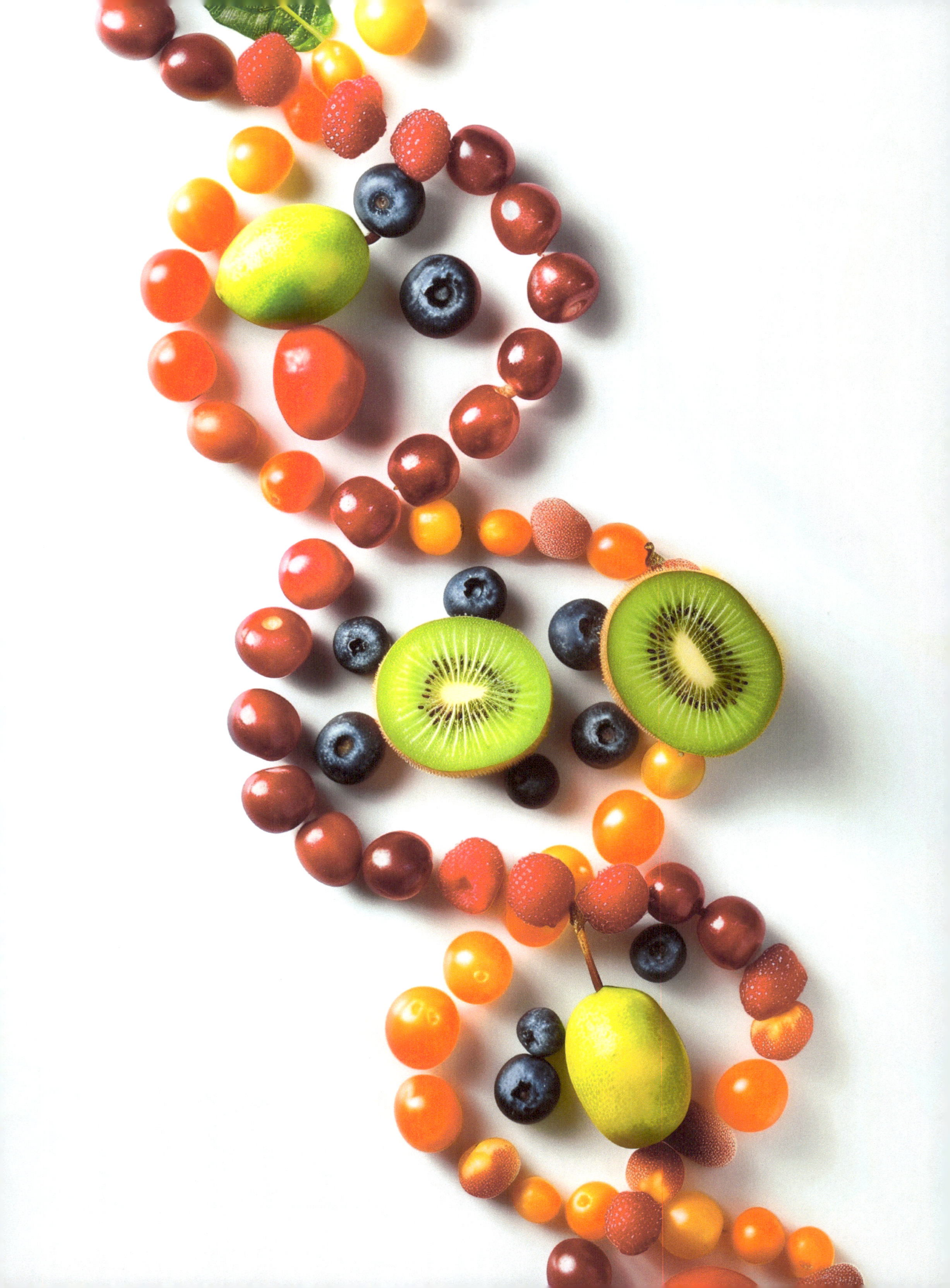

SECTION 6

PERSONALIZED Nutrition

Welcome to the Personalized Nutrition section of "The Evolutionary Plate: From Taste to Transformation." Achieving optimal health and well-being starts with understanding that everyone's nutritional needs are unique. This section provides comprehensive guidance on how to tailor your nutrition to support your specific goals. By considering factors such as your body type, lifestyle, and personal preferences, you can develop a personalized approach to nutrition that promotes long-term wellness.

In the subsections that follow, you'll find detailed guidelines on customizing your meal plan, understanding your body type, and applying principles like the 80/20 rule. You'll also have access to self-assessment tools to identify your body type, practical tips for meal customization, and insights into how different nutrients impact your health. This holistic approach ensures that your nutrition plan is not only effective but also enjoyable and sustainable.

CUSTOMIZED NUTRITION Guidelines

Everyone's nutritional needs are unique, influenced by factors such as age, gender, body type, activity level, and health goals. Customized nutrition ensures your dietary choices support your specific needs, promoting optimal health and well-being.

Understanding your body type—whether you're an ectomorph, mesomorph, or endomorph—plays a key role in this customization. Each body type has different nutritional needs and responds differently to various foods.

Use the comprehensive 4-week meal plan provided in this book as a foundation to create meals that offer variety and balance, ensuring you get a broad spectrum of nutrients from whole, unprocessed foods. As you proceed, you'll learn how to adjust these meals to fit your specific nutritional needs and health goals.

Adopting a diet rich in whole, natural foods is a powerful way to manage your calorie intake and achieve a calorie deficit. A calorie deficit occurs when you consume fewer calories than your body needs to maintain its current weight, leading to weight loss. Whole foods, such as fruits, vegetables, lean proteins, and whole grains, are typically lower in calories and higher in nutrients compared to processed foods. By replacing high-calorie, processed foods with nutrient-dense whole foods, you naturally reduce your calorie intake without feeling deprived. This shift not only helps you lose weight but also enhances your overall health. Additionally, eating whole foods can change your palate, making overly salty and sweet processed foods less appealing over time. Keeping a food log for a week can help you identify and understand your eating habits, allowing you to make more informed dietary choices and effectively create a calorie deficit.

PRIORITIZING PROTEIN FOR OPTIMAL HEALTH

Incorporating adequate protein into your diet is essential for several reasons. Eating more lean protein can help satiate you for longer periods, which is key to weight loss as it helps curb cravings and prevents overeating. Protein also plays an essential role in sustaining muscle mass, especially when combined with regular exercise.

DAILY PROTEIN REQUIREMENTS

To give your body the necessary nutrients, aim to prioritize protein in your meals. Here are some general baseline guidelines:

- **Women**: Aim for at least 46 grams of protein per day.
- **Men**: Aim for at least 56 grams of protein per day.

However, these numbers can vary based on individual needs, activity levels, and specific health goals. For those looking to lose weight, build muscle, or maintain muscle mass, a higher protein intake may be beneficial. Refer to the macronutrient guidelines for each body type to determine the optimal protein intake for your specific situation.

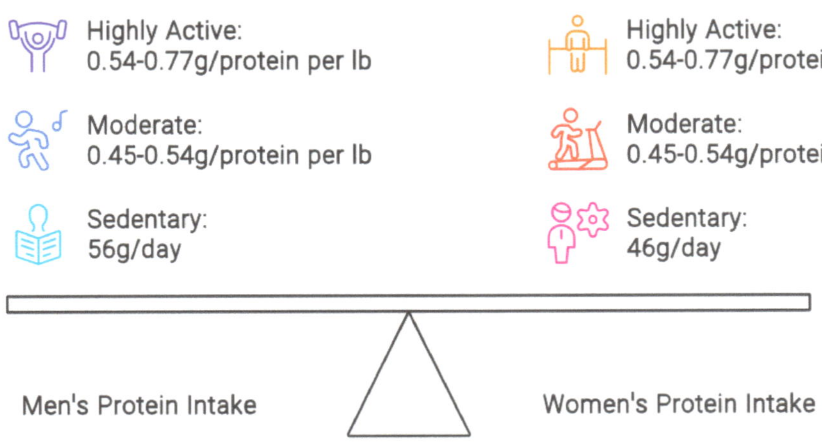

Protein Intake for Men and Women Based on Activity Level

PROTEIN IN YOUR 4-WEEK MEAL PLAN

The 4-week meal plan in this book incorporates balanced meals with a focus on nutrient-dense foods, including adequate protein. This structured approach helps eliminate guesswork, making it easier to stick to healthy eating habits and meet your protein needs.

By starting with this comprehensive plan, you build a strong foundation that prepares you for the more tailored approach of the customized meal plans provided later in the book. These customized plans consider your unique body type and goals, ensuring that you get the most out of your diet.

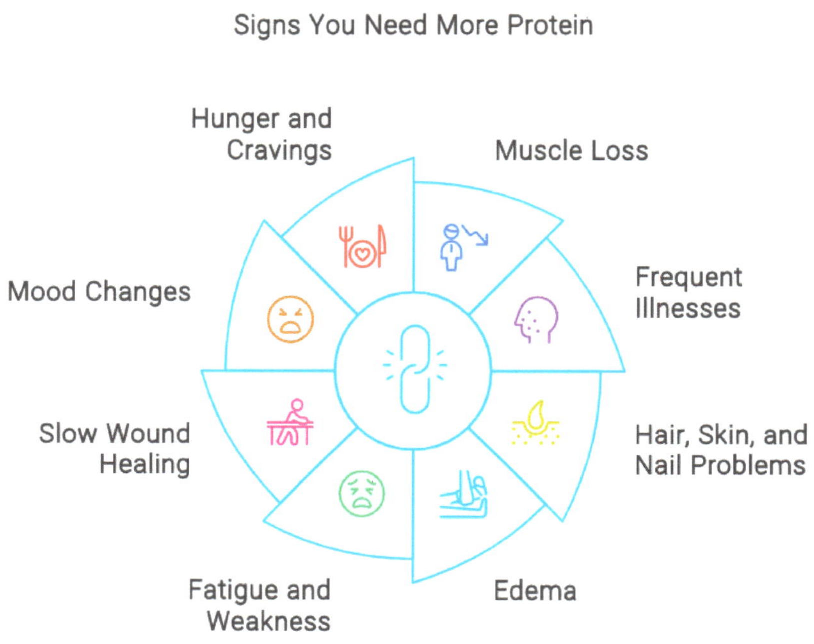
Signs You Need More Protein
Hunger and Cravings
Muscle Loss
Frequent Illnesses
Hair, Skin, and Nail Problems
Edema
Fatigue and Weakness
Slow Wound Healing
Mood Changes

INTEGRATING PROTEIN INTO YOUR DIET

To seamlessly incorporate more protein into your diet, consider the following tips:

- **Choose lean protein sources:** Opt for chicken, turkey, fish, lean beef, eggs, and plant-based proteins like beans and lentils.
- **Include protein in every meal:** Make sure each meal contains a source of protein to help balance your diet and keep you full.
- **Snack wisely:** Choose protein-rich snacks like Greek yogurt, cottage cheese, nuts, and seeds to keep your energy levels stable throughout the day.

By prioritizing protein intake, you support your overall health, sustain muscle mass, and curb cravings, making it easier to achieve and maintain a balanced diet.

STEPS TO CUSTOMIZE YOUR MEAL PLAN

This guidance will help you identify your body type and tailor your diet accordingly:

1. **Identify Your Body Type:**
   - Use the self-assessment quiz provided to determine whether you are an ectomorph, mesomorph, or endomorph.

2. **Set Your Health Goals:**
   - Define what you want to achieve: weight loss, muscle gain, improved energy levels, or overall wellness.

3. **Understand Your Nutritional Needs:**
   - Learn the recommended macronutrient ratios for your body type and health goals. For example, ectomorphs may need higher carbohydrate intake, while endomorphs might benefit from a higher protein and fat intake.

4. **Adjust the Meal Plan:**
   - Modify the provided 4-week meal plan to align with your body type's nutritional needs. This could involve increasing protein portions for muscle gain or adjusting carbohydrate sources for better energy levels.
   - Incorporate the recipes that best suit your taste preferences and dietary requirements, but ensure they meet the macronutrient guidelines for your body type.

5. **Listen to Your Body:**
   - Pay attention to how different foods make you feel. Adjust portions and food choices based on your hunger and fullness cues.

6. **Use the 80/20 Rule:**
   - Aim for 80% of your meals to consist of wholesome, nutritious foods, while allowing 20% for your favorite indulgences. This balanced approach supports sustainable healthy eating.

7. **Reflect and Adjust:**
   - Regularly review your progress and how you feel. Make necessary adjustments to your meal plan to continue supporting your health goals.

INTEGRATING PROTEIN INTO YOUR DIET

To seamlessly incorporate more protein into your diet, consider the following tips:

- Choose lean protein sources: Opt for chicken, turkey, fish, lean beef, eggs, and plant-based proteins like beans and lentils.

- Include protein in every meal: Make sure each meal contains a source of protein to help balance your diet and keep you full.
- Snack wisely: Choose protein-rich snacks like Greek yogurt, cottage cheese, nuts, and seeds to keep your energy levels stable throughout the day.

By prioritizing protein intake, you support your overall health, sustain muscle mass, and curb cravings, making it easier to achieve and maintain a balanced diet. By following these steps, you can effectively customize the provided meal plan to meet your unique nutritional needs and achieve your health goals. This approach ensures that you build a strong foundation with the 4-week meal plan, preparing you for the more tailored approach of the customized meal plans provided later in the book. These customized plans consider your unique body type and goals, ensuring that you get the most out of your diet.

"Wellness Insights: *Did You Know?*"

» ***Did you know...*** that deficiencies in magnesium, selenium, and zinc can lead to a variety of health issues? For example, low levels of magnesium can cause muscle cramps and fatigue, insufficient selenium can impact thyroid function, and a lack of zinc can weaken your immune system and reduce your sense of taste and smell.

» ***Did you know...*** that essential fatty acids, such as omega-3s found in fish, can improve heart health and support brain function?

INTRODUCTION TO Different Body Types

Understanding your body type can significantly influence how you approach both nutrition and exercise. Recognizing the unique characteristics and needs of your body type allows for more informed and effective decisions, ultimately supporting your overall health and fitness goals. The three main body types are:

Ectomorph:

- Characteristics: Lean, long, and often struggle to gain weight or muscle.
- Nutritional Needs: Higher intake of carbohydrates and proteins to support energy and muscle growth. Focus on nutrient-dense foods to meet high metabolic demands.
- Exercise Recommendations: Emphasize strength training to build muscle mass. Include compound movements like squats, deadlifts, and bench presses. Incorporate moderate cardio to support cardiovascular health without excessive calorie burning.
- Potential Challenges: Difficulty in gaining weight and muscle mass. May need to consume more calories and protein to achieve fitness goals.

Mesomorph:

- Characteristics: Naturally muscular, easy to gain muscle and maintain a healthy weight.
- Nutritional Needs: Balanced intake of carbohydrates, proteins, and fats. Ensure adequate protein for muscle maintenance and moderate carbohydrates for energy.
- Exercise Recommendations: A mix of strength training and cardio exercises. Include both compound and isolation movements to enhance muscle definition. High-intensity interval training (HIIT) can be beneficial for cardiovascular health and fat burning.
- Potential Challenges: Maintaining a balanced diet to avoid gaining excess weight. Monitoring portion sizes and macronutrient intake can help sustain a healthy physique.

Endomorph:

- Characteristics: Naturally higher body fat, easily gain weight.
- Nutritional Needs: Controlled intake of carbohydrates with a focus on proteins and healthy fats. Emphasize portion control and nutrient-dense foods to support metabolism.
- Exercise Recommendations: Prioritize cardio exercises to aid in fat loss. Include strength training to build muscle and boost metabolism. Regular low to moderate intensity cardio, like walking or cycling, can be effective.
- Potential Challenges: Managing carbohydrate intake and portion sizes. Maintaining consistency in both diet and exercise is key to achieving and sustaining weight loss goals.

SELF-ASSESSMENT QUIZ to Identify Body Type

To help you determine your body type and tailor your nutritional needs accordingly, take this self-assessment quiz. Answer the following questions to determine your body type:

1. **What is your natural build?**
    - A. Lean and tall (Ectomorph)
    - B. Muscular and athletic (Mesomorph)
    - C. Round and soft (Endomorph)

2. **How easily do you gain weight?**
    - A. Difficult to gain weight (Ectomorph)
    - B. Gain weight moderately (Mesomorph)
    - C. Easily gain weight (Endomorph)

3. **How easily do you gain muscle?**
    - A. Difficult to gain muscle (Ectomorph)
    - B. Easily gain muscle (Mesomorph)
    - C. Gain muscle slowly (Endomorph)

4. **What is your energy level like?**
    - A. High energy, but get tired quickly (Ectomorph)
    - B. Consistent and balanced energy (Mesomorph)
    - C. Lower energy, but can sustain activities (Endomorph)
5. **How does your body respond to exercise?**
    - A. Burn calories quickly, struggle to build muscle (Ectomorph)
    - B. Build muscle easily, stay fit (Mesomorph)
    - C. Burn calories slowly, gain muscle and fat easily (Endomorph)

Scoring:

- Mostly A's: Ectomorph
- Mostly B's: Mesomorph
- Mostly C's: Endomorph

CALORIE INTAKE AND Macros by Body Type and Goals

(for Men and Women)

To achieve your health and fitness goals, it's essential to understand the right calorie intake and macronutrient distribution for your specific body type and objectives. These guidelines offer a starting point, but individual needs can vary based on factors such as gender, age, activity level, and specific goals. Adjusting your eating habits according to these needs can help you optimize your energy levels, support muscle growth, and promote overall well-being.
Understanding the Range

The provided calorie ranges are designed to cater to both men and women, as well as different ages and activity levels. For example, a sedentary woman might aim for the lower end of the range, while an active man might need the higher end. These are general recommendations to help you find what works best for you. Consulting with a nutritionist can provide more personalized advice.

Ectomorph

- **Calories:** 2500-3000 calories per day
- **Macronutrients:**
  - 50-60% carbohydrates (1250-1800 calories or 312-450 grams)
  - 20-30% protein (500-900 calories or 125-225 grams)
  - 20-30% fat (500-900 calories or 56-100 grams)

Mesomorph

- **Calories:** 2000-2500 calories per day
- **Macronutrients:**
  - 40-50% carbohydrates (800-1250 calories or 200-312 grams)
  - 30-40% protein (600-1000 calories or 150-250 grams)
  - 20-30% fat (400-750 calories or 44-83 grams)

Endomorph

- **Calories:** 1500-2000 calories per day
- **Macronutrients:**
  - 30-40% carbohydrates (450-800 calories or 112-200 grams)
  - 30-40% protein (450-800 calories or 112-200 grams)
  - 30-40% fat (450-800 calories or 50-89 grams)

These ranges are recommendations and should be adjusted based on your individual needs. For example, if you're highly active, you may need to consume more calories to fuel your activities. Conversely, if you have a lower activity level, you may need fewer calories.

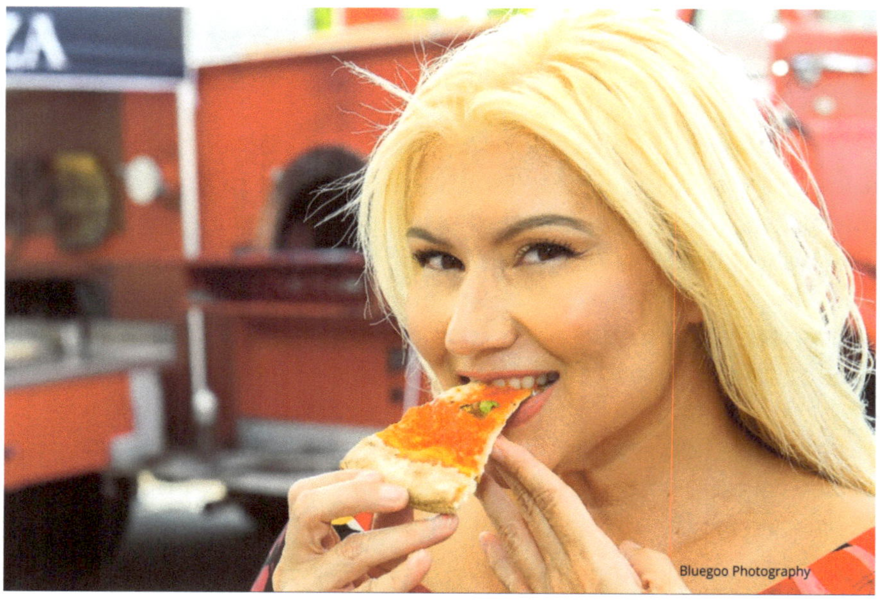

Embracing the 80/20 rule: Enjoying a slice of margarita pizza as part of a balanced and healthy lifestyle.

APPLYING THE 80/20 RULE

The 80/20 rule is a practical way to maintain a balanced diet by emphasizing nutritious foods while still enjoying occasional treats. Here's how you can integrate this approach into your daily eating habits effectively:

1. **80% Nutritious Foods**
2. **20% Indulgent Foods**

EXAMPLE:

Daily Plan for an Ectomorph. Total Daily Intake, 2500 calories:

- Carbohydrates: 50-60% (1250-1500 calories or 312-375 grams)
- Protein: 20-30% (500-750 calories or 125-188 grams)
- Fats: 20-30% (500-750 calories or 56-83 grams)

80% Nutritious Foods:

- Breakfast: High-protein smoothie with oats, spinach, and banana (400 calories)
- Lunch: Quinoa salad with chickpeas, avocado, and mixed greens (600 calories)
- Dinner: Grilled salmon with sweet potato and steamed broccoli (700 calories)
- Snacks: Nuts and dried fruit (300 calories), Greek yogurt with honey (300 calories)

20% Indulgent Foods:

- Indulgence: A small piece of chocolate (200 calories)

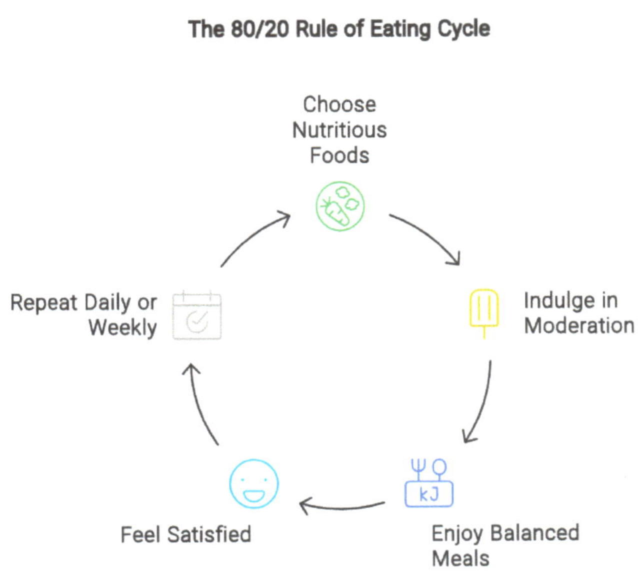

By following these guidelines, you can adapt your meals to your body type, meet your nutritional needs, and maintain a balanced and healthy lifestyle with the flexibility of the 80/20 rule.

As you progress, regularly reflect on how you feel and make adjustments as needed. The goal is to develop a positive relationship with food, where healthy eating becomes a natural part of your lifestyle. By making mindful choices and enjoying the process, you can achieve a balanced and healthy lifestyle that supports your overall well-being.

MEAL RECOMMENDATIONS Based on Body Type

Achieving your health and fitness goals starts with understanding that different body types have unique nutritional needs. This section provides tailored meal plans based on the three main body types—Ectomorph, Mesomorph, and Endomorph. These examples demonstrate how to adjust your existing 4-week meal plan to meet your specific nutritional requirements.

KEY DIFFERENCES:

- **Portion Sizes:** Adjusted according to the caloric needs of each body type.
- **Macronutrient Ratios:** Different ratios of proteins, carbs, and fats to align with the metabolic and energy requirements of each body type.
- **Frequency of Meals:** Ectomorphs may have more frequent, higher-carb meals to support a faster metabolism, while endomorphs may have fewer, protein- and fat-focused meals to support slower metabolism and weight management.

When looking at the plans, there are key differences:

1. **Ectomorphs:**
    - Higher carb intake for energy.
    - More frequent meals to support a faster metabolism.
    - Example: Blueberry Bliss Protein Smoothie with extra oats and banana for added carbs.

2. **Mesomorphs:**
    - Balanced macronutrient distribution.
    - Moderate portion sizes to maintain muscle and energy levels.
    - Example: Blueberry Bliss Protein Smoothie with balanced portions of protein, carbs, and fats.

3. **Endomorphs:**
    - Lower carb, higher protein and fat for sustained energy.
    - Fewer meals to manage caloric intake.
    - Example: Blueberry Bliss Protein Smoothie with reduced carbs and increased protein and fat.

By understanding and applying these necessary adjustments to your meal plans based on your body type, you can ensure you get the most out of your nutrition plan.

CUSTOMIZED MEAL PLANS
Based on Body Type

After learning how to adjust your existing meal plans based on your body type, the following are customized meal plans designed to support your nutritional needs and health goals, whether you are an ectomorph, mesomorph, or endomorph. These plans aim to optimize energy levels, support muscle growth, and promote well-being by aligning with your body's natural tendencies.

Knowing your physique will help you make the most of these plans. The meal recommendations use recipes from the book and show the subtle differences in adjustments for each body type. For the same meals, you will see how the variations cater to the unique needs of ectomorphs, mesomorphs, and endomorphs.

These plans provide you with detailed, ready-to-follow meal recommendations, guiding you toward achieving your health and fitness objectives efficiently and effectively. Enjoy the journey to a more balanced approach to eating, designed to complement your unique physique.

WEEK 1

Day 1

Meal	Ectomorph	Mesomorph	Endomorph
Breakfast: Blueberry Bliss Protein Smoothie	1 cup almond milk, 1 banana, 1 cup blueberries, 1 scoop protein powder	3/4 cup almond milk, 1/2 banana, 3/4 cup blueberries, 3/4 scoop protein powder	1/2 cup almond milk, 1/2 banana, 1/2 cup blueberries, 1/2 scoop protein powder
Lunch: Mediterranean Orzo Pasta Salad	1 cup cooked orzo, 1/2 cup cherry tomatoes, 1/2 cup cucumber, 1/4 cup feta, 2 tbsp olive oil	3/4 cup cooked orzo, 1/3 cup cherry tomatoes, 1/3 cup cucumber, 2 tbsp feta, 1.5 tbsp olive oil	1/2 cup cooked orzo, 1/4 cup cherry tomatoes, 1/4 cup cucumber, 1 tbsp feta, 1 tbsp olive oil
Dinner: Pan-Seared Salmon with Lemon Dill Sauce and Sautéed Asparagus	1 large salmon fillet, 1 tbsp lemon dill sauce, 1 cup asparagus	1 medium salmon fillet, 3/4 tbsp lemon dill sauce, 3/4 cup asparagus	1 small salmon fillet, 1/2 tbsp lemon dill sauce, 1/2 cup asparagus
Snack: Homemade Organic Granola	1 cup granola	3/4 cup granola	1/2 cup granola

Day 2

Meal	Ectomorph	Mesomorph	Endomorph
Breakfast: Spinach and Veggie Egg Bites	3 eggs, 1 cup mixed vegetables	2 eggs, 3/4 cup mixed vegetables	2 eggs, 1/2 cup mixed vegetables
Lunch: Chipotle Chicken Salad Bowl	1 cup chicken, 1/2 cup black beans, 1/2 cup corn, 1/4 avocado, 2 tbsp chipotle dressing	3/4 cup chicken, 1/3 cup black beans, 1/3 cup corn, 1/4 avocado, 1.5 tbsp chipotle dressing	1/2 cup chicken, 1/4 cup black beans, 1/4 cup corn, 1/4 avocado, 1 tbsp chipotle dressing
Dinner: Sweet and Spicy Crispy Pork Stir Fry with Rice Noodles	1 cup pork, 1 cup rice noodles, 1 cup mixed vegetables, 2 tbsp sweet and spicy sauce	3/4 cup pork, 3/4 cup rice noodles, 3/4 cup mixed vegetables, 1.5 tbsp sweet and spicy sauce	1/2 cup pork, 1/2 cup rice noodles, 1/2 cup mixed vegetables, 1 tbsp sweet and spicy sauce
Snack: Dark Chocolate Cacao Cookies	2 cookies	1.5 cookies	1 cookie

Day 3

Meal	Ectomorph	Mesomorph	Endomorph
Breakfast: High-Protein Sweet Banana Nut Overnight Oats	1 cup oats, 1 banana, 1 cup almond milk, 2 tbsp nuts	3/4 cup oats, 1 banana, 3/4 cup almond milk, 1.5 tbsp nuts	1/2 cup oats, 1/2 banana, 1/2 cup almond milk, 1 tbsp nuts
Lunch: Savory Lettuce Wraps with Peanut Sauce	1 cup chicken, 4 large lettuce leaves, 2 tbsp peanut sauce, 1/2 cup shredded carrots	3/4 cup chicken, 3 large lettuce leaves, 1.5 tbsp peanut sauce, 1/3 cup shredded carrots	1/2 cup chicken, 2 large lettuce leaves, 1 tbsp peanut sauce, 1/4 cup shredded carrots
Dinner: Shrimp Tacos with Creamy Citrus Sauce	3 tacos, 1 cup shrimp, 3 small corn tortillas, 2 tbsp creamy citrus sauce	2 tacos, 3/4 cup shrimp, 2 small corn tortillas, 1.5 tbsp creamy citrus sauce	2 tacos, 1/2 cup shrimp, 2 small corn tortillas, 1 tbsp creamy citrus sauce
Snack: Strawberry Chia Yogurt Parfait	1 cup Greek yogurt, 1/2 cup strawberries, 1 tbsp chia seeds	3/4 cup Greek yogurt, 1/3 cup strawberries, 1/2 tbsp chia seeds	1/2 cup Greek yogurt, 1/4 cup strawberries, 1/2 tbsp chia seeds

Day 4

Meal	Ectomorph	Mesomorph	Endomorph
Breakfast: Avocado Toast with Jammy Eggs	2 slices whole-grain bread, 1 avocado, 2 eggs	1 slice whole-grain bread, 1/2 avocado, 1 egg	1 slice whole-grain bread, 1/2 avocado, 1 egg
Lunch: Quinoa Bowl with Roasted Eggplant and Hummus	1 cup cooked quinoa, 1 cup roasted eggplant, 2 tbsp hummus	3/4 cup cooked quinoa, 3/4 cup roasted eggplant, 1.5 tbsp hummus	1/2 cup cooked quinoa, 1/2 cup roasted eggplant, 1 tbsp hummus
Dinner: Baked Cod in Luscious Tomato Sauce	1 large cod fillet, 1 cup tomato sauce, 1 tbsp olive oil, 1/2 cup mixed vegetables	1 medium cod fillet, 3/4 cup tomato sauce, 3/4 tbsp olive oil, 1/3 cup mixed vegetables	1 small cod fillet, 1/2 cup tomato sauce, 1/2 tbsp olive oil, 1/4 cup mixed vegetables
Snack: Creamy Chocolate Protein Mousse with Cacao Powder	1 cup mousse, 2 tbsp cacao powder	3/4 cup mousse, 1.5 tbsp cacao powder	1/2 cup mousse, 1 tbsp cacao powder

Day 5

Meal	Ectomorph	Mesomorph	Endomorph
Breakfast: Bagels & Lox Protein Deluxe	1 bagel, 3 oz smoked salmon, 1 tbsp cream cheese	1/2 bagel, 2 oz smoked salmon, 1/2 tbsp cream cheese	1/2 bagel, 1 oz smoked salmon, 1/2 tbsp cream cheese
Lunch: Savory Chicken & Spinach Tortilla Wrap	1 large tortilla, 1 cup chicken, 1 cup spinach, 1 tbsp dressing	1 medium tortilla, 3/4 cup chicken, 3/4 cup spinach, 1/2 tbsp dressing	1 small tortilla, 1/2 cup chicken, 1/2 cup spinach, 1/2 tbsp dressing
Dinner: Sensational Shakshuka	2 eggs, 1 cup tomato sauce, 1/2 cup mixed vegetables	1.5 eggs, 3/4 cup tomato sauce, 1/3 cup mixed vegetables	1 egg, 1/2 cup tomato sauce, 1/4 cup mixed vegetables
Snack: Granola Breakfast Bowl	1 cup granola, 1 cup milk, 1/2 cup mixed berries	3/4 cup granola, 3/4 cup milk, 1/3 cup mixed berries	1/2 cup granola, 1/2 cup milk, 1/4 cup mixed berries

Day 6

Meal	Ectomorph	Mesomorph	Endomorph
Breakfast: Peanut Butter & Jelly Toast	2 slices whole-grain bread, 2 tbsp peanut butter, 2 tbsp jelly	1 slice whole-grain bread, 1.5 tbsp peanut butter, 1.5 tbsp jelly	1 slice whole-grain bread, 1 tbsp peanut butter, 1 tbsp jelly
Lunch: Greek Chicken Souvlaki Wraps with Tzatziki Sauce	1 large wrap, 1 cup chicken, 2 tbsp tzatziki sauce, 1 cup mixed greens	1 medium wrap, 3/4 cup chicken, 1.5 tbsp tzatziki sauce, 3/4 cup mixed greens	1 small wrap, 1/2 cup chicken, 1 tbsp tzatziki sauce, 1/2 cup mixed greens
Dinner: Mediterranean Salmon with Quinoa & Green Pea Purée	1 large salmon fillet, 1 cup quinoa, 1/2 cup green pea purée	1 medium salmon fillet, 3/4 cup quinoa, 1/3 cup green pea purée	1 small salmon fillet, 1/2 cup quinoa, 1/4 cup green pea purée
Snack: Blueberry Cobbler	1 cup cobbler	3/4 cup cobbler	1/2 cup cobbler

Day 7

Meal	Ectomorph	Mesomorph	Endomorph
Breakfast: Protein Packed Belgian Waffle	1 large waffle, 2 tbsp syrup, 1/2 cup berries	1 medium waffle, 1.5 tbsp syrup, 1/3 cup berries	1 small waffle, 1 tbsp syrup, 1/4 cup berries
Lunch: Falafel Bowl with Zesty Tahini Dressing	1 cup falafel, 1 cup mixed greens, 2 tbsp tahini dressing	3/4 cup falafel, 3/4 cup mixed greens, 1.5 tbsp tahini dressing	1/2 cup falafel, 1/2 cup mixed greens, 1 tbsp tahini dressing
Dinner: Golden Seafood and Chicken Paella	1 cup seafood and chicken, 1 cup rice, 1 cup mixed vegetables	3/4 cup seafood and chicken, 3/4 cup rice, 3/4 cup mixed vegetables	1/2 cup seafood and chicken, 1/2 cup rice, 1/2 cup mixed vegetables
Snack: Raspberry Chia Yogurt Cups	1 cup yogurt, 1/2 cup raspberries, 1 tbsp chia seeds	3/4 cup yogurt, 1/3 cup raspberries, 1/2 tbsp chia seeds	1/2 cup yogurt, 1/4 cup raspberries, 1/2 tbsp chia seeds

WEEK 2

Day 1

Meal	Ectomorph	Mesomorph	Endomorph
Breakfast: High-Protein Sweet Banana Nut Overnight Oats	1 cup oats, 1 banana, 1 cup almond milk, 2 tbsp nuts	3/4 cup oats, 1/2 banana, 3/4 cup almond milk, 1.5 tbsp nuts	1/2 cup oats, 1/2 banana, 1/2 cup almond milk, 1 tbsp nuts
Lunch: Savory Lettuce Wraps with Peanut Sauce	1 cup chicken, 4 large lettuce leaves, 2 tbsp peanut sauce, 1/2 cup shredded carrots	3/4 cup chicken, 3 large lettuce leaves, 1.5 tbsp peanut sauce, 1/3 cup shredded carrots	1/2 cup chicken, 2 large lettuce leaves, 1 tbsp peanut sauce, 1/4 cup shredded carrots
Dinner: Shrimp Tacos with Creamy Citrus Sauce	3 tacos, 1 cup shrimp, 3 small corn tortillas, 2 tbsp creamy citrus sauce	2 tacos, 3/4 cup shrimp, 2 small corn tortillas, 1.5 tbsp creamy citrus sauce	2 tacos, 1/2 cup shrimp, 2 small corn tortillas, 1 tbsp creamy citrus sauce
Snack: Strawberry Chia Yogurt Parfait	1 cup Greek yogurt, 1/2 cup strawberries, 1 tbsp chia seeds	3/4 cup Greek yogurt, 1/3 cup strawberries, 1/2 tbsp chia seeds	1/2 cup Greek yogurt, 1/4 cup strawberries, 1/2 tbsp chia seeds

Day 2

Meal	Ectomorph	Mesomorph	Endomorph
Breakfast: Avocado Toast with Jammy Eggs	2 slices whole-grain bread, 1 avocado, 2 eggs	1 slice whole-grain bread, 1/2 avocado, 1 egg	1 slice whole-grain bread, 1/2 avocado, 1 egg
Lunch: Quinoa Bowl with Roasted Eggplant and Hummus	1 cup cooked quinoa, 1 cup roasted eggplant, 2 tbsp hummus	3/4 cup cooked quinoa, 3/4 cup roasted eggplant, 1.5 tbsp hummus	1/2 cup cooked quinoa, 1/2 cup roasted eggplant, 1 tbsp hummus
Dinner: Baked Cod in Luscious Tomato Sauce	1 large cod fillet, 1 cup tomato sauce, 1 tbsp olive oil, 1/2 cup mixed vegetables	1 medium cod fillet, 3/4 cup tomato sauce, 3/4 tbsp olive oil, 1/3 cup mixed vegetables	1 small cod fillet, 1/2 cup tomato sauce, 1/2 tbsp olive oil, 1/4 cup mixed vegetables
Snack: Creamy Chocolate Protein Mousse with Cacao Powder	1 cup mousse, 2 tbsp cacao powder	3/4 cup mousse, 1.5 tbsp cacao powder	1/2 cup mousse, 1 tbsp cacao powder

Day 3

Meal	Ectomorph	Mesomorph	Endomorph
Breakfast: Bagels & Lox Protein Deluxe	1 bagel, 3 oz smoked salmon, 1 tbsp cream cheese	1/2 bagel, 2 oz smoked salmon, 1/2 tbsp cream cheese	1/2 bagel, 1 oz smoked salmon, 1/2 tbsp cream cheese
Lunch: Savory Chicken & Spinach Tortilla Wrap	1 large tortilla, 1 cup chicken, 1 cup spinach, 1 tbsp dressing	1 medium tortilla, 3/4 cup chicken, 3/4 cup spinach, 1/2 tbsp dressing	1 small tortilla, 1/2 cup chicken, 1/2 cup spinach, 1/2 tbsp dressing
Dinner: Beef Stir Fry with Brown Rice and Bell Peppers	1 cup beef, 1 cup brown rice, 1 cup bell peppers	3/4 cup beef, 3/4 cup brown rice, 3/4 cup bell peppers	1/2 cup beef, 1/2 cup brown rice, 1/2 cup bell peppers
Snack: Granola Breakfast Bowl	1 cup granola, 1 cup milk, 1/2 cup mixed berries	3/4 cup granola, 3/4 cup milk, 1/3 cup mixed berries	1/2 cup granola, 1/2 cup milk, 1/4 cup mixed berries

Day 4

Meal	Ectomorph	Mesomorph	Endomorph
1/2 bagel, 1 oz smoked salmon, 1/2 tbsp cream cheese	2 slices whole-grain bread, 2 tbsp peanut butter, 2 tbsp jelly	1 slice whole-grain bread, 1.5 tbsp peanut butter, 1.5 tbsp jelly	1 slice whole-grain bread, 1 tbsp peanut butter, 1 tbsp jelly
1 small tortilla, 1/2 cup chicken, 1/2 cup spinach, 1/2 tbsp dressing	1 large wrap, 1 cup chicken, 2 tbsp tzatziki sauce, 1 cup mixed greens	1 medium wrap, 3/4 cup chicken, 1.5 tbsp tzatziki sauce, 3/4 cup mixed greens	1 small wrap, 1/2 cup chicken, 1 tbsp tzatziki sauce, 1/2 cup mixed greens
1/2 cup beef, 1/2 cup brown rice, 1/2 cup bell peppers	2 eggs, 1 cup tomato sauce, 1/2 cup mixed vegetables	1.5 eggs, 3/4 cup tomato sauce, 1/3 cup mixed vegetables	1 egg, 1/2 cup tomato sauce, 1/4 cup mixed vegetables
1/2 cup granola, 1/2 cup milk, 1/4 cup mixed berries	1 cup blueberries, 1/2 cup oats, 2 tbsp honey	3/4 cup blueberries, 1/3 cup oats, 1.5 tbsp honey	1/2 cup blueberries, 1/4 cup oats, 1 tbsp honey

Day 5

Meal	Ectomorph	Mesomorph	Endomorph
Breakfast: High-Protein Sweet Banana Nut Overnight Oats	1 cup oats, 1 banana, 1 cup almond milk, 2 tbsp nuts	3/4 cup oats, 1/2 banana, 3/4 cup almond milk, 1.5 tbsp nuts	1/2 cup oats, 1/2 banana, 1/2 cup almond milk, 1 tbsp nuts
Lunch: Quinoa Bowl with Roasted Eggplant and Hummus	1 cup cooked quinoa, 1 cup roasted eggplant, 2 tbsp hummus	3/4 cup cooked quinoa, 3/4 cup roasted eggplant, 1.5 tbsp hummus	1/2 cup cooked quinoa, 1/2 cup roasted eggplant, 1 tbsp hummus
Dinner: Grilled Salmon with Lemon Dill Sauce and Sautéed Asparagus	1 large salmon fillet, 1 tbsp lemon dill sauce, 1 cup sautéed asparagus	1 medium salmon fillet, 3/4 tbsp lemon dill sauce, 3/4 cup sautéed asparagus	1 small salmon fillet, 1/2 tbsp lemon dill sauce, 1/2 cup sautéed asparagus
Snack: Dark Chocolate Cacao Cookies	2 cookies	1.5 cookies	1 cookie

Day 6

Meal	Ectomorph	Mesomorph	Endomorph
Breakfast: Avocado Toast with Jammy Eggs	2 slices whole-grain bread, 1 avocado, 2 eggs	1 slice whole-grain bread, 1/2 avocado, 1 egg	1 slice whole-grain bread, 1/2 avocado, 1 egg
Lunch: Savory Lettuce Wraps with Peanut Sauce	1 cup chicken, 4 large lettuce leaves, 2 tbsp peanut sauce, 1/2 cup shredded carrots	3/4 cup chicken, 3 large lettuce leaves, 1.5 tbsp peanut sauce, 1/3 cup shredded carrots	1/2 cup chicken, 2 large lettuce leaves, 1 tbsp peanut sauce, 1/4 cup shredded carrots
Dinner: Baked Cod in Luscious Tomato Sauce	1 large cod fillet, 1 cup tomato sauce, 1 tbsp olive oil, 1/2 cup mixed vegetables	1 medium cod fillet, 3/4 cup tomato sauce, 3/4 tbsp olive oil, 1/3 cup mixed vegetables	1 small cod fillet, 1/2 cup tomato sauce, 1/2 tbsp olive oil, 1/4 cup mixed vegetables
Snack: Strawberry Chia Yogurt Parfait	1 cup Greek yogurt, 1/2 cup strawberries, 1 tbsp chia seeds	3/4 cup Greek yogurt, 1/3 cup strawberries, 1/2 tbsp chia seeds	1/2 cup Greek yogurt, 1/4 cup strawberries, 1/2 tbsp chia seeds

Day 7

Meal	Ectomorph	Mesomorph	Endomorph
Breakfast: High-Protein Sweet Banana Nut Overnight Oats	1 cup oats, 1 banana, 1 cup almond milk, 2 tbsp nuts	3/4 cup oats, 1/2 banana, 3/4 cup almond milk, 1.5 tbsp nuts	1/2 cup oats, 1/2 banana, 1/2 cup almond milk, 1 tbsp nuts
Lunch: Quinoa Bowl with Roasted Eggplant and Hummus	1 cup cooked quinoa, 1 cup roasted eggplant, 2 tbsp hummus	3/4 cup cooked quinoa, 3/4 cup roasted eggplant, 1.5 tbsp hummus	1/2 cup cooked quinoa, 1/2 cup roasted eggplant, 1 tbsp hummus
Dinner: Grilled Salmon with Lemon Dill Sauce and Sautéed Asparagus	1 large salmon fillet, 1 tbsp lemon dill sauce, 1 cup sautéed asparagus	1 medium salmon fillet, 3/4 tbsp lemon dill sauce, 3/4 cup sautéed asparagus	1 small salmon fillet, 1/2 tbsp lemon dill sauce, 1/2 cup sautéed asparagus
Snack: Dark Chocolate Cacao Cookies	2 cookies	1.5 cookies	1 cookie

WEEK 3

Day 1

Meal	Ectomorph	Mesomorph	Endomorph
Breakfast: Bagels & Lox Protein Deluxe	1 bagel, 3 oz smoked salmon, 1 tbsp cream cheese	1/2 bagel, 2 oz smoked salmon, 1/2 tbsp cream cheese	1/2 bagel, 1 oz smoked salmon, 1/2 tbsp cream cheese
Lunch: Mediterranean Orzo Pasta Salad	1 cup orzo, 1/2 cup cherry tomatoes, 1/4 cup olives, 1/4 cup feta	3/4 cup orzo, 1/3 cup cherry tomatoes, 3 tbsp olives, 3 tbsp feta	1/2 cup orzo, 1/4 cup cherry tomatoes, 2 tbsp olives, 2 tbsp feta
Dinner: Shrimp Tacos with Creamy Citrus Sauce	3 tacos, 1 cup shrimp, 3 small corn tortillas, 2 tbsp creamy citrus sauce	2 tacos, 3/4 cup shrimp, 2 small corn tortillas, 1.5 tbsp creamy citrus sauce	2 tacos, 1/2 cup shrimp, 2 small corn tortillas, 1 tbsp creamy citrus sauce
Snack: Blueberry Cobbler	1 cup blueberries, 1/2 cup oats, 2 tbsp honey	3/4 cup blueberries, 1/3 cup oats, 1.5 tbsp honey	1/2 cup blueberries, 1/4 cup oats, 1 tbsp honey

Day 2

Meal	Ectomorph	Mesomorph	Endomorph
Breakfast: High-Protein Sweet Banana Nut Overnight Oats	1 cup oats, 1 banana, 1 cup almond milk, 2 tbsp nuts	3/4 cup oats, 1/2 banana, 3/4 cup almond milk, 1.5 tbsp nuts	1/2 cup oats, 1/2 banana, 1/2 cup almond milk, 1 tbsp nuts
Lunch: Greek Chicken Souvlaki Wraps with Tzatziki Sauce	1 large wrap, 1 cup chicken, 2 tbsp tzatziki sauce, 1 cup mixed greens	1 medium wrap, 3/4 cup chicken, 1.5 tbsp tzatziki sauce, 3/4 cup mixed greens	1 small wrap, 1/2 cup chicken, 1 tbsp tzatziki sauce, 1/2 cup mixed greens
Dinner: Baked Cod in Luscious Tomato Sauce	1 large cod fillet, 1 cup tomato sauce, 1 tbsp olive oil, 1/2 cup mixed vegetables	1 medium cod fillet, 3/4 cup tomato sauce, 3/4 tbsp olive oil, 1/3 cup mixed vegetables	1 small cod fillet, 1/2 cup tomato sauce, 1/2 tbsp olive oil, 1/4 cup mixed vegetables
Snack: Strawberry Chia Yogurt Parfait	1 cup Greek yogurt, 1/2 cup strawberries, 1 tbsp chia seeds	3/4 cup Greek yogurt, 1/3 cup strawberries, 1/2 tbsp chia seeds	1/2 cup Greek yogurt, 1/4 cup strawberries, 1/2 tbsp chia seeds

Day 3

Meal	Ectomorph	Mesomorph	Endomorph
Breakfast: Peanut Butter & Jelly Toast	2 slices whole-grain bread, 2 tbsp peanut butter, 2 tbsp jelly	1 slice whole-grain bread, 1.5 tbsp peanut butter, 1.5 tbsp jelly	1 slice whole-grain bread, 1 tbsp peanut butter, 1 tbsp jelly
Lunch: Quinoa Bowl with Roasted Eggplant and Hummus	1 cup cooked quinoa, 1 cup roasted eggplant, 2 tbsp hummus	3/4 cup cooked quinoa, 3/4 cup roasted eggplant, 1.5 tbsp hummus	1/2 cup cooked quinoa, 1/2 cup roasted eggplant, 1 tbsp hummus
Dinner: Sensational Shakshuka	2 eggs, 1 cup tomato sauce, 1/2 cup mixed vegetables	1.5 eggs, 3/4 cup tomato sauce, 1/3 cup mixed vegetables	1 egg, 1/2 cup tomato sauce, 1/4 cup mixed vegetables
Snack: Granola Breakfast Bowl	1 cup granola, 1 cup milk, 1/2 cup mixed berries	3/4 cup granola, 3/4 cup milk, 1/3 cup mixed berries	1/2 cup granola, 1/2 cup milk, 1/4 cup mixed berries

Day 4

Meal	Ectomorph	Mesomorph	Endomorph
Breakfast: Avocado Toast with Jammy Eggs	2 slices whole-grain bread, 1 avocado, 2 eggs	1 slice whole-grain bread, 1/2 avocado, 1 egg	1 slice whole-grain bread, 1/2 avocado, 1 egg
Lunch: Mediterranean Orzo Pasta Salad	1 cup orzo, 1/2 cup cherry tomatoes, 1/4 cup olives, 1/4 cup feta	3/4 cup orzo, 1/3 cup cherry tomatoes, 3 tbsp olives, 3 tbsp feta	1/2 cup orzo, 1/4 cup cherry tomatoes, 2 tbsp olives, 2 tbsp feta
Dinner: Shrimp Tacos with Creamy Citrus Sauce	3 tacos, 1 cup shrimp, 3 small corn tortillas, 2 tbsp creamy citrus sauce	2 tacos, 3/4 cup shrimp, 2 small corn tortillas, 1.5 tbsp creamy citrus sauce	2 tacos, 1/2 cup shrimp, 2 small corn tortillas, 1 tbsp creamy citrus sauce
Snack: Blueberry Cobbler	1 cup blueberries, 1/2 cup oats, 2 tbsp honey	3/4 cup blueberries, 1/3 cup oats, 1.5 tbsp honey	1/2 cup blueberries, 1/4 cup oats, 1 tbsp honey

Day 5

Meal	Ectomorph	Mesomorph	Endomorph
Breakfast: High-Protein Sweet Banana Nut Overnight Oats	1 cup oats, 1 banana, 1 cup almond milk, 2 tbsp nuts	3/4 cup oats, 1/2 banana, 3/4 cup almond milk, 1.5 tbsp nuts	1/2 cup oats, 1/2 banana, 1/2 cup almond milk, 1 tbsp nuts
Lunch: Greek Chicken Souvlaki Wraps with Tzatziki Sauce	1 large wrap, 1 cup chicken, 2 tbsp tzatziki sauce, 1 cup mixed greens	1 medium wrap, 3/4 cup chicken, 1.5 tbsp tzatziki sauce, 3/4 cup mixed greens	1 small wrap, 1/2 cup chicken, 1 tbsp tzatziki sauce, 1/2 cup mixed greens
Dinner: Baked Cod in Luscious Tomato Sauce	1 large cod fillet, 1 cup tomato sauce, 1 tbsp olive oil, 1/2 cup mixed vegetables	1 medium cod fillet, 3/4 cup tomato sauce, 3/4 tbsp olive oil, 1/3 cup mixed vegetables	1 small cod fillet, 1/2 cup tomato sauce, 1/2 tbsp olive oil, 1/4 cup mixed vegetables
Snack: Strawberry Chia Yogurt Parfait	1 cup Greek yogurt, 1/2 cup strawberries, 1 tbsp chia seeds	3/4 cup Greek yogurt, 1/3 cup strawberries, 1/2 tbsp chia seeds	1/2 cup Greek yogurt, 1/4 cup strawberries, 1/2 tbsp chia seeds

Day 6

Meal	Ectomorph	Mesomorph	Endomorph
Breakfast: Peanut Butter & Jelly Toast	2 slices whole-grain bread, 2 tbsp peanut butter, 2 tbsp jelly	1 slice whole-grain bread, 1.5 tbsp peanut butter, 1.5 tbsp jelly	1 slice whole-grain bread, 1 tbsp peanut butter, 1 tbsp jelly
Lunch: Savory Lettuce Wraps with Peanut Sauce	1 cup chicken, 4 large lettuce leaves, 2 tbsp peanut sauce, 1/2 cup shredded carrots	3/4 cup chicken, 3 large lettuce leaves, 1.5 tbsp peanut sauce, 1/3 cup shredded carrots	1/2 cup chicken, 2 large lettuce leaves, 1 tbsp peanut sauce, 1/4 cup shredded carrots
Dinner: Sweet and Spicy Crispy Pork Stir Fry with Rice Noodles	1 cup pork, 1 cup rice noodles, 1 cup mixed vegetables, 2 tbsp sweet and spicy sauce	3/4 cup pork, 3/4 cup rice noodles, 3/4 cup mixed vegetables, 1.5 tbsp sweet and spicy sauce	1/2 cup pork, 1/2 cup rice noodles, 1/2 cup mixed vegetables, 1 tbsp sweet and spicy sauce
Snack: Dark Chocolate Cacao Cookies	2 cookies	1.5 cookies	1 cookie

Day 7

Meal	Ectomorph	Mesomorph	Endomorph
Breakfast: Bagels & Lox Protein Deluxe	1 bagel, 3 oz smoked salmon, 1 tbsp cream cheese	1/2 bagel, 2 oz smoked salmon, 1/2 tbsp cream cheese	1/2 bagel, 1 oz smoked salmon, 1/2 tbsp cream cheese
Lunch: Mediterranean Orzo Pasta Salad	1 cup orzo, 1/2 cup cherry tomatoes, 1/4 cup olives, 1/4 cup feta	3/4 cup orzo, 1/3 cup cherry tomatoes, 3 tbsp olives, 3 tbsp feta	1/2 cup orzo, 1/4 cup cherry tomatoes, 2 tbsp olives, 2 tbsp feta
Dinner: Grilled Salmon with Lemon Dill Sauce and Sautéed Asparagus	1 large salmon fillet, 1 tbsp lemon dill sauce, 1 cup sautéed asparagus	1 medium salmon fillet, 3/4 tbsp lemon dill sauce, 3/4 cup sautéed asparagus	1 small salmon fillet, 1/2 tbsp lemon dill sauce, 1/2 cup sautéed asparagus
Snack: Granola Breakfast Bowl	1 cup granola, 1 cup milk, 1/2 cup mixed berries	3/4 cup granola, 3/4 cup milk, 1/3 cup mixed berries	1/2 cup granola, 1/2 cup milk, 1/4 cup mixed berries

WEEK 4

Day 1

Meal	Ectomorph	Mesomorph	Endomorph
Breakfast: Protein Packed Belgian Waffle	2 waffles, 1/2 cup berries, 2 tbsp syrup	1.5 waffles, 1/3 cup berries, 1.5 tbsp syrup	1 waffle, 1/4 cup berries, 1 tbsp syrup
Lunch: Falafel Bowl with Zesty Tahini Dressing	1 cup falafel, 1 cup mixed greens, 2 tbsp tahini dressing	3/4 cup falafel, 3/4 cup mixed greens, 1.5 tbsp tahini dressing	1/2 cup falafel, 1/2 cup mixed greens, 1 tbsp tahini dressing
Dinner: Mediterranean Salmon with Quinoa & Green Pea Purée	1 large salmon fillet, 1 cup quinoa, 1 cup green pea purée	1 medium salmon fillet, 3/4 cup quinoa, 3/4 cup green pea purée	1 small salmon fillet, 1/2 cup quinoa, 1/2 cup green pea purée
Snack: Protein-Rich Dreamy Hot Chocolate	1 cup milk, 1 tbsp cocoa powder, 1 tbsp protein powder	3/4 cup milk, 3/4 tbsp cocoa powder, 3/4 tbsp protein powder	1/2 cup milk, 1/2 tbsp cocoa powder, 1/2 tbsp protein powder

Day 2

Meal	Ectomorph	Mesomorph	Endomorph
Breakfast: Breakfast Tacos with Chorizo, Eggs, and Salsa	2 tacos, 2 eggs, 1/2 cup chorizo, 1/4 cup salsa	1.5 tacos, 1.5 eggs, 1/3 cup chorizo, 3 tbsp salsa	1 taco, 1 egg, 1/4 cup chorizo, 2 tbsp salsa
Lunch: Hearty Cinnamon Spiced Sweet Potato Hash	1 large sweet potato, 1 cup mixed vegetables, 2 tbsp cinnamon	3/4 large sweet potato, 3/4 cup mixed vegetables, 1.5 tbsp cinnamon	1/2 large sweet potato, 1/2 cup mixed vegetables, 1 tbsp cinnamon
Dinner: Golden Seafood and Chicken Paella	1 cup seafood, 1 cup chicken, 1 cup rice, 1/2 cup mixed vegetables	3/4 cup seafood, 3/4 cup chicken, 3/4 cup rice, 1/3 cup mixed vegetables	1/2 cup seafood, 1/2 cup chicken, 1/2 cup rice, 1/4 cup mixed vegetables
Snack: Raspberry Chia Yogurt Cups	1 cup Greek yogurt, 1/2 cup raspberries, 1 tbsp chia seeds	3/4 cup Greek yogurt, 1/3 cup raspberries, 1/2 tbsp chia seeds	1/2 cup Greek yogurt, 1/4 cup raspberries, 1/2 tbsp chia seeds

Day 3

Meal	Ectomorph	Mesomorph	Endomorph
Breakfast: Blueberry Bliss Protein Smoothie	1 cup blueberries, 1 cup milk, 1 banana, 2 tbsp protein powder	3/4 cup blueberries, 3/4 cup milk, 1/2 banana, 1.5 tbsp protein powder	1/2 cup blueberries, 1/2 cup milk, 1/2 banana, 1 tbsp protein powder
Lunch: Mediterranean Orzo Pasta Salad	1 cup orzo, 1/2 cup cherry tomatoes, 1/4 cup olives, 1/4 cup feta	3/4 cup orzo, 1/3 cup cherry tomatoes, 3 tbsp olives, 3 tbsp feta	1/2 cup orzo, 1/4 cup cherry tomatoes, 2 tbsp olives, 2 tbsp feta
Dinner: Shrimp Tacos with Creamy Citrus Sauce	3 tacos, 1 cup shrimp, 3 small corn tortillas, 2 tbsp creamy citrus sauce	2 tacos, 3/4 cup shrimp, 2 small corn tortillas, 1.5 tbsp creamy citrus sauce	2 tacos, 1/2 cup shrimp, 2 small corn tortillas, 1 tbsp creamy citrus sauce
Snack: Dark Chocolate Cacao Cookies	2 cookies	1.5 cookies	1 cookie

Day 4

Meal	Ectomorph	Mesomorph	Endomorph
Breakfast: Peanut Butter & Jelly Toast	2 slices whole-grain bread, 2 tbsp peanut butter, 2 tbsp jelly	1 slice whole-grain bread, 1.5 tbsp peanut butter, 1.5 tbsp jelly	1 slice whole-grain bread, 1 tbsp peanut butter, 1 tbsp jelly
Lunch: Greek Chicken Souvlaki Wraps with Tzatziki Sauce	1 large wrap, 1 cup chicken, 2 tbsp tzatziki sauce, 1 cup mixed greens	1 medium wrap, 3/4 cup chicken, 1.5 tbsp tzatziki sauce, 3/4 cup mixed greens	1 small wrap, 1/2 cup chicken, 1 tbsp tzatziki sauce, 1/2 cup mixed greens
Dinner: Baked Cod in Luscious Tomato Sauce	1 large cod fillet, 1 cup tomato sauce, 1 tbsp olive oil, 1/2 cup mixed vegetables	1 medium cod fillet, 3/4 cup tomato sauce, 3/4 tbsp olive oil, 1/3 cup mixed vegetables	1 small cod fillet, 1/2 cup tomato sauce, 1/2 tbsp olive oil, 1/4 cup mixed vegetables
Snack: Strawberry Chia Yogurt Parfait	1 cup Greek yogurt, 1/2 cup strawberries, 1 tbsp chia seeds	3/4 cup Greek yogurt, 1/3 cup strawberries, 1/2 tbsp chia seeds	1/2 cup Greek yogurt, 1/4 cup strawberries, 1/2 tbsp chia seeds

Day 5

Meal	Ectomorph	Mesomorph	Endomorph
Breakfast: Bagels & Lox Protein Deluxe	1 bagel, 3 oz smoked salmon, 1 tbsp cream cheese	1/2 bagel, 2 oz smoked salmon, 1/2 tbsp cream cheese	1/2 bagel, 1 oz smoked salmon, 1/2 tbsp cream cheese
Lunch: Savory Lettuce Wraps with Peanut Sauce	1 cup chicken, 4 large lettuce leaves, 2 tbsp peanut sauce, 1/2 cup shredded carrots	3/4 cup chicken, 3 large lettuce leaves, 1.5 tbsp peanut sauce, 1/3 cup shredded carrots	1/2 cup chicken, 2 large lettuce leaves, 1 tbsp peanut sauce, 1/4 cup shredded carrots
Dinner: Sweet and Spicy Crispy Pork Stir Fry with Rice Noodles	1 cup pork, 1 cup rice noodles, 1 cup mixed vegetables, 2 tbsp sweet and spicy sauce	3/4 cup pork, 3/4 cup rice noodles, 3/4 cup mixed vegetables, 1.5 tbsp sweet and spicy sauce	1/2 cup pork, 1/2 cup rice noodles, 1/2 cup mixed vegetables, 1 tbsp sweet and spicy sauce
Snack: Blueberry Cobbler	1 cup blueberries, 1/2 cup oats, 2 tbsp honey	3/4 cup blueberries, 1/3 cup oats, 1.5 tbsp honey	1/2 cup blueberries, 1/4 cup oats, 1 tbsp honey

Day 6

Meal	Ectomorph	Mesomorph	Endomorph
Breakfast: Avocado Toast with Jammy Eggs	2 slices whole-grain bread, 1 avocado, 2 eggs	1 slice whole-grain bread, 1/2 avocado, 1 egg	1 slice whole-grain bread, 1/2 avocado, 1 egg
Lunch: Quinoa Bowl with Roasted Eggplant and Hummus	1 cup cooked quinoa, 1 cup roasted eggplant, 2 tbsp hummus	3/4 cup cooked quinoa, 3/4 cup roasted eggplant, 1.5 tbsp hummus	1/2 cup cooked quinoa, 1/2 cup roasted eggplant, 1 tbsp hummus
Dinner: Golden Seafood and Chicken Paella	1 cup seafood, 1 cup chicken, 1 cup rice, 1/2 cup mixed vegetables	3/4 cup seafood, 3/4 cup chicken, 3/4 cup rice, 1/3 cup mixed vegetables	1/2 cup seafood, 1/2 cup chicken, 1/2 cup rice, 1/4 cup mixed vegetables
Snack: Dark Chocolate Cacao Cookies	2 cookies	1.5 cookies	1 cookie

Day 7

Meal	Ectomorph	Mesomorph	Endomorph
Breakfast: Blueberry Bliss Protein Smoothie	1 cup blueberries, 1 cup milk, 1 banana, 2 tbsp protein powder	3/4 cup blueberries, 3/4 cup milk, 1/2 banana, 1.5 tbsp protein powder	1/2 cup blueberries, 1/2 cup milk, 1/2 banana, 1 tbsp protein powder
Lunch: Greek Chicken Souvlaki Wraps with Tzatziki Sauce	1 large wrap, 1 cup chicken, 2 tbsp tzatziki sauce, 1 cup mixed greens	1 medium wrap, 3/4 cup chicken, 1.5 tbsp tzatziki sauce, 3/4 cup mixed greens	1 small wrap, 1/2 cup chicken, 1 tbsp tzatziki sauce, 1/2 cup mixed greens
Dinner: Grilled Salmon with Lemon Dill Sauce and Sautéed Asparagus	1 large salmon fillet, 1 tbsp lemon dill sauce, 1 cup sautéed asparagus	1 medium salmon fillet, 3/4 tbsp lemon dill sauce, 3/4 cup sautéed asparagus	1 small salmon fillet, 1/2 tbsp lemon dill sauce, 1/2 cup sautéed asparagus
Snack: Granola Breakfast Bowl	1 cup granola, 1 cup milk, 1/2 cup mixed berries	3/4 cup granola, 3/4 cup milk, 1/3 cup mixed berries	1/2 cup granola, 1/2 cup milk, 1/4 cup mixed berries

"Wellness Insights: *Did You Know?*"

» ***Did you know...*** that after the age of 40, the risk of insulin resistance increases due to changes in metabolism, hormonal shifts, and potential decreases in physical activity? Maintaining a balanced diet with whole grains, lean proteins, and plenty of vegetables can help manage blood sugar levels and reduce the risk of insulin resistance.

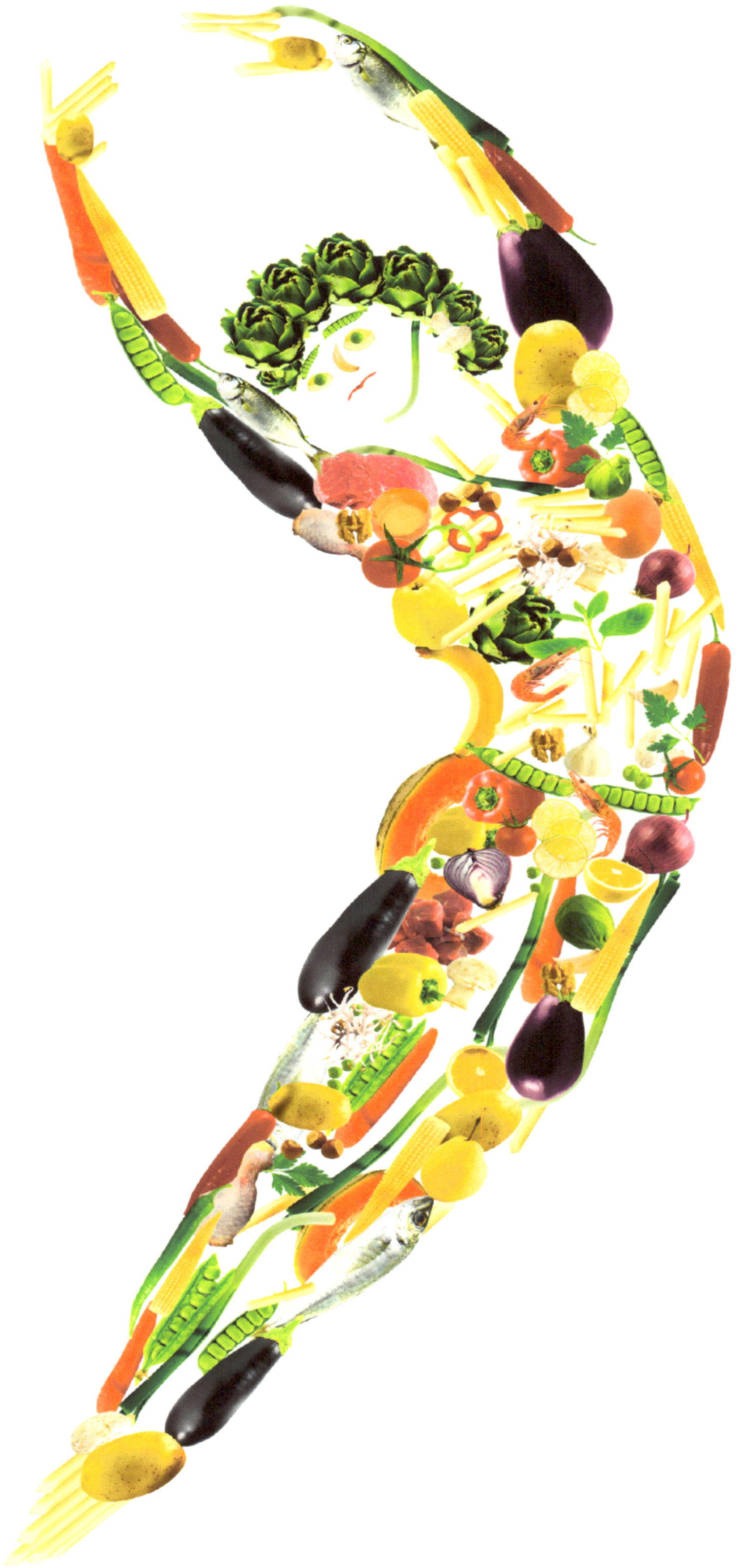

SECTION 7

MINDFUL Eating Practices

Engaging deeply with the experience of eating can transform your relationship with food. This section of "The Evolutionary Plate: From Taste to Transformation" delves into the art of mindful eating, offering insights and techniques to help you savor your meals and make more thoughtful dietary choices.

Mindful eating encourages you to be present and fully immersed in the act of eating. It involves appreciating the sensory experiences—flavors, textures, aromas—and tuning into your body's signals of hunger and fullness. By adopting mindful eating practices, you can improve digestion, manage portions more effectively, and find greater enjoyment in your meals.

In the following subsections, you'll find practical techniques to incorporate mindful eating into your daily routine, tips for developing a positive relationship with food, and an exploration of the numerous benefits that mindful eating can bring to your overall wellness. Embrace this approach to create a more balanced and fulfilling eating experience.

TECHNIQUES FOR PRACTICING Mindful Eating

Mindful eating is about fully engaging with the experience of eating and drinking, paying close attention to the sensations, thoughts, and feelings associated with each meal. It helps you develop a healthier relationship with food, enhances your enjoyment of meals, and supports better nutrition choices. Here are some techniques to help you practice mindful eating:

Eat Without Distractions: It's common to eat while multitasking. To practice mindful eating, make a conscious effort to turn off the TV, put away your phone, and focus solely on your meal. Creating a calm, distraction-free environment allows you to be present and fully appreciate the food in front of you.

Savor Your Food: Take time to truly enjoy your meals by appreciating the colors, textures, and aromas of your food. Chew slowly and thoroughly, paying attention to the flavors and sensations with each bite. This not only enhances your dining experience but also aids digestion.

Listen to Your Body: One of the key aspects of mindful eating is tuning into your body's hunger and fullness cues. Eat when you're hungry and stop when you're satisfied, avoiding the temptation to overeat. By listening to your body, you can better regulate your intake and maintain a healthy relationship with food.

Reflect on Your Food Choices: Consider the nutritional value of the foods you choose and how they make you feel. Opt for meals that nourish both your body and mind. This reflection helps you make informed choices that support your overall well-being.

Practice Gratitude: Take a moment before eating to express gratitude for your food and the effort that went into preparing it. Acknowledge the sources of your food, such as the farmers who grew it and the natural resources that made it possible. This practice fosters a deeper appreciation for your meals.

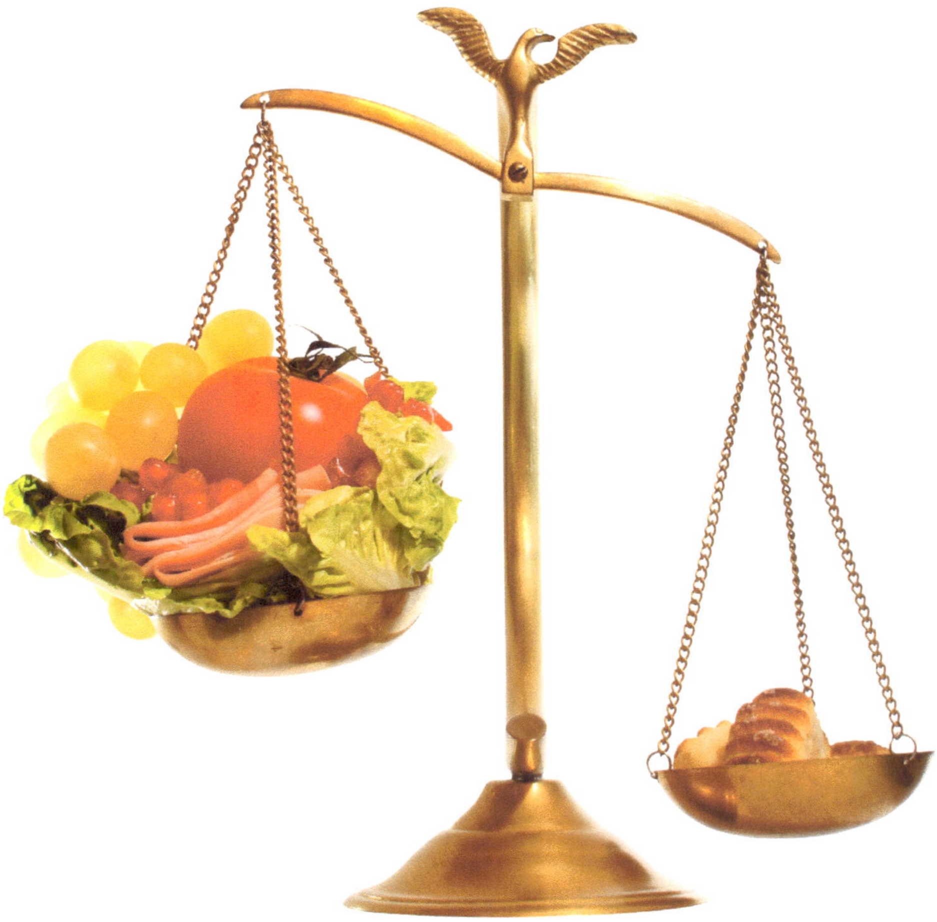

"Wellness Insights: *Did You Know?*"

- **_Did you know..._** that practicing mindful eating can create a new habit to help you reduce overeating and improve your relationship with food?
- **_Did you know..._** that listening to your body's hunger and fullness cues can help you improve digestion and maintain a healthy weight, allowing you to focus on how you feel rather than counting calories or weighing yourself frequently?

TIPS FOR ENHANCING YOUR Relationship with Food

Creating a healthy relationship with food is key to your well-being. It means enjoying your meals, making thoughtful choices, and understanding the role of food in your life. Here are some tips to help you enhance your connection with what you eat:

Embrace Food Freedom:

- Allow yourself to enjoy all types of food without guilt.
- Focus on balance and moderation instead of labeling foods as "good" or "bad."
- This approach reduces stress and promotes a healthier mindset towards eating.

Honor Your Cravings:

- Listen to your body's cravings and find healthy ways to satisfy them.
- Indulge mindfully and appreciate every bite.
- Prevent feelings of deprivation and maintain a balanced diet.

Respect Your Body's Needs:

- Appreciate your body's signals and needs.
- Nourish it with foods that make you feel good and provide energy.
- Encourages a positive self-image and healthy eating habits.

Celebrate Cooking and Eating:

- Find joy in cooking and experimenting with new recipes.
- Share meals with loved ones to enhance the eating experience.
- Transform mealtimes into enjoyable and fulfilling moments.

Empower Yourself with Knowledge:

- Learn about nutrition and how different foods impact your health.
- Make informed food choices and understand the benefits of various nutrients.
- Supports a more mindful approach to eating.

BENEFITS OF MINDFUL EATING
On Overall Wellness

Mindful eating brings a wide range of benefits that go beyond just physical health, enhancing your mental and emotional well-being as well. By being present and attentive during meals, you can transform your eating habits and improve your overall quality of life. Here are some key benefits of mindful eating:

Improved Digestion
Eating slowly and chewing thoroughly aids digestion and enhances nutrient absorption. When you take your time with meals, your body can process food more efficiently, reducing digestive issues.

Better Portion Control
Listening to your hunger and fullness cues helps prevent overeating and maintains healthy portion sizes. This natural sense of portion control supports weight management and overall health.

Enhanced Enjoyment
Focusing on the sensory experience of eating increases your enjoyment of meals. By paying attention to the flavors, textures, and aromas, you can fully appreciate each bite and derive more satisfaction from your food.

Reduced Stress
Mindful eating can alleviate stress and anxiety related to food and eating habits. Creating a calm and focused eating environment helps ease mealtime pressures and fosters a more relaxed approach to food.

Healthier Relationship with Food
Developing a mindful approach to eating helps reduce emotional eating and food-related guilt. This healthier relationship supports overall well-being and encourages nutritious eating habits.

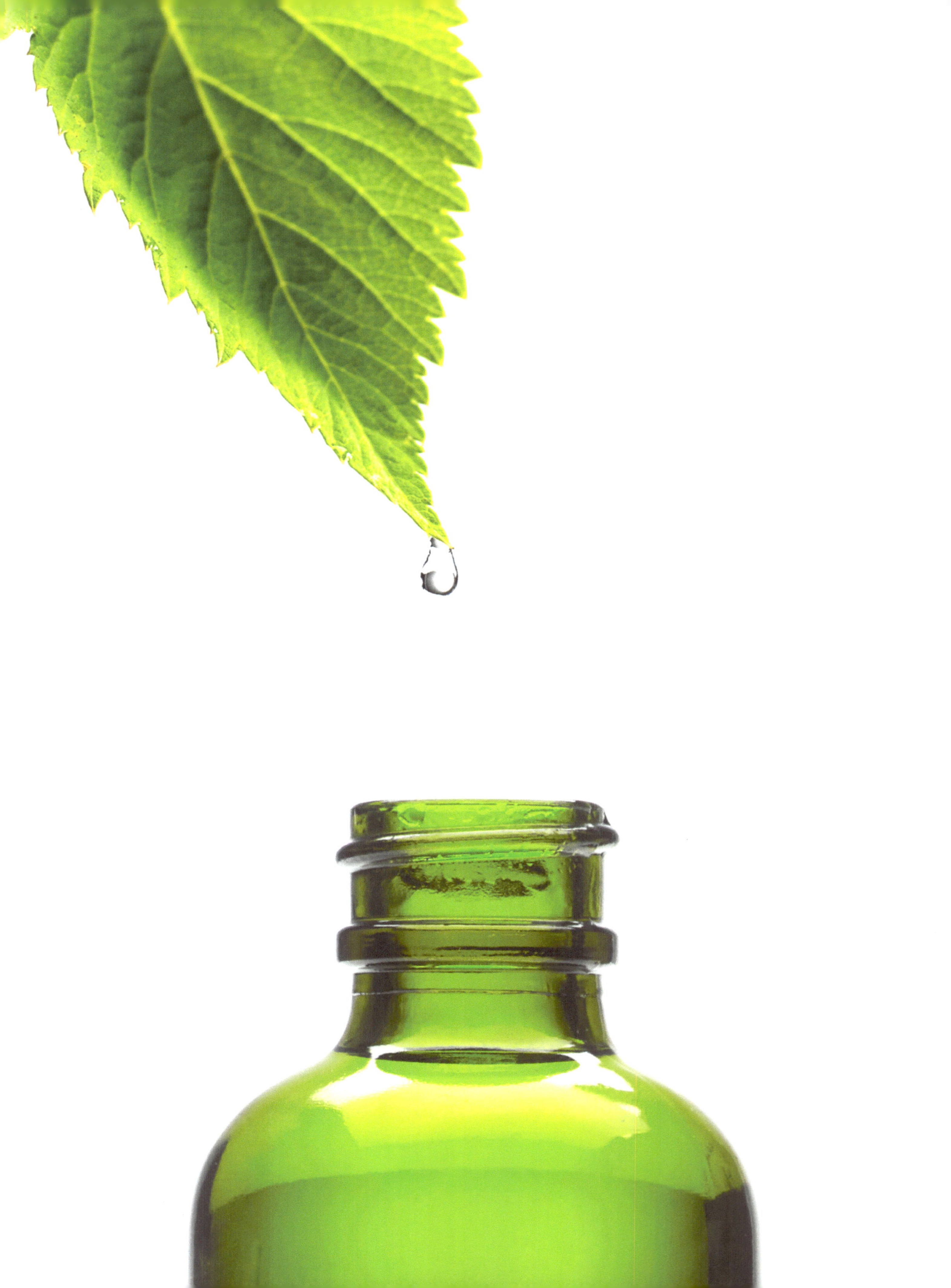

SECTION 8

DETOXIFICATION

Detoxification is about supporting your body's innate ability to cleanse and heal itself. When addressing issues like Candida overgrowth and parasite infections, it's important to focus on natural methods that enhance the functioning of your liver, kidneys, and other organs, helping to eliminate harmful toxins and restore balance. Candida, a type of yeast, can proliferate in the body, leading to a range of health issues such as digestive problems, fatigue, skin issues, and weakened immunity. Similarly, parasites can cause a host of health problems, often exacerbating existing conditions. Stress plays a significant role in both Candida overgrowth and parasite infections, as elevated cortisol levels can compromise immune function and create an environment where these pathogens can thrive.

As you undergo detoxification, you might experience what's known as a Herxheimer reaction (Herx reaction), which occurs when toxins are released faster than the body can eliminate them. Symptoms may include headaches, fatigue, joint or muscle pain, and flu-like symptoms. These are temporary and typically a sign that your body is effectively eliminating toxins.

By following a structured detoxification protocol, you can help your body combat these issues, reduce stress, and support overall well-being. It's important to consult with a healthcare provider before beginning any detox program, especially if you have existing health conditions or are taking medication. This section explores the processes and benefits of detoxifying from parasites, Candida, supporting liver and kidney health, and removing heavy metals from your body. Embrace these practices to maintain a vibrant and balanced state of well-being.

Lab Testing and Analysis:
For comprehensive functional lab testing for your whole body and overall health, you can visit:

1. Everlywell
2. Genova Diagnostics.

These platforms offer a range of tests to help you understand various aspects of your health and wellness.

Detoxification and Protocols:
For more detailed guidance and personalized advice on detoxification and managing parasites, consider consulting the following resource:

Dr. Clark Store | The Leader in Pure Vitamins and Supplements (drclarkstore.com)

This resource offers comprehensive support for body cleanses and detox protocols.

DETOXIFICATION AND Parasites

Detoxification is not a commonly understood concept, especially when it involves parasites. Natural detoxification supports the liver and kidneys through a healthy diet, staying hydrated, and reducing exposure to toxins, including parasites. Removing potential sources of parasites from your environment and diet is essential to support your body's natural detox processes and maintain overall health.

UNDERSTANDING PARASITES

Parasites are organisms that live in or on another organism (the host) and benefit at the host's expense. Many people think parasites are only a problem in third-world countries, but this is not the case. In reality, parasites can affect anyone, regardless of where they live. They are not just a result of poor hygiene or living conditions; they can be contracted through various means, including:

- **Contaminated Water and Food:** Consuming unfiltered water or undercooked meat can introduce parasites.
- **Travel:** Visiting regions where parasites are more common can increase exposure.
- **Pets:** Animals can carry parasites that transfer to humans.
- **Personal Contact:** Some parasites spread through physical contact or sharing items like towels.

Common symptoms of parasitic infections include digestive issues, fatigue, and unexplained weight changes. Maintaining a clean environment and being mindful of what you consume can help prevent parasitic infections.

HOW TO DETOX FROM PARASITES

Detoxification from parasites can be significantly supported by understanding the right foods, herbs, and nutrients. Nature has provided us with many holistic remedies to help our bodies in this process:

1. **Dietary Adjustments (Follow for at least 4-6 weeks):**
    - Garlic and Onions: Known for their anti-parasitic properties.
    - Pumpkin Seeds: Effective against certain types of parasites.
    - Probiotics: Support gut health and can help fight off parasites.
    - Papaya Seeds: Have shown effectiveness in eliminating certain parasites.

2. **Herbal Supplements (Use for 2-4 weeks):**
    - Wormwood: Known for its anti-parasitic effects.
    - Black Walnut: Used in traditional medicine to eliminate parasites.
    - Clove: Contains compounds that help eliminate parasites and eggs.

3. **Hydration:**
    - Drink plenty of water daily, to help flush out toxins and support kidney function.

4. **Environmental Cleanliness:**
    - Regularly clean and disinfect your living environment.
    - Practice good hygiene, such as washing hands thoroughly and regularly.

5. **Consult a Professional:**
    - Seek advice from a healthcare provider or a specialist in parasitology for appropriate testing and treatment options.

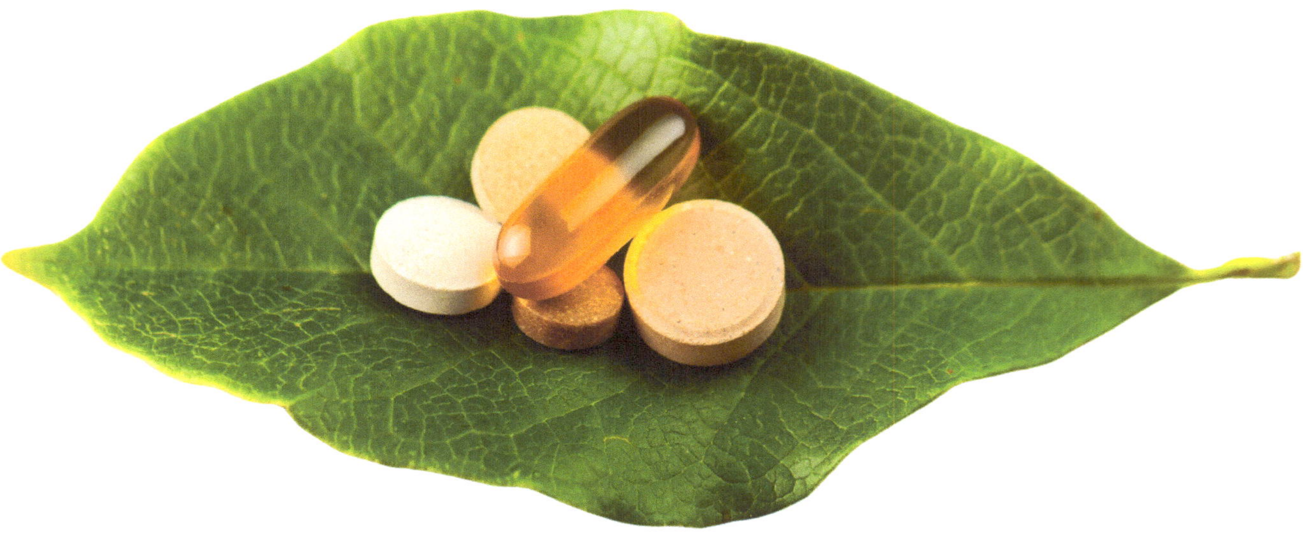

DETOXIFICATION and Candida

Detoxification is about supporting your body's innate ability to cleanse and heal itself. When addressing Candida overgrowth, it's important to focus on natural methods that enhance the functioning of your liver, kidneys, and other organs, helping to eliminate harmful toxins and restore balance. Candida, a type of yeast, can proliferate in the body, leading to a range of health issues such as digestive problems, fatigue, skin issues, and weakened immunity. Stress plays a significant role in exacerbating Candida overgrowth, as elevated cortisol levels can compromise immune function and create an environment where Candida can thrive. By following a structured detoxification protocol, you can help your body combat Candida, reduce stress, and support overall well-being.

HOW TO DETOX FROM CANDIDA OVERGROWTH

1. **Dietary Adjustments (Follow for at least 6-8 weeks):**

- **Avoid Sugary and Processed Foods:** These can feed Candida and promote its growth. Eliminate sugars, refined grains, and processed foods from your diet.
- **Incorporate Anti-Candida Foods:** Focus on foods that combat Candida, such as:
    - **Garlic and Onions:** Known for their antifungal properties.
    - **Coconut Oil:** Contains caprylic acid, which helps kill Candida cells.
    - **Leafy Greens:** Alkaline foods like spinach, kale, and arugula help balance the body's pH levels.
    - **Probiotics:** Support gut health by introducing beneficial bacteria that can outcompete Candida. Include fermented foods like sauerkraut, kimchi, and kefir.
    - **Apple Cider Vinegar:** Helps restore the body's pH balance and has antifungal properties.

2. **Herbal Supplements (Use for 4-6 weeks):**

- **Oregano Oil:** Known for its powerful antifungal properties. Take as directed on the product label.
- **Pau D'Arco Tea:** Drink 1-2 cups per day to benefit from its antifungal and immune-boosting properties.
- **Berberine:** A compound found in several plants that has been shown to inhibit Candida growth. Take as per the recommended dosage.

3. **Hydration:**

- **Drink Plenty of Water:** Aim for at least 8 glasses of water daily to help flush out toxins and support kidney function.
- **Herbal Teas:** Incorporate teas like dandelion or nettle tea, which support liver and kidney detoxification.

4. **Stress Reduction:**

- **Mindfulness Practices:** Engage in activities that reduce stress and lower cortisol levels, such as yoga, meditation, and deep breathing exercises.
- **Regular Exercise:** Helps to reduce stress and improve overall immune function. Aim for at least 30 minutes of moderate exercise most days of the week.
- **Adequate Sleep:** Ensure you get 7-9 hours of quality sleep each night to help your body recover and manage stress effectively.

5. **Environmental Cleanliness:**

- Maintain a Clean Living Environment: Regularly clean and disinfect your living space to reduce exposure to potential sources of Candida.
- **Personal Hygiene:** Practice good hygiene, including thorough hand washing and regular showering.

6. **Consult a Professional:**

- **Medical Advice:** Seek guidance from a healthcare provider or a specialist in functional medicine for personalized advice and appropriate testing.

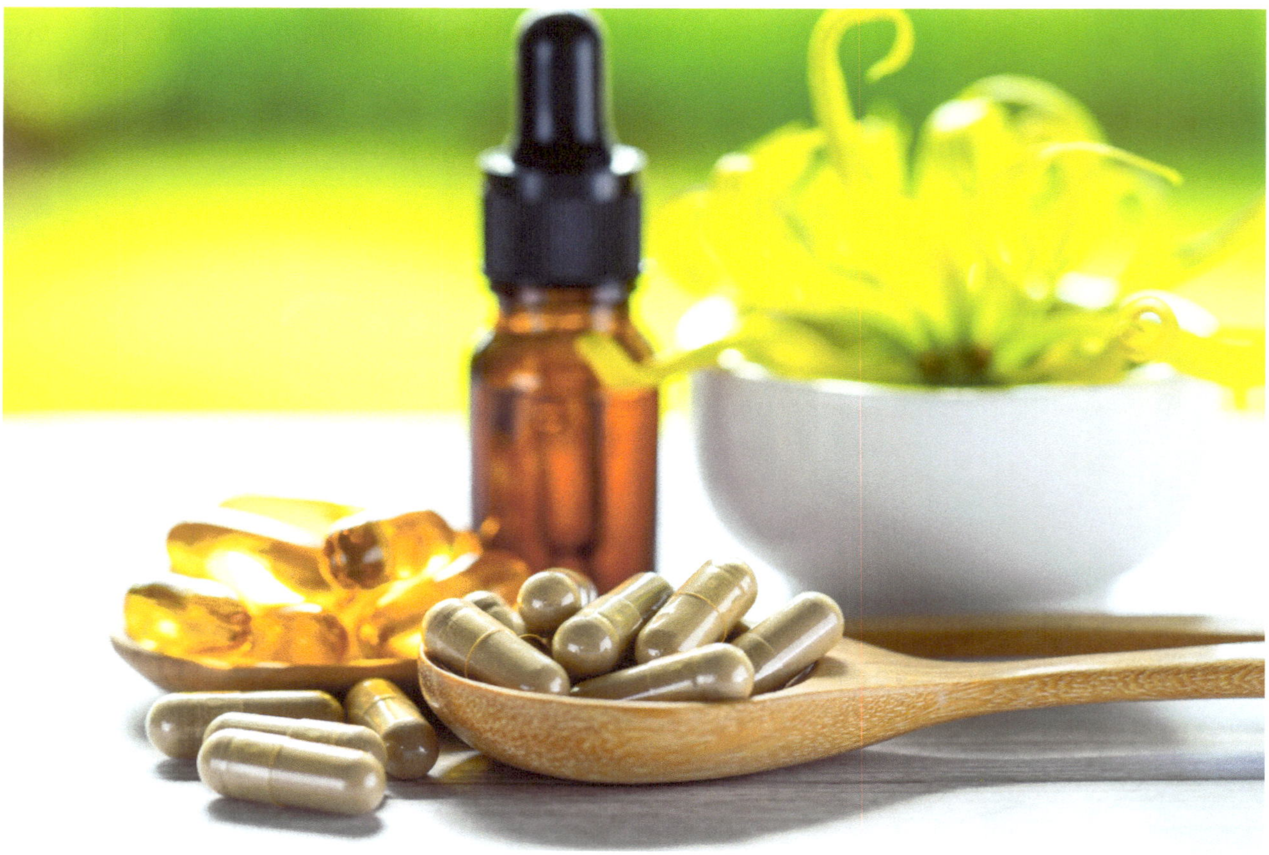

LIVER DETOXIFICATION

Liver detoxification supports the liver through a healthy diet, hydration, and reducing exposure to toxins. The liver is essential for detoxifying the body, processing everything from alcohol to environmental pollutants.

HOW TO DETOX THE LIVER

1. **Dietary Adjustments (Follow for 4-6 weeks):**
    - **Leafy Greens:** Incorporate foods like spinach, kale, and arugula into your meals. These help increase bile production, aiding in the removal of waste.
    - **Citrus Fruits:** Lemons, limes, and oranges help stimulate the liver. Drink lemon water first thing in the morning.
    - **Cruciferous Vegetables:** Eat broccoli, cauliflower, and Brussels sprouts regularly to enhance liver detoxification.
    - **Beets and Carrots:** Add these to your diet several times a week, either raw, roasted, or juiced.

2. **Herbal Supplements (Use for 2-4 weeks):**
    - **Milk Thistle:** Take a milk thistle supplement daily to support liver health.
    - **Dandelion Root:** Drink dandelion root tea 1-2 times per day to aid liver function.
    - **Turmeric:** Add turmeric to your cooking or take a turmeric supplement. Ensure it contains black pepper to enhance absorption.

3. **Hydration:**
    - **Adequate Water Intake:** Drink at least 8 glasses of water daily to help your body flush out toxins.
    - **Lemon Water:** Start your day with a glass of warm water with lemon to help stimulate the liver.

4. **Reducing Exposure to Toxins:**
    - **Minimize Alcohol Intake:** Reduce or eliminate alcohol consumption to lessen the liver's workload.
    - **Choose Organic Foods:** Opt for organic produce to avoid pesticides and other chemicals.
    - **Avoid Processed Foods:** Limit consumption of processed foods that contain additives and preservatives.

5. **Consult a Professional:**
    - **Liver Function Tests:** Schedule regular check-ups with a healthcare provider to monitor liver health.

KIDNEY DETOXIFICATION

Supporting kidney function is essential for overall health, as kidneys filter waste from the blood.

HOW TO DETOX THE KIDNEYS

1. **Dietary Adjustments (Follow for 4-6 weeks):**
   - Berries: Eat a serving of blueberries, strawberries, or cranberries daily.
   - Leafy Greens: Include spinach, kale, and Swiss chard in your meals regularly.
   - Apples: Have an apple a day as a snack or part of a meal.
   - Cabbage: Use cabbage in salads, soups, or as a side dish.

2. **Herbal Supplements (Use for 2-4 weeks):**
   - Cranberry Extract: Take a cranberry supplement daily to support kidney health.
   - Marshmallow Root Tea: Drink a cup of marshmallow root tea daily to support the urinary tract.
   - Parsley: Brew fresh parsley in hot water and drink it 1-2 times per day as a diuretic.

3. **Hydration:**
   - Drink Plenty of Water: Aim for at least 8 glasses of water daily to help the kidneys flush out toxins.
   - Herbal Teas: Incorporate teas like dandelion or nettle tea into your daily routine for kidney support.

4. **Reducing Exposure to Toxins:**
   - Avoid High-Sodium Foods: Limit foods that are high in sodium to reduce the strain on your kidneys.
   - Reduce Sugar Intake: Lower your intake of sugary foods and drinks to prevent kidney damage.

5. **Consult a Professional:**
   - Kidney Function Tests: Schedule regular check-ups with a healthcare provider to monitor kidney health.

HEAVY METAL Detoxification

Heavy metals can accumulate in the body and lead to various health issues. Detoxifying from heavy metals involves supporting the body's natural elimination processes.

HOW TO DETOX FROM HEAVY METALS

1. **Dietary Adjustments (Follow for at least 6-8 weeks):**
   - Cilantro: Add a handful of fresh cilantro to your daily smoothie to help chelate heavy metals.
   - Chlorella: Take a chlorella supplement daily as per the product's instructions.
   - Garlic: Incorporate fresh garlic into your meals daily to support detoxification.
   - Spirulina: Include spirulina in your diet through supplements or by adding it to smoothies.

2. **Herbal Supplements (Use for 4-6 weeks):**
   - Cilantro Extract: Take a cilantro supplement daily to support heavy metal detoxification.
   - Activated Charcoal: Use activated charcoal according to the product's instructions to bind and remove toxins.
   - Zeolite Clay: Take zeolite clay as directed to help remove heavy metals from the body.

3. **Hydration:**
   - Drink Water Throughout the Day: Ensure you drink at least 8 glasses of water daily to aid in flushing out toxins.
   - Detoxifying Drinks: Make green juices or smoothies that include detoxifying ingredients like cilantro and parsley.

4. **Reducing Exposure to Toxins:**
   - Avoid Contaminated Fish: Limit intake of fish high in mercury, such as swordfish and tuna.
   - Use Filtered Water: Drink filtered water to avoid heavy metals present in tap water.

5. **Consult a Professional:**
   - Heavy Metal Testing: Seek advice from a healthcare provider for appropriate testing and detoxification protocols.

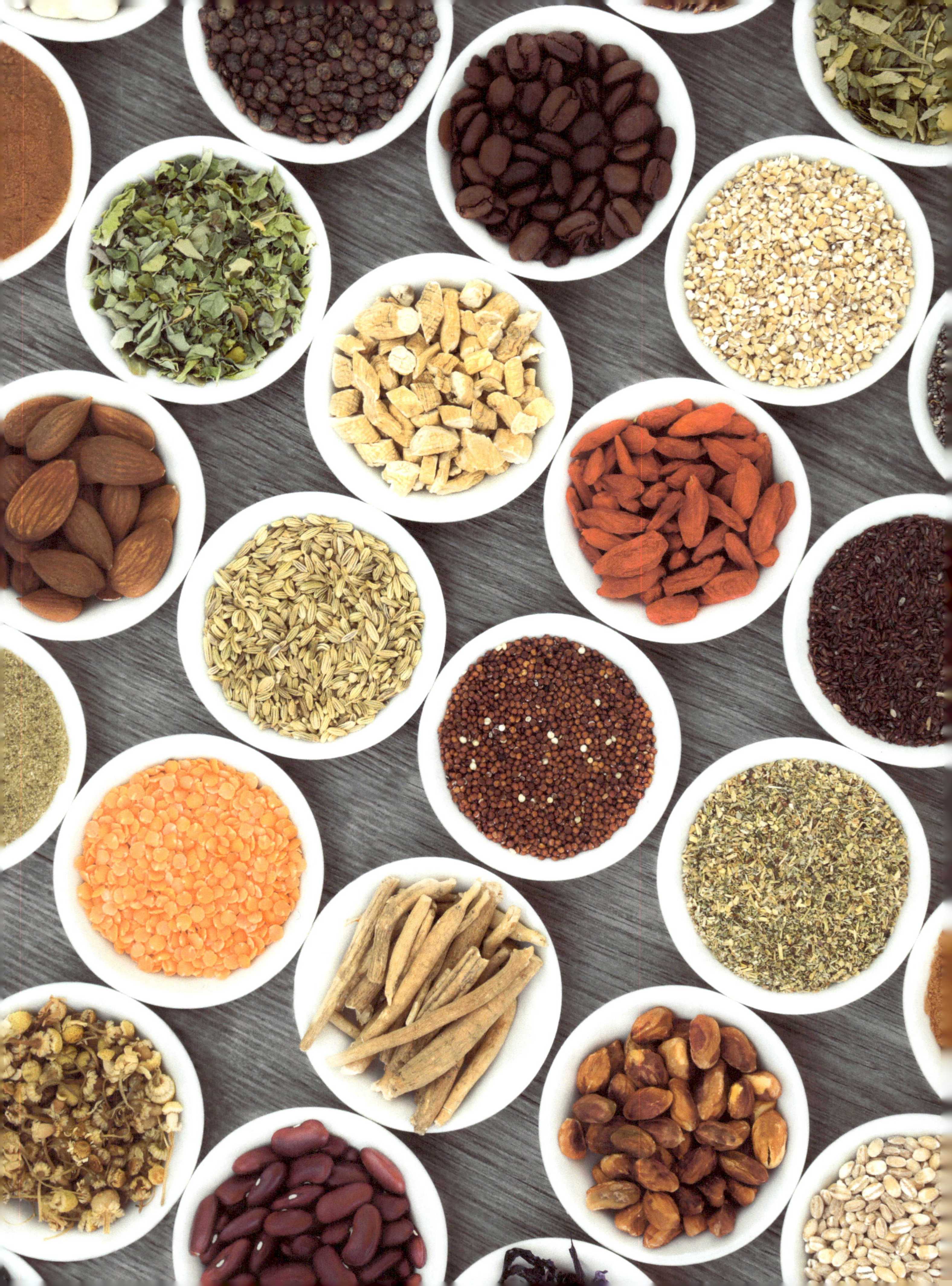

SECTION 9

HERBS AND Supplements

Exploring the power of nature through herbs and supplements can be a transformative journey for your health. This section delves into the potent benefits of various herbs and essential supplements, illustrating how they can enhance your overall wellness. From boosting your immune system to improving mental clarity, these natural elements are key to achieving a balanced and vibrant life. Discover how to integrate these powerful allies into your daily routine for optimal health.

Resources for Further Information

For more detailed guidance and personalized advice on:

Starwest Botanicals | Learn more about their commitment to quality and sustainability.

For more detailed guidance and personalized advice on detoxification and managing parasites, consider consulting the following resource:

Supreme Nutrition Products | Founded to provide pure herbal supplements with no fillers or binders. 100% natural.

HERBS, BENEFITS and Deficiencies

Herbs and supplements are essential components of holistic wellness, supporting a variety of bodily functions and preventing nutritional deficiencies. Gaining insight into the powerful benefits of common herbs and supplements can help you make informed choices to enhance your health and well-being. Understanding the role of these natural elements empowers you to address deficiencies and optimize your overall wellness.

COMMON HERBS AND THEIR BENEFITS:

1. Ashwagandha (Withania somnifera):
Benefits: Reduces stress and anxiety, supports adrenal health, boosts energy, enhances cognitive function.
Deficiency Disorders: Increased stress, cortisol imbalance, anxiety, adrenal fatigue.

2. Chamomile (Matricaria chamomilla):
Benefits: Calming, aids sleep, anti-inflammatory, supports digestive health.
Deficiency Disorders: Sleep disturbances, digestive issues.
3. Chasteberry (Vitex agnus-castus):
Benefits: Balances hormones, supports menstrual health, reduces PMS symptoms, helps manage symptoms of PCOS and other hormonal imbalances.
Deficiency Disorders: Hormonal imbalances, menstrual irregularities, severe PMS symptoms, PCOS symptoms.

4. Echinacea (Echinacea purpurea):
Benefits: Boosts immune system, reduces duration of colds, anti-inflammatory, antioxidant.
Deficiency Disorders: Increased susceptibility to colds and infections.

5. Garlic (Allium sativum):
Benefits: Antimicrobial, supports cardiovascular health, boosts immune system, anti-inflammatory.
Deficiency Disorders: Weakened immune response, increased risk of infections, cardiovascular issues.

6. Ginger (Zingiber officinale):
Benefits: Aids digestion, reduces nausea, anti-inflammatory, supports cardiovascular health, boosts immunity.
Deficiency Disorders: Digestive issues, increased inflammation, weakened immune response.

7. Ginseng (Panax ginseng):
Benefits: Boosts energy, enhances cognitive function, supports immune health, anti-inflammatory.
Deficiency Disorders: Fatigue, cognitive decline, weakened immune response.

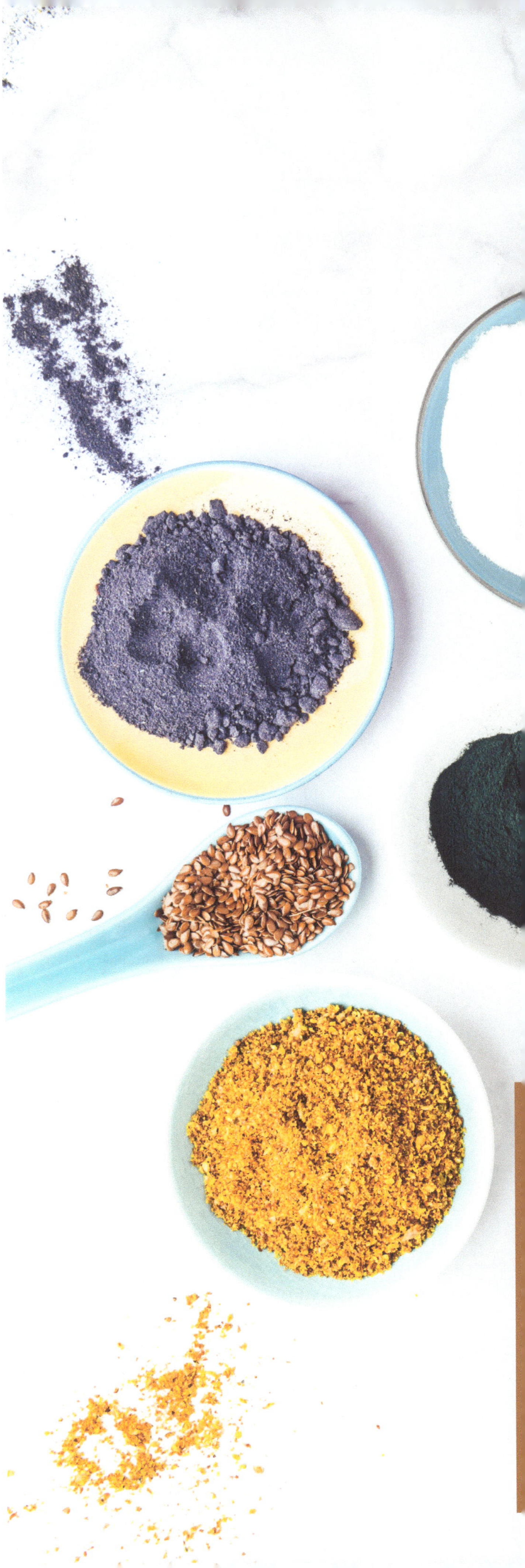

8. Lavender (Lavandula angustifolia):
Benefits: Reduces anxiety, promotes relaxation, aids sleep, anti-inflammatory.
Deficiency Disorders: Increased anxiety, sleep disturbances.

9. Lion's Mane (Hericium erinaceus):
Benefits: Supports cognitive function, enhances nerve growth, boosts immune system, reduces inflammation.
Deficiency Disorders: Cognitive decline, weakened immune response, increased inflammation.

10. Maca (Lepidium meyenii):
Benefits: Boosts energy, enhances mood, supports hormone balance, improves fertility.
Deficiency Disorders: Fatigue, hormonal imbalances, reduced fertility.

11. Milk Thistle (Silybum marianum):
Benefits: Supports liver health, detoxification, antioxidant, anti-inflammatory.
Deficiency Disorders: Liver issues, reduced detoxification efficiency.

12. Peppermint (Mentha piperita):
Benefits: Aids digestion, relieves headaches, anti-inflammatory, antimicrobial.
Deficiency Disorders: Digestive issues, increased susceptibility to headaches.

13. Reishi Mushroom (Ganoderma lucidum):
Benefits: Boosts immune system, reduces inflammation, supports liver health, enhances mood.
Deficiency Disorders: Weakened immune response, increased inflammation, liver issues.

14. Turmeric (Curcuma longa):
Benefits: Anti-inflammatory, antioxidant, supports joint health, aids digestion, boosts immune system.
Deficiency Disorders: Increased inflammation, joint pain, weakened immune response.

While herbs offer powerful benefits on their own, combining them with other natural supplements can amplify their effects and support holistic health. One such supplement is omega-3 fatty acids, which are essential for maintaining overall well-being.

OMEGA-3 FATTY ACIDS AND THEIR BENEFITS

Omega-3 fatty acids are essential polyunsaturated fats that play a critical role in human health. Since they cannot be synthesized by the body, they must be obtained through diet. There are three main types of omega-3 fatty acids: Alpha-linolenic acid (ALA) found in plant oils such as flaxseed, chia seeds, and walnuts; Eicosapentaenoic acid (EPA) found in marine sources like fatty fish and fish oil; and Docosahexaenoic acid (DHA) also found in marine sources and particularly important for brain health.

Health Benefits of Omega-3 Fatty Acids: Heart Health:

- *Reduces Triglycerides:* Omega-3s can significantly reduce blood triglyceride levels, lowering the risk of heart disease.
- *Lowers Blood Pressure:* Regular intake of omega-3s can help reduce blood pressure in people with hypertension.
- *Prevents Plaque Formation:* Omega-3s help prevent the formation of arterial plaque, improving blood flow and reducing the risk of cardiovascular events.
- *Reduces Arrhythmias:* They can help prevent irregular heartbeats, reducing the risk of sudden cardiac death.

Brain Health:

- *Supports Cognitive Function:* DHA is a major structural component of the brain and is integral for maintaining cognitive function and brain health throughout life.
- *Reduces Depression and Anxiety:* Studies suggest that omega-3 supplements can help reduce symptoms of depression and anxiety.
- *May Improve ADHD Symptoms:* Some research indicates that omega-3 supplements can reduce the symptoms of ADHD in children.

Inflammation Reduction:

- *Anti-inflammatory Properties:* Omega-3s have anti-inflammatory effects, which can help manage chronic inflammation and reduce the risk of chronic diseases like arthritis.

Eye Health:

- *Prevents Macular Degeneration:* DHA is also a major component of the retina, and adequate intake of omega-3s can help prevent macular degeneration, a leading cause of vision impairment and blindness.

Prenatal and Infant Health:

- *Supports Brain and Eye Development:* Adequate intake of DHA during pregnancy is vital for fetal brain and eye development.
- *May Improve Pregnancy Outcomes:* Omega-3 intake during pregnancy has been associated with reduced risk of preterm birth and may benefit the baby's birth weight.

Bone and Joint Health:

- *Improves Bone Strength:* Omega-3s can improve bone strength by increasing the calcium in bones, which may help prevent osteoporosis.
- *Reduces Symptoms of Rheumatoid Arthritis*: They can also help reduce symptoms of rheumatoid arthritis by reducing joint pain and stiffness.

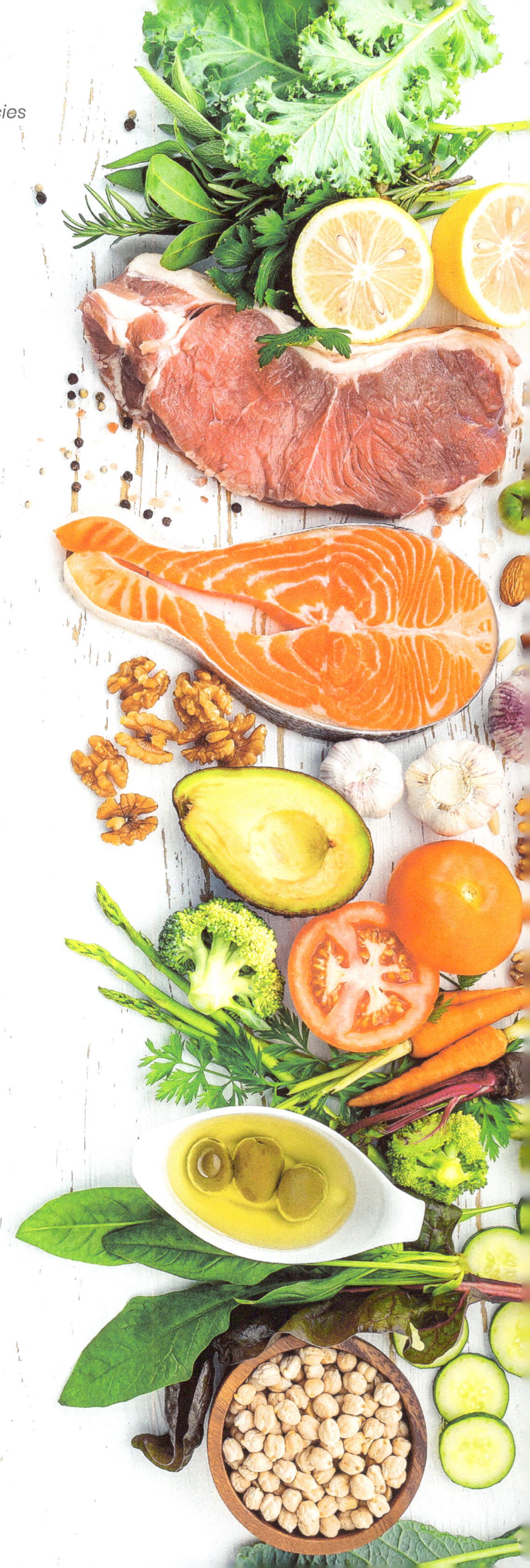

Skin Health:

- ***Improves Skin Hydration:*** Omega-3s help maintain skin hydration and may protect against sun damage.
- ***Reduces Acne:*** Their anti-inflammatory properties can help reduce acne.

Sources of Omega-3 Fatty Acids:

- ***Fatty Fish:*** Salmon, mackerel, sardines, and trout
- ***Plant Oils:*** Flaxseed oil, chia seeds, and walnuts
- ***Algal Oil:*** A plant-based source of DHA, suitable for vegetarians and vegans
- ***Supplements***: Fish oil capsules, krill oil, and flaxseed oil supplements

Incorporating omega-3-rich foods into your diet or taking supplements can help you reap these numerous health benefits. By combining omega-3s with certain herbs, you can maximize their positive effects on your health. This synergy between herbs and omega-3s can lead to enhanced overall well-being. Similarly, many other herbs can be paired together to amplify their benefits, providing a more comprehensive approach to holistic health.

HARNESSING SYNERGY for Enhanced Health

Understanding how herbs work synergistically can amplify their health benefits. Synergy refers to the combined effects of different substances that result in a greater effect than the sum of their individual effects. This principle extends across many herb combinations, offering comprehensive support for various aspects of your well-being.

Explore Synergistic Herb Pairings:

- **Black Pepper and Turmeric:** Enhances absorption of curcumin, maximizing anti-inflammatory and antioxidant effects.
- **Garlic and Ginger:** Combined antimicrobial and anti-inflammatory properties, supports digestion and immune health.
- **Lavender and Chamomile:** Combined calming effects, promotes relaxation and aids in sleep quality.
- **Ginseng* and Ginkgo Biloba:** Boosts cognitive function and mental clarity, enhances energy levels and circulation.
- **Milk Thistle and Dandelion:** Supports liver health and detoxification, enhances antioxidant effects.
- **Echinacea and Goldenseal:** Boosts immune function and fights infections, supports overall immune system health.
- **Ashwaghanda* and Rhodiola*:** Enhances stress resilience, supports adrenal health, and boosts energy levels.
- **Cinnamon and Honey:** Combined anti-inflammatory and antimicrobial properties, supports digestion and immune health.
- **Turmeric and Ginger:** Joint pain relief, anti-inflammatory properties, and digestive support.
- **Oregano and Thyme:** Combined antimicrobial and antioxidant properties, supports respiratory and digestive health.
- **Peppermint and Lemon Balm:** Calming effects, aids digestion, and promotes relaxation.
- **Rosemary and Sage:** Cognitive function support, antioxidant properties, and digestive health.
- **Holy Basil* and Licorice Root*:** Stress management, adrenal support, and immune system modulation.

*Adaptogens are marked with an asterisk.

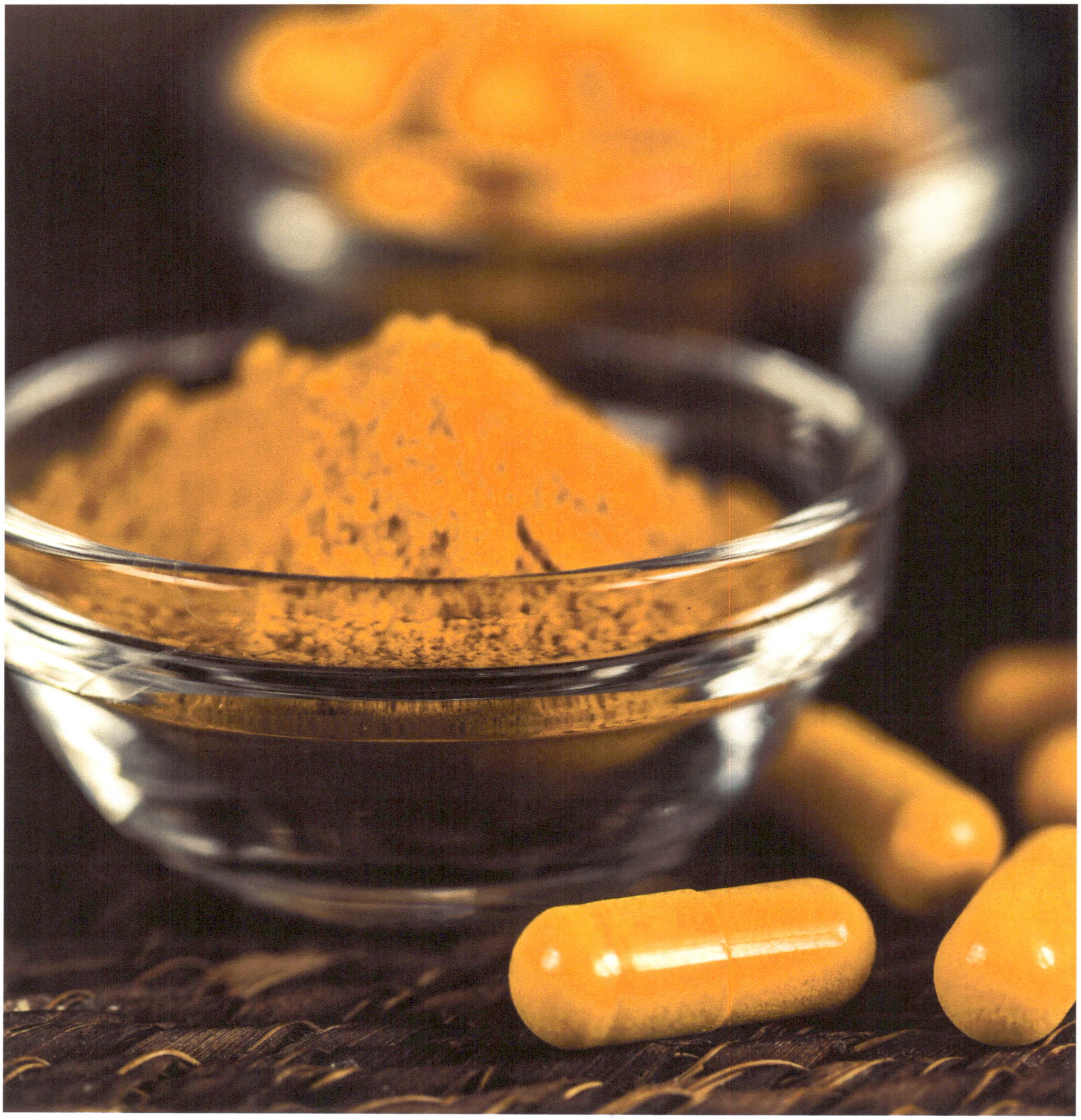

"Wellness Insights: *Did You Know?*"

- ***Did you know...*** that pairing turmeric with black pepper increases the absorption of curcumin by up to 2,000%, enhancing its anti-inflammatory and antioxidant benefits?
- ***Did you know...*** that adaptogens are natural substances that help your body adapt to stress, boost energy levels, and improve overall balance?

SUPPLEMENTS, BENEFITS and Deficiencies

Supplements can be an essential part of maintaining overall health and wellness. They help fill nutritional gaps, support bodily functions, and address specific health concerns. Here, you'll find a list of common supplements, their benefits, and the disorders associated with deficiencies, guiding you in making informed choices for your health needs.

1. Vitamin D:
Benefits: Supports bone health, boosts immune system, reduces inflammation, enhances mood.
Deficiency Disorders: Osteoporosis, weakened immune response, depression.

2. Omega-3 Fatty Acids:
Benefits: Supports cardiovascular health, reduces inflammation, enhances cognitive function, supports joint health.
Deficiency Disorders: Cardiovascular issues, increased inflammation, cognitive decline.

3. Probiotics:
Benefits: Supports digestive health, boosts immune system, reduces inflammation, balances gut flora.
Deficiency Disorders: Digestive issues, weakened immune response, increased inflammation.

4. Magnesium:
Benefits: Supports muscle and nerve function, promotes relaxation, aids sleep, supports bone health.
Deficiency Disorders: Muscle cramps, sleep disturbances, anxiety, bone health issues.

5. Vitamin B12:
Benefits: Supports energy production, enhances cognitive function, supports nervous system health.
Deficiency Disorders: Fatigue, cognitive decline, neurological issues.

6. Iron:
Benefits: Supports red blood cell production, boosts energy, enhances cognitive function.
Deficiency Disorders: Anemia, fatigue, cognitive decline.

7. Calcium:
Benefits: Supports bone health, aids muscle function, supports cardiovascular health.
Deficiency Disorders: Osteoporosis, muscle cramps, cardiovascular issues.

8. Zinc:
Benefits: Boosts immune system, supports wound healing, enhances cognitive function.
Deficiency Disorders: Weakened immune response, delayed wound healing, cognitive decline.

9. Coenzyme Q10:
Benefits: Supports cardiovascular health, boosts energy, reduces oxidative stress.
Deficiency Disorders: Cardiovascular issues, fatigue, increased oxidative stress.

10. Curcumin:
Benefits: Anti-inflammatory, antioxidant, supports joint health, boosts immune system.
Deficiency Disorders: Increased inflammation, joint pain, weakened immune response.

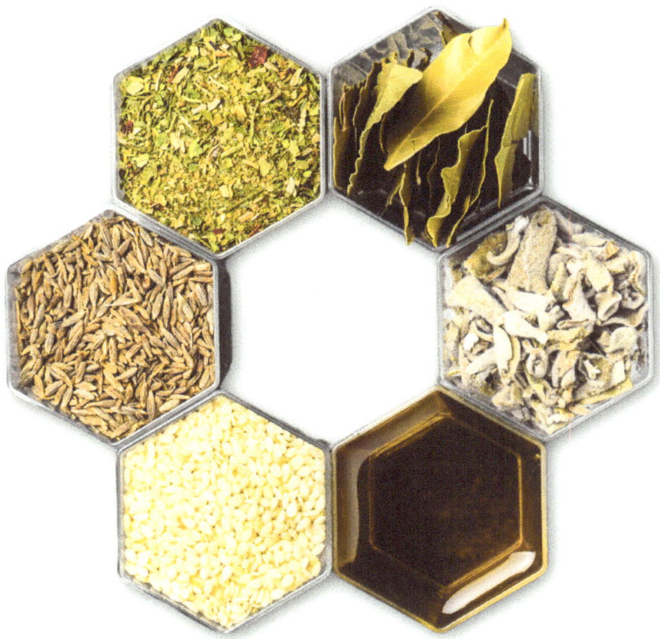

"Wellness Insights: *Did You Know?*"

» ***Did you know...*** that magnesium supports over 300 biochemical reactions in the body, including muscle and nerve function, blood glucose control, and blood pressure regulation?

» ***Did you know...*** that probiotics are beneficial bacteria that can improve your digestive health and boost your immune system?

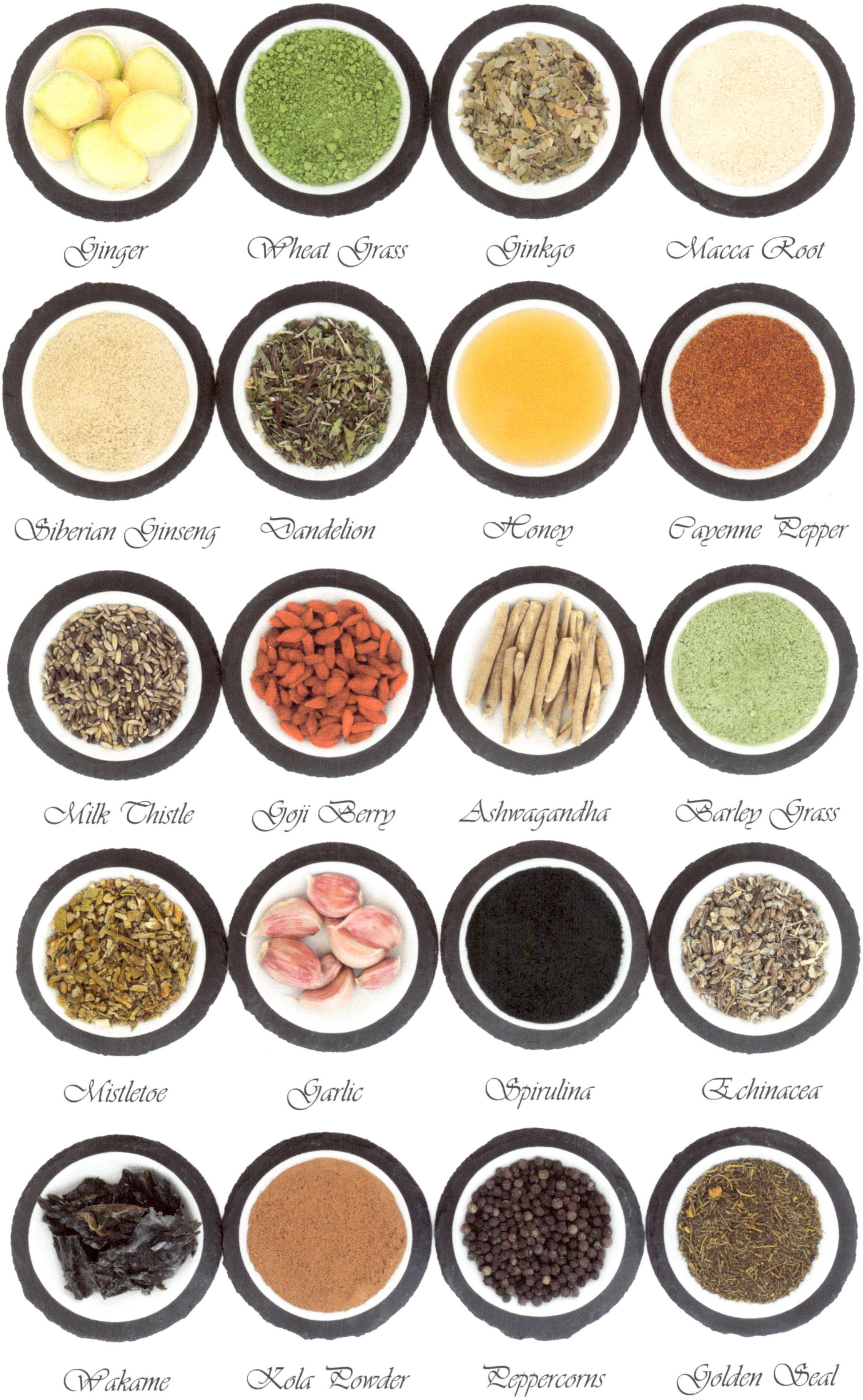
Ginger
Wheat Grass
Ginkgo
Macca Root
Siberian Ginseng
Dandelion
Honey
Cayenne Pepper
Milk Thistle
Goji Berry
Ashwagandha
Barley Grass
Mistletoe
Garlic
Spirulina
Echinacea
Wakame
Kola Powder
Peppercorns
Golden Seal

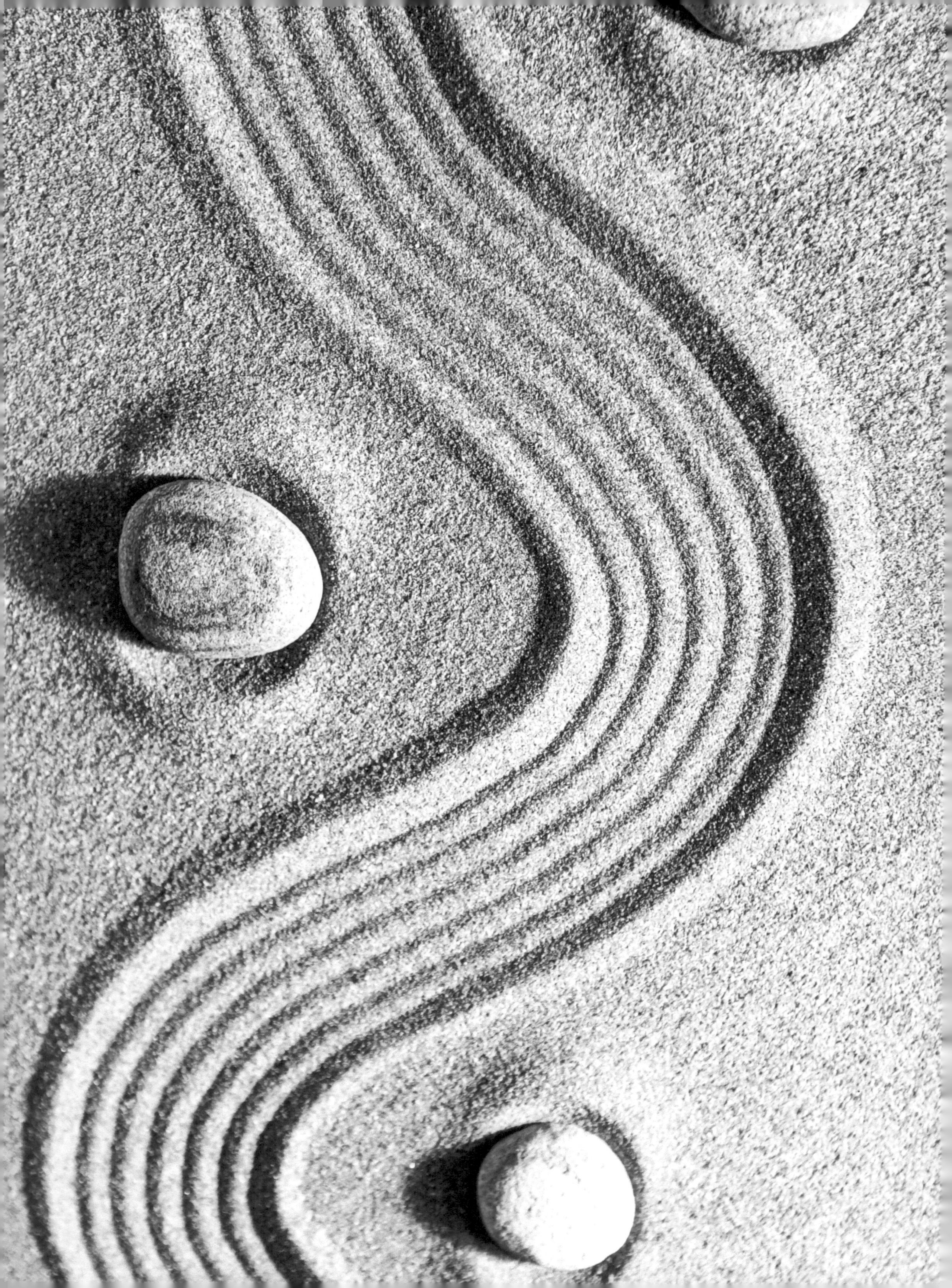

SECTION 10

HOLISTIC
Wellness Practices

OVERVIEW OF HOLISTIC Health Practices

Holistic wellness is about achieving balance in all aspects of life, encompassing physical, mental, emotional, and spiritual well-being. Holistic health practices focus on the interconnectedness of the body, mind, and spirit. By integrating key practices into your daily routine, you can create a harmonious and balanced approach to wellness for a more fulfilling life.

Physical Wellness: This involves taking care of your body through regular exercise, proper nutrition, adequate sleep, and preventive healthcare. Physical wellness practices include:

1. **Regular Exercise:** Engaging in physical activities that you enjoy, such as walking, yoga, strength training, or dancing, to maintain a healthy body.
2. **Balanced Nutrition:** Eating a variety of nutrient-dense foods that provide the energy and nutrients your body needs to function optimally.
3. **Adequate Sleep:** Ensuring you get enough restful sleep each night to support your body's recovery and overall health.
4. **Preventive Healthcare:** Regular check-ups, screenings, and self-care practices to prevent illness and maintain good health.

Mental Wellness: Mental wellness is about maintaining a healthy mind through practices that enhance cognitive function, reduce stress, and promote emotional stability. Key practices include:

1. **Mindfulness and Meditation:** Incorporating mindfulness and meditation into your daily routine to reduce stress, improve focus, and enhance emotional resilience.
2. **Continuous Learning:** Engaging in activities that stimulate your mind, such as reading, puzzles, or learning new skills, to keep your brain active and healthy.
3. **Stress Management:** Identifying and managing sources of stress through techniques like deep breathing, time management, and relaxation exercises.

Emotional Wellness: Emotional wellness involves understanding and managing your emotions in a healthy way, fostering positive relationships, and maintaining a positive outlook on life. Practices include:

1. **Self-Reflection:** Taking time to reflect on your thoughts and feelings, and understanding how they impact your behavior and well-being.
2. **Healthy Relationships:** Building and maintaining supportive relationships with family, friends, and loved ones.
3. **Positive Affirmations:** Using positive affirmations to boost self-esteem and cultivate a positive mindset.

Spiritual Wellness: Spiritual wellness is about finding purpose and meaning in life, connecting with something greater than yourself, and nurturing your soul. Practices include:

1. **Spiritual Practices:** Engaging in spiritual activities that resonate with you, such as prayer, meditation, or spending time in nature.
2. **Purpose and Meaning:** Identifying and pursuing your life purpose and passions, and finding meaning in your daily activities.
3. **Community and Service:** Participating in community activities and volunteer work to connect with others and give back.

4. KEY HEALTH CONSIDERATIONS:

In addition to these wellness practices, there are specific health considerations that play an essential role in overall well-being. Understanding and addressing these factors can significantly enhance your holistic wellness journey:

1. **Cortisol and Stress:** Cortisol is a hormone released in response to stress. Chronic stress can lead to cortisol imbalances, causing weight gain, fatigue, and other health issues. Reducing stress through mindfulness, exercise, and proper sleep can help balance cortisol levels.
2. **Thyroid Health:** The thyroid gland regulates metabolism, and imbalances can lead to weight fluctuations, fatigue, and mood changes. A balanced diet rich in iodine, selenium, and zinc supports thyroid health.
3. **Gut Health:** Maintaining a healthy gut microbiome with probiotics, prebiotics, and fiber is essential for digestion, immunity, and overall well-being. Foods like yogurt, sauerkraut, and whole grains are beneficial.
4. **Sleep Health:** Quality sleep impacts overall health, influencing mood, cognitive function, and physical health. Establishing a regular sleep routine and creating a restful environment are key strategies.
5. **Hydration:** Staying hydrated is vital for bodily functions, including digestion, temperature regulation, and cognitive performance. Aim to drink plenty of water throughout the day.
6. **Mental Health:** Beyond stress management, addressing anxiety and depression through professional help, self-care practices, and social support is essential for mental well-being.

7. **Hormonal Balance:** Hormones like estrogen, testosterone, and insulin play vital roles in health. Maintaining a balanced diet, regular exercise, and stress management supports hormonal health.
8. **Immune System Support:** A strong immune system is supported by a healthy diet, regular exercise, adequate sleep, and stress management. Foods rich in vitamins C and D, zinc, and antioxidants are beneficial.
9. **Detoxification:** Natural detoxification involves supporting the liver and kidneys through a healthy diet, hydration, and reducing exposure to toxins. Focus on eliminating chemicals, pollutants, heavy metals, and parasites. This process is supported by specific foods, herbs, and supplements like leafy greens, citrus fruits, garlic, cilantro, milk thistle, dandelion root, pumpkin seeds, black walnut, and clove. Proper hydration and avoiding processed foods are also essential.
10. **Chronic Inflammation:** Chronic inflammation can lead to various health issues and disease. An anti-inflammatory diet rich in omega-3 fatty acids, fruits, vegetables, and whole grains helps reduce inflammation.
11. **Bone Health:** Calcium, vitamin D, and weight-bearing exercises are critical for maintaining bone density and preventing osteoporosis.
12. **Heart Health:** Maintaining cardiovascular health involves regular exercise, a balanced diet low in saturated fats, and managing stress. Foods like leafy greens, berries, and nuts are heart-healthy choices.

Achieving Gut Health: A Key to Overall Wellbeing

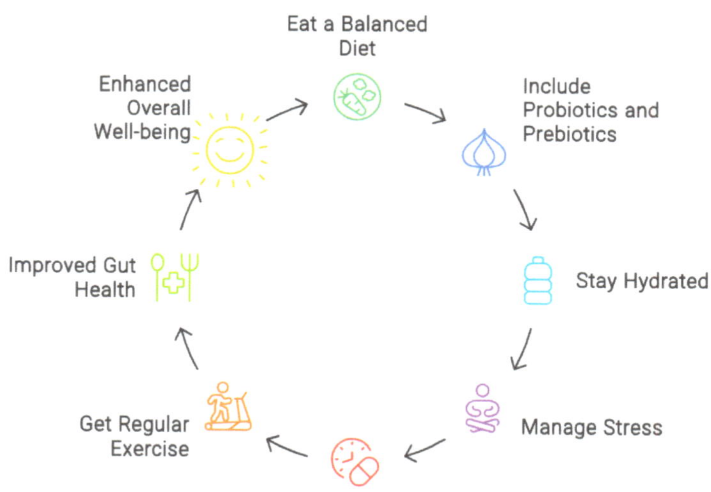
Eat a Balanced Diet
Include Probiotics and Prebiotics
Stay Hydrated
Manage Stress
Get Regular Exercise
Improved Gut Health
Enhanced Overall Well-being

"Wellness Insights: *Did You Know?*"

- ***Did you know...*** that regular meditation can reduce levels of the stress hormone cortisol and improve overall mental well-being?
- ***Did you know...*** that facial mapping can help you identify internal health issues based on where you experience breakouts or skin changes?

IMPORTANCE OF INTEGRATING Body, Mind, and Spirit

Achieving holistic wellness involves harmonizing the body, mind, and spirit. When these elements are balanced, you'll experience a deeper sense of fulfillment and overall well-being. Let's explore why each aspect is important and how you can nurture them in your everyday life:

Body:

A healthy body is the foundation for an active and energetic life. By taking care of your physical health, you'll find it easier to engage fully in all aspects of life.

1. **Stay Active:** Regular physical activity, like walking, dancing, or practicing yoga, keeps your muscles strong and your heart healthy. Find something you enjoy and make it a part of your routine.
2. **Eat Well:** Focus on a balanced diet filled with whole foods—think colorful fruits and veggies, lean proteins, and healthy fats. Nourishing your body with the right foods boosts energy and supports overall health.
3. **Get Enough Sleep:** Quality sleep is essential for recovery and mental clarity. Aim for 7-9 hours each night to help your body recharge and function at its best.

Mind:

A healthy mind is key to emotional stability and mental clarity. By nurturing your mental health, you'll enhance cognitive function and emotional well-being.

1. **Practice Mindfulness:** Simple mindfulness exercises, like deep breathing or meditation, can reduce stress and improve focus. Just a few minutes each day can make a big difference.
2. **Keep Learning:** Engage your mind with new challenges—read books, explore new hobbies, or take up a class. Lifelong learning keeps your brain sharp and your spirits high.
3. **Emotional Check-ins:** Take time to understand your emotions. Whether it's journaling, talking with a friend, or seeking professional help, acknowledging your feelings is vital for mental health.

Spirit:

Nurturing your spirit provides a sense of purpose and connection. By paying attention to your spiritual health, you'll find greater meaning and joy in everyday life.

1. **Find Your Practice:** Whether it's meditation, prayer, or spending time in nature, find activities that connect you to your inner self and bring peace.
2. **Connect with Others:** Building relationships through community activities or social gatherings fosters a sense of belonging and purpose.
3. **Seek Meaning:** Reflect on what truly brings you joy and fulfillment. Set intentions and goals that resonate with your values and incorporate them into your daily life.

Integrating body, mind, and spirit creates a holistic approach to health that enhances your quality of life. Remember, the journey to holistic wellness is personal and ongoing. Embrace the process, make adjustments as you grow, and celebrate your achievements along the way.

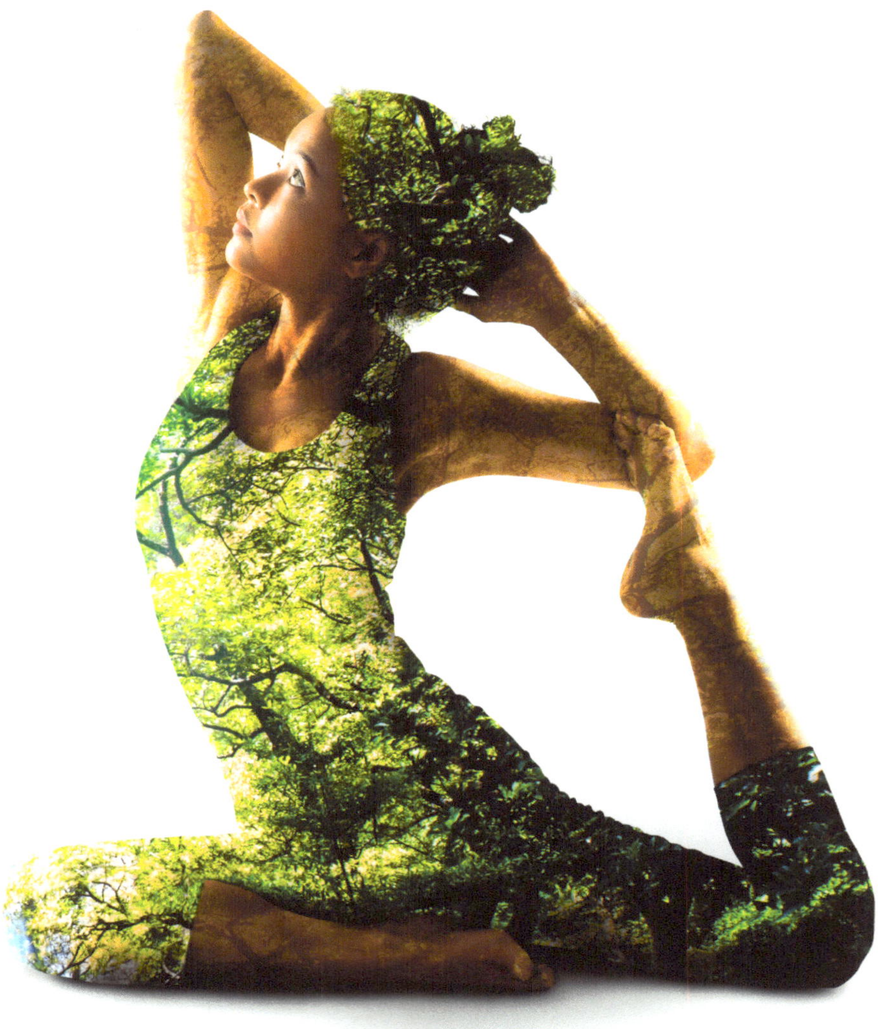

ACHIEVING HOLISTIC Wellness

By integrating the holistic health principles discussed in this book, you can unlock a range of positive transformations in your life. These principles can help you achieve better physical, mental, and emotional well-being. Here are some potential benefits you may experience:

Increased Energy Levels
Boost your energy and help combat chronic fatigue by following a balanced diet and regular exercise routine.

Weight Management
Support healthy weight loss and maintenance through mindful eating practices and personalized nutrition plans.

Improved Digestion
Alleviate digestive issues and promote better gut health with holistic dietary changes.

Enhanced Mental Well-Being
Improve your mental clarity and emotional resilience through mindfulness, meditation, and stress management techniques.

Stronger Connection to Body and Mind
Deepen your connection to your body and overall well-being by engaging in regular physical activity and mindfulness practices.

Balanced Lifestyle
Achieve a more balanced and fulfilling lifestyle by integrating body, mind, and spirit.

To help you effectively implement these principles and ease into a routine, refer to the 4-Week Wellness Transformation Plan in the Self-Care Practices section. This plan will guide you in establishing a solid foundation for your wellness journey before moving on to more customized meal and workout plans tailored to your specific goals.

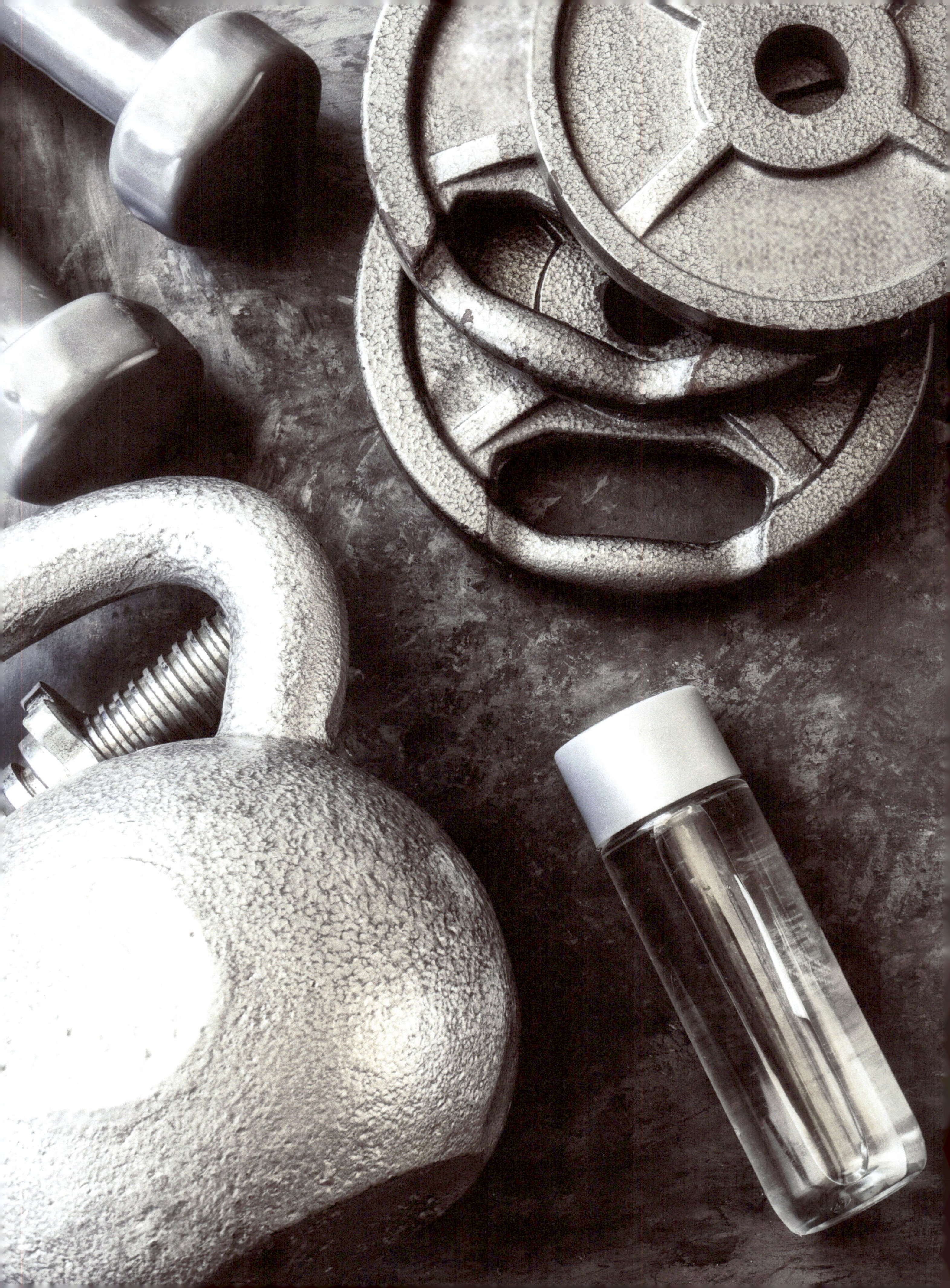

SECTION 11

WORKOUT Plans

INTRODUCTION TO Workout Plans

Welcome to the Workout Plans section of this guide. In this chapter, you'll find a variety of dynamic workout plans tailored to different body types, exercise recommendations, and routines. Whether you're looking to build muscle, tone up, lose weight, or simply incorporate more movement into your daily life, these plans are designed to help you achieve your fitness goals.

Starting a new fitness routine can be daunting, especially with the busy schedules and numerous responsibilities that most of us juggle. However, making time for regular exercise is essential for maintaining physical health, boosting energy levels, and improving overall well-being. The key is to approach fitness as a new, enjoyable activity rather than a chore.

One common misconception about fitness is that it requires long hours at the gym or strict workout regimens. In reality, the most important aspect of any fitness plan is consistency. Starting small and gradually increasing your activity level can lead to sustainable habits and significant improvements over time. Even just a few minutes of exercise each day can make a difference. Incorporating regular physical activity is not only beneficial for physical health but also serves as a form of self-care and self-respect, honoring your commitment to your well-being.

This section provides workout plans specifically designed for different body types—ectomorph, mesomorph, and endomorph. Each plan includes a variety of exercises to suit different fitness levels and goals. You'll also find tips on how to make exercise a regular part of your routine, whether you're new to fitness or a seasoned gym-goer.

STRENGTH TRAINING AND BODY COMPOSITION

Strength training is essential for changing your body composition. While cardio can help you lose weight by burning calories, it primarily reduces both fat and muscle mass. To truly reshape your body, you need to incorporate weight training. Strength training builds lean muscle mass, which not only enhances your strength but also boosts your metabolism. More muscle means your body burns more calories at rest, leading to more effective fat loss. Additionally, weight training can target specific areas, allowing you to sculpt and define your body in ways cardio alone cannot achieve.

Strength training significantly impacts body composition by reducing adipose tissue, commonly known as body fat. Adipose tissue is stored all over your body, not just in areas like the thighs, hips, buttocks, back, and abdomen. When you engage in strength training, your body uses energy from fat stores, leading to fat loss from all over, not just targeted areas. This means you can see changes throughout your entire body, including areas you might not have initially focused on. By building lean muscle, you enhance your metabolism, which further aids in reducing adipose tissue and creating a more toned and defined physique.

While there is no such thing as spot reduction—losing fat in just one specific area—strength training helps reduce overall body fat and build muscle. However, it's important to avoid overworking certain muscle groups, as this can lead to imbalances. For example, focusing too much on the chest and neglecting the back can cause poor posture and potential injuries. To get it right, aim for a balanced strength training routine that targets all major muscle groups: legs, back, chest, arms, and core. Incorporate a variety of exercises to ensure even muscle development and prevent imbalances. This approach will not only help you achieve a well-proportioned physique but also improve overall strength, stability, and flexibility.

ADENOSINE TRIPHOSPHATE (ATP) AND MUSCLE FUNCTION

physical activity, your muscles require ATP to contract and perform movements.

Here's why ATP matters in your fitness journey:

1. **Energy Source:** ATP provides the energy needed for muscle contractions. During exercises like weight-lifting or resistance training, ATP is broken down to release energy, which powers muscle contractions.
2. **Immediate Energy Supply:** Muscles only store a small amount of ATP. Therefore, during intense or pro-longed exercise, ATP must be rapidly replenished to sustain muscle function. This is achieved through metabolic processes that convert stored energy sources like glucose or fat into ATP.
3. **Role in Strength and Endurance:** The availability and efficient use of ATP influence your strength and endurance levels. Regular strength training not only increases muscle mass but also enhances your body's ability to produce and utilize ATP, leading to improved performance and stamina over time.

Understanding ATP helps you appreciate how your body fuels movement and adapts to exercise. By optimizing ATP production and utilization through consistent training, you can enhance your physical performance and achieve your fitness goals effectively.

My own fitness journey began with small steps. When I first started exercising, I felt overwhelmed by the idea of committing to a routine. But I discovered that starting with just 10 minutes of walking each day made a significant impact. Over time, I gradually increased my activity, eventually walking for an hour and sometimes even twice a day. This simple yet consistent approach, combined with changes in my eating habits, led to noticeable improvements in my health and well-being.

If you're brand new to fitness, start as I did with walking. Begin with 5-10 minutes for a week or two until the habit forms, then add on in slow increments. This gradual approach, coupled with new eating habits, will make achieving improvements and weight loss feel less overwhelming, and your confidence will improve.

You don't have to be in a gym to see results. Walking with a walking pad at home is a great investment, as is a pair of adjustable dumbbells and a yoga mat to get started. If you do go to the gym, start off slow to get comfortable. Use the initial training session that often comes with a new gym membership to get a tour of the gym and learn how the equipment works. You can always decide to go it on your own or get a trainer to help you get started.

As my confidence and stamina grew, I became more active at the gym and embraced strength training. Despite the common misconception among women that weightlifting will lead to bulkiness, it remains one of the most effective methods for toning and sculpting the body. Building muscle not only enhances physical appearance but also boosts metabolism and improves overall strength. Personally, lifting weights transformed my body and empowered me in ways that cardio alone couldn't achieve.

Remember, the goal of these workout plans is to support a healthy lifestyle. It's not about quick fixes or drastic changes but rather about finding a balance that works for you. Take it one day at a time, stay consistent, and enjoy the process of becoming stronger and healthier. Your journey to fitness is a personal one, and these plans are here to guide and support you along the way.

Let's get started on this exciting path to a healthier, more active you. Enjoy the workout plans and embrace the positive changes that regular exercise can bring to your life.

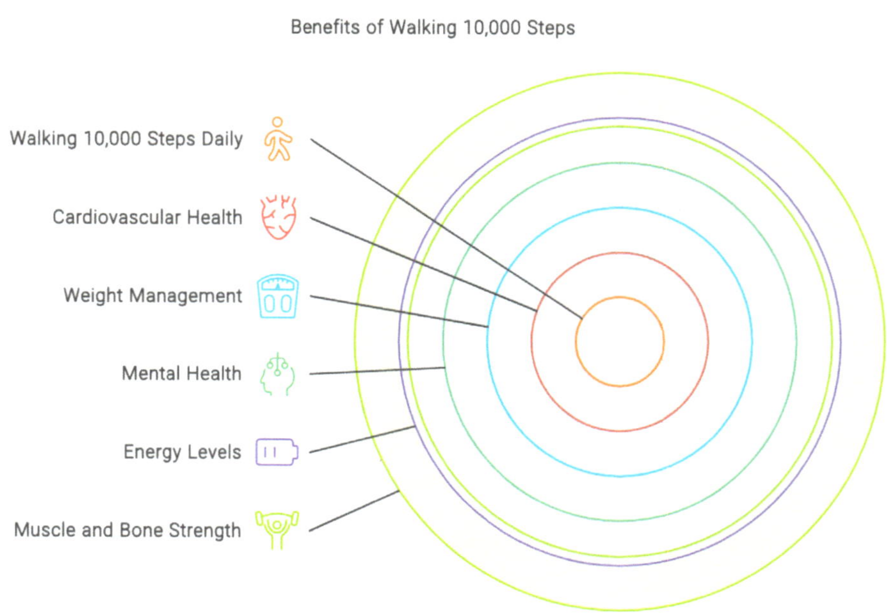

DYNAMIC WORKOUT
Plans Tailored to Body Types

A well-rounded workout plan is essential for achieving holistic wellness, as it enhances physical fitness, boosts mental health, and contributes to overall well-being. This section provides dynamic workout plans tailored to different body types, helping you achieve your fitness goals effectively.

Understanding your body type can help you select the most effective workout routine. Here are exercise recommendations for each body type:

Ectomorph:

Ectomorphs are typically lean and have a harder time gaining weight and muscle. The focus for ectomorphs should be on strength training to build muscle mass and increase overall strength. After the initial workout plan, you'll find additional plans tailored specifically for ectomorphs to address goals like muscle gain, toning, and weight management.

ECTOMORPH: MUSCLE GAIN AND INCREASED WEIGHT

This workout plan is designed to help Ectomorphs gain muscle and increase weight effectively. It includes a focused strength training routine to build muscle mass, coupled with dietary guidance for a calorie surplus. Adequate rest and recovery are also emphasized to support muscle growth and weight gain.

Strength Training Routine:

- **Frequency:** 3-4 days a week.
- **Duration:** 45-60 minutes per session.
- **Exercises:** Focus on compound movements like squats, deadlifts, bench presses, and rows. Aim for 3-4 sets of 8-12 repetitions.
- **Rest:** Allow 48 hours of rest between working the same muscle group.

Dietary Guidance:

- Consume a calorie surplus to support muscle gain.
- Prioritize lean proteins, complex carbohydrates, and healthy fats.
- Consider protein shakes or weight gainer supplements.
- Macro Ratio:
    - Protein: 30-40% of total daily calories
    - Carbohydrates: 40-50% of total daily calories
    - Fats: 20-30% of total daily calories

Recovery and Rest:

- Stay well-hydrated throughout the day.
- Ensure 7-9 hours of quality sleep per night.
- Include active recovery days with light activities like walking or yoga.

ECTOMORPH WORKOUT PLAN: MUSCLE GAIN AND INCREASED WEIGHT

Goal: Build Lean Muscle Mass
Ectomorphs, this workout plan is your blueprint for building lean muscle mass effectively. It provides a structured routine targeting all major muscle groups.

Weekly Workout Schedule:

Day 1: Full-Body Strength Training

- Squats: 3 sets of 8-10 reps
- Bench Press: 3 sets of 8-10 reps
- Bent-Over Rows: 3 sets of 8-10 reps
- Dumbbell Lunges: 3 sets of 10 reps per leg
- Planks: 3 sets of 30-60 seconds

Day 2: Rest or Low-Intensity Activity

Day 3: Upper Body Strength

- Pull-Ups or Lat Pulldowns: 3 sets of 8-10 reps
- Push-Ups or Chest Flyes: 3 sets of 8-10 reps
- Dumbbell Bicep Curls: 3 sets of 10-12 reps
- Tricep Dips: 3 sets of 10-12 reps

Day 4: Rest or Low-Intensity Activity

Day 5: Lower Body Strength

- Deadlifts: 3 sets of 8-10 reps
- Leg Press: 3 sets of 8-10 reps
- Leg Curls: 3 sets of 10 reps
- Standing Calf Raises: 3 sets of 12-15 reps

Day 6: Rest or Low-Intensity Activity

Day 7: Full-Body Strength Training (Different Exercises)

- Romanian Deadlifts: 3 sets of 8-10 reps
- Incline Bench Press: 3 sets of 8-10 reps
- Pull-Ups or Lat Pulldowns: 3 sets of 8-10 reps
- Leg Press: 3 sets of 8-10 reps
- Planks: 3 sets of 30-60 seconds

Workout Tips:

- Focus on compound exercises that target multiple muscle groups.
- Lift with proper form and gradually increase weights as you progress.
- Perform each exercise with controlled movements and a full range of motion.
- Rest for 1-2 minutes between sets.
- Stay hydrated and ensure adequate nutrition to support muscle growth.

Additional Tips:

- Consume a protein-rich diet to support muscle recovery and growth.
- Ensure you are in a slight calorie surplus to facilitate muscle gain.
- Get enough sleep to aid recovery and muscle repair.
- Consider consulting a fitness professional for personalized guidance.

ECTOMORPH: BUILDING STRENGTH AND TONING

This workout plan is designed to help Ectomorphs build strength and achieve a toned physique. It includes a structured strength training routine, dietary guidance for maintaining balance, and a focus on recovery for optimal strength development.

Strength Training Routine:

- **Frequency:** 3-4 days a week.
- **Duration:** 45-60 minutes per session.
- **Exercises:** Focus on compound movements like squats, deadlifts, bench presses, and rows. Aim for 3-4 sets of 8-12 repetitions.
- **Rest:** Allow 48 hours of rest between working the same muscle group.

Dietary Guidance:

- Maintain a balanced diet with a focus on lean proteins, complex carbohydrates, and healthy fats.
- Monitor calorie intake to support strength gains without a significant surplus.
- Macro Ratio:
    - Protein: 30-40% of total daily calories
    - Carbohydrates: 40-50% of total daily calories
    - Fats: 20-30% of total daily calories

Recovery and Rest:

- Stay well-hydrated throughout the day.
- Ensure 7-9 hours of quality sleep per night.
- Incorporate active recovery days with light activities like walking or yoga.

ECTOMORPH WORKOUT PLAN: BUILDING STRENGTH AND TONING

Goal: Build Strength and Achieve Toning
Ectomorphs, your quest to strength and toning starts here. This specialized workout plan emphasizes strength-building exercises with a focus on compound movements.

Weekly Workout Schedule:

Day 1: Full-Body Strength Training
- Squats: 4 sets of 6-8 reps
- Bench Press: 4 sets of 6-8 reps
- Bent-Over Rows: 4 sets of 6-8 reps
- Leg Press: 3 sets of 10 reps
- Planks: 3 sets of 30-60 seconds

Day 2: Rest or Low-Intensity Activity

Day 3: Upper Body Strength
- Pull-Ups: 4 sets of 6-8 reps
- Push-Ups: 4 sets of 6-8 reps
- Dumbbell Bicep Curls: 3 sets of 8-10 reps
- Tricep Dips: 3 sets of 8-10 reps

Day 4: Rest or Low-Intensity Activity

Day 5: Lower Body Strength
- Deadlifts: 4 sets of 6-8 reps
- Leg Press: 4 sets of 6-8 reps
- Leg Curls: 3 sets of 8-10 reps
- Standing Calf Raises: 3 sets of 10-12 reps

Day 6: Rest or Low-Intensity Activity

Day 7: Full-Body Strength Training (Different Exercises)
- Romanian Deadlifts: 4 sets of 6-8 reps
- Incline Bench Press: 4 sets of 6-8 reps
- Pull-Ups: 4 sets of 6-8 reps
- Leg Press: 4 sets of 6-8 reps
- Planks: 3 sets of 30-60 seconds

Workout Tips:
- Focus on compound exercises that target multiple muscle groups.
- Lift with proper form and gradually increase weights as you progress.
- Perform each exercise with controlled movements and a full range of motion.
- Rest for 1-2 minutes between sets.
- Stay hydrated and ensure adequate nutrition to support strength development.

Additional Tips:

- Consume a protein-rich diet to support muscle recovery and growth.
- Ensure you are in a slight calorie surplus or maintenance level.
- Get enough sleep to aid recovery and muscle repair.
- Consider consulting a fitness professional for personalized guidance.

ECTOMORPH: WEIGHT MANAGEMENT AND FAT LOSS

This workout plan is designed to help Ectomorphs effectively manage their weight and reduce body fat. It combines cardio and strength training to enhance calorie burn, along with dietary guidance for calorie control. Proper hydration and recovery are emphasized for successful weight management and fat loss.

Cardio and Strength Training:

- **Frequency**: 4-6 days a week.
- **Duration**: 30-60 minutes per session.
- **Exercises**: Combine cardio workouts like running, cycling, or swimming with strength training exercises. Include compound movements for full-body workouts.
- **Intensity**: Aim for a mix of moderate-intensity cardio and strength exercises.

Dietary Guidance

- Maintain a balanced diet with portion control and emphasis on whole, nutrient-dense foods.
- Create a calorie deficit to support weight management and fat loss.
- Macros Ratio:
  - Protein: 30-40% of total daily calories
  - Carbohydrates: 30-40% of total daily calories
  - Fats: 30-40% of total daily calories

Rest and Recovery:

- Stay well-hydrated throughout the day.
- Allow at least 24 hours of rest between high-intensity workouts.

ECTOMORPH WORKOUT PLAN: WEIGHT MANAGEMENT AND FAT LOSS

Goal: *Effective Weight Management and Fat Loss*
For Ectomorphs looking to manage their weight and reduce body fat, this plan combines cardio and strength training for optimal calorie burn.

Weekly Workout Schedule:

Day 1: Cardio and Strength Training

- 30 minutes of moderate-intensity cardio (e.g., running, cycling)
- Followed by 30 minutes of strength training focusing on full body exercises
- Squats: 3 sets of 10-12 reps
- Push-Ups: 3 sets of 10-12 reps
- Planks: 3 sets of 30 seconds

Day 2: Rest or Low-Intensity Activity

Day 3: Cardio and Strength Training

- 30 minutes of moderate-intensity cardio (e.g., brisk walking, swimming, elliptical machine)
- Followed by 30 minutes of strength training targeting all major muscle groups
- Deadlifts: 3 sets of 10-12 reps
- Pull-Ups: 3 sets of 10-12 reps
- Leg Press: 3 sets of 10-12 reps

Day 4: Rest or Low-Intensity Activity

Day 5: Cardio and Full-Body Strength Training

- 30 minutes of moderate-intensity cardio (e.g., elliptical)
- Followed by 30 minutes of strength training emphasizing compound movements
- Bench Press: 3 sets of 10-12 reps
- Bent-Over Rows: 3 sets of 10-12 reps
- Lunges: 3 sets of 12-15 reps

Day 6: Rest or Low-Intensity Activity

Day 7: Cardio and Strength Training (Different Exercises)

- 30 minutes of moderate-intensity cardio (e.g., stationary bike)
- Followed by 30 minutes of strength training, incorporating isolation exercises for specific muscle groups
- Dumbbell Bicep Curls: 3 sets of 10-12 reps
- Tricep Dips: 3 sets of 10-12 reps
- Standing Calf Raises: 3 sets of 12-15 reps

Workout Tips:

- Incorporate both steady-state cardio and high-intensity interval training (HIIT) for effective fat burning.
- Perform strength training exercises with controlled movements and a full range of motion.
- Rest for 1-2 minutes between strength training sets.
- Stay well-hydrated throughout the day.
- Focus on maintaining a calorie deficit through diet for successful weight management and fat loss.

Additional Tips:

- Follow a balanced diet with portion control and emphasis on whole, nutrient-dense foods.
- Monitor portion sizes and avoid excessive calorie consumption.
- Ensure 7-9 hours of quality sleep per night.
- Include active recovery days with low-intensity activities like walking or yoga.

Mesomorph

Mesomorphs tend to have a naturally athletic build, making it easier to gain muscle and lose fat. The focus should be on a balanced mix of strength training and cardiovascular exercise to maintain muscle mass and keep body fat in check. Following the initial workout plan, there are customized plans designed to enhance muscle gain, strength building, and effective weight management.

MESOMORPH: BUILDING STRENGTH AND TONING

This workout plan helps Mesomorphs build strength and tone their physique effectively through a balanced approach to training, nutrition, and recovery. Customize it based on individual preferences and progress.

Mixed Training Plan:

- **Frequency**: 3-5 days a week.
- **Duration:** 30-60 minutes per session.
- Exercises: Combine strength training with aerobic exercises like running or cycling. Include compound exercises for full-body workouts.
- **Repetitions**: 3-4 sets of 8-15 repetitions.

Balanced Diet:

- Maintain a balanced diet with a slight calorie surplus or maintenance level.
- Include a variety of nutrients from lean proteins, whole grains, fruits, and vegetables.
- Macros Ratio:
    - Protein: 25-35% of total daily calories
    - Carbohydrates: 40-50% of total daily calories
    - Fats: 20-30% of total daily calories

Flexibility and Recovery:

- Stay well-hydrated throughout the day.
- Add stretching and flexibility exercises to your routine.
- Allow at least 48 hours of rest between intense strength workouts.

MESOMORPH WORKOUT PLAN: BUILDING STRENGTH AND TONING

Goal: Build Strength and Achieve Toned Physique
Mesomorphs, this plan is designed to help you build strength and achieve a toned physique effectively.

Weekly Workout Schedule:

Day 1: Full-Body Strength and Toning
- Squats: 4 sets of 8-10 reps
- Bench Press: 4 sets of 8-10 reps
- Pull-Ups or Lat Pulldowns: 3 sets of 8-10 reps
- Lunges: 3 sets of 10 reps per leg
- Planks: 3 sets of 30-60 seconds

Day 2: Rest or Low-Intensity Activity

Day 3: Upper Body Strength and Toning
- Push-Ups or Chest Flyes: 4 sets of 8-10 reps
- Bent-Over Rows: 4 sets of 8-10 reps
- Dumbbell Bicep Curls: 3 sets of 10-12 reps
- Tricep Dips: 3 sets of 10-12 reps

Day 4: Rest or Low-Intensity Activity

Day 5: Lower Body Strength and Toning
- Deadlifts: 4 sets of 8-10 reps
- Leg Press: 4 sets of 8-10 reps
- Leg Curls: 3 sets of 10 reps
- Standing Calf Raises: 3 sets of 12-15 reps

Day 6: Rest or Low-Intensity Activity

Day 7: Full-Body Strength and Toning (Different Exercises)
- Romanian Deadlifts: 4 sets of 8-10 reps
- Incline Bench Press: 4 sets of 8-10 reps
- Pull-Ups or Lat Pulldowns: 3 sets of 8-10 reps
- Leg Press: 3 sets of 8-10 reps
- Planks: 3 sets of 30-60 seconds

Workout Tips:
- Emphasize compound exercises that engage multiple muscle groups.
- Ensure proper form and gradually increase weights as you progress.
- Perform exercises with controlled movements and a full range of motion.
- Allow 1-2 minutes of rest between sets.

- Maintain proper hydration and ensure adequate nutrition to support muscle growth.

Additional Tips:

- Consume a balanced diet with a slight calorie surplus or maintenance level.
- Include a variety of nutrients from lean proteins, whole grains, fruits, and vegetables.
- Stay well-hydrated throughout the day.
- Incorporate stretching and flexibility exercises into your routine.
- Allow at least 48 hours of rest between intense strength workouts.

MESOMORPH: MUSCLE GAIN AND INCREASED WEIGHT

This workout plan is designed to help Mesomorphs gain muscle and increase weight effectively. It includes a structured strength training routine, dietary guidance for a calorie surplus, and a focus on recovery for optimal muscle growth. Customize it to fit individual preferences and progress.

Strength Training Routine:

- **Frequency**: 4-5 days a week.
- **Duration**: 45-60 minutes per session.
- **Exercises**: Focus on compound movements and muscle isolation exercises.
- **Sets and Repetitions:** Aim for 4-5 sets of 6-10 repetitions.
- **Rest**: Allow 48 hours of rest between working the same muscle group.

Dietary Guidance:

- Consume a calorie surplus to support muscle gain.
- Prioritize lean proteins, complex carbohydrates, and healthy fats.
- Consider protein shakes or weight gainer supplements.
- Macros Ratio:
  - Protein: 25-35% of total daily calories
  - Carbohydrates: 40-50% of total daily calories
  - Fats: 20-30% of total daily calories

Recovery and Rest:

- Stay well-hydrated throughout the day.
- Ensure 7-9 hours of quality sleep per night.
- Include active recovery days with light activities like walking or yoga.

MESOMORPH WORKOUT PLAN: MUSCLE GAIN AND INCREASED WEIGHT

Goal: Build Muscle Mass and Increase Weight
Mesomorphs, this structured workout plan is your ticket to gaining muscle mass and increasing weight effectively.

Weekly Workout Schedule:

Day 1: Full-Body Strength and Muscle Building

- Squats: 4 sets of 6-8 reps
- Bench Press: 4 sets of 6-8 reps
- Pull-Ups or Lat Pulldowns: 4 sets of 6-8 reps
- Lunges: 3 sets of 8 reps per leg
- Planks: 3 sets of 30-60 seconds

Day 2: Rest or Low-Intensity Activity

Day 3: Upper Body Strength and Muscle Building

- Push-Ups or Chest Flyes: 4 sets of 6-8 reps
- Bent-Over Rows: 4 sets of 6-8 reps
- Dumbbell Bicep Curls: 3 sets of 8-10 reps
- Tricep Dips: 3 sets of 8-10 reps

Day 4: Rest or Low-Intensity Activity

Day 5: Lower Body Strength and Muscle Building

- Deadlifts: 4 sets of 6-8 reps
- Leg Press: 4 sets of 6-8 reps
- Leg Curls: 3 sets of 8 reps
- Standing Calf Raises: 3 sets of 10-12 reps

Day 6: Rest or Low-Intensity Activity

Day 7: Full-Body Strength and Muscle Building (Different Exercises)

- Romanian Deadlifts: 4 sets of 6-8 reps
- Incline Bench Press: 4 sets of 6-8 reps
- Pull-Ups or Lat Pulldowns: 4 sets of 6-8 reps
- Leg Press: 3 sets of 8-10 reps
- Planks: 3 sets of 30-60 seconds

Workout Tips:

- Focus on compound exercises that target multiple muscle groups.
- Lift with proper form and gradually increase weights as you progress.
- Perform each exercise with controlled movements and a full range of motion.
- Allow 1-2 minutes of rest between sets.
- Stay well-hydrated throughout the day.
- Ensure adequate nutrition to support muscle growth.

Additional Tips:

- Consume a calorie surplus to facilitate muscle gain and weight increase.
- Prioritize lean proteins, complex carbohydrates, and healthy fats in your diet.
- Consider incorporating protein shakes or weight gainer supplements.

- Ensure 7-9 hours of quality sleep per night.
- Include active recovery days with light activities like walking or yoga.

MESOMORPH: WEIGHT MANAGEMENT AND FAT LOSS

This plan is designed to help Mesomorphs effectively manage their weight and reduce body fat. It combines cardio and strength training to enhance calorie burn, along with dietary guidance for calorie control. Proper hydration and recovery are emphasized for successful weight management and fat loss. Customize the plan to align with individual preferences and goals.

Cardio and Strength Training Routine:

- **Frequency**: 4-6 days a week.
- **Duration**: Alternate between 30-45 minutes of cardiovascular exercise (e.g., running, cycling) and 30-45 minutes of strength training on different days.
- **Cardio Intensity:** Include both steady-state and high-intensity interval training (HIIT) sessions for fat burning.

Dietary Guidance:

- Consume a calorie deficit to support fat loss.
- Emphasize lean proteins, vegetables, and whole grains.
- Monitor portion sizes and avoid excessive calorie consumption.
- Macros Ratio:
  - Protein: 25-35% of total daily calories
  - Carbohydrates: 30-40% of total daily calories
  - Fats: 30-40% of total daily calories

Recovery and Rest:

- Stay well-hydrated throughout the day.
- Ensure 7-9 hours of quality sleep per night.
- Incorporate active recovery days with low-intensity activities like walking or yoga.

MESOMORPH WORKOUT PLAN: WEIGHT MANAGEMENT AND FAT LOSS

Goal: Effective Weight Management and Fat Loss
Mesomorphs, with your balanced physique, you can effectively manage your weight and reduce body fat with this structured workout plan.

Weekly Workout Schedule:

Day 1: Cardio and Strength Training

- Warm-up: 10 minutes of light jogging or cycling
- Cardio: 30 minutes of moderate-intensity running or cycling

- Strength Training:
    - Push-Ups or Chest Press: 3 sets of 10-12 reps
    - Bent-Over Rows: 3 sets of 10-12 reps
    - Bodyweight Squats: 3 sets of 12-15 reps
- Cool-down: 5 minutes of stretching

Day 2: Rest or Low-Intensity Activity

Day 3: Cardio and Strength Training

- Warm-up: 10 minutes of light jogging or cycling
- Cardio: 30 minutes of high-intensity interval training (HIIT) alternating between sprinting and walking or cycling
- Strength Training:
    - Pull-Ups or Lat Pulldowns: 3 sets of 10-12 reps
    - Dumbbell Lunges: 3 sets of 10 reps per leg
    - Planks: 3 sets of 30-60 seconds
- Cool-down: 5 minutes of stretching

Day 4: Rest or Low-Intensity Activity

Day 5: Cardio and Strength Training

- Warm-up: 10 minutes of light jogging or cycling
- Cardio: 30 minutes of steady-state running or cycling at a moderate pace
- Strength Training:
    - Leg Press: 3 sets of 10-12 reps
    - Dumbbell Bicep Curls: 3 sets of 12-15 reps
    - Tricep Dips: 3 sets of 12-15 reps
- Cool-down: 5 minutes of stretching

Day 6: Rest or Low-Intensity Activity

Day 7: Active Recovery

- Engage in low-intensity activities like walking, swimming, or yoga for 30-45 minutes to aid recovery and promote flexibility.

Workout Tips:

- Alternate between cardiovascular exercises and strength training for effective fat burning.
- Maintain proper form and technique during strength exercises.
- Gradually increase the intensity of cardio workouts.
- Incorporate HIIT sessions to boost metabolism and fat loss.
- Allow 1-2 minutes of rest between strength training sets.
- Stay well-hydrated throughout the day.
- Monitor portion sizes and maintain a calorie deficit for weight management.

Additional Tips:

- Follow a balanced diet emphasizing lean proteins, vegetables, and whole grains.
- Avoid excessive calorie consumption and practice portion control.
- Ensure 7-9 hours of quality sleep per night.
- Include active recovery days for overall well-being.
- Consult with a fitness professional for personalized guidance if needed.

Endomorph

Endomorphs typically have a higher body fat percentage and may find it more challenging to lose weight. The focus for endomorphs should be on a combination of strength training and cardio to boost metabolism, burn calories, and improve overall fitness. Beyond the initial workout plan, there are additional plans for endomorphs that focus on building strength, toning, and achieving sustainable fat loss.

ENDOMORPH: MUSCLE GAIN AND INCREASED WEIGHT

This plan is designed to help Endomorphs gain muscle and increase weight effectively. It includes a structured strength training routine, dietary guidance for a calorie surplus, and a focus on recovery for optimal muscle growth. Customize it to fit individual preferences and progress.

Strength Training Routine:

- **Frequency**: 4-5 days a week.
- **Duration**: 45-60 minutes per session.
- **Exercises:** Focus on compound movements and muscle isolation exercises.
- **Sets and Repetitions:** Aim for 4-5 sets of 6-10 repetitions.
- **Rest**: Allow 48 hours of rest between working the same muscle group.

Dietary Guidance:

- Consume a calorie surplus to support muscle gain.
- Prioritize lean proteins, complex carbohydrates, and healthy fats.
- Consider protein shakes or weight gainer supplements.
- Macros Ratio:
    - Protein: 20-30% of total daily calories
    - Carbohydrates: 40-50% of total daily calories
    - Fats: 30-40% of total daily calories

Recovery and Rest:

- Stay well-hydrated throughout the day.
- Ensure 7-9 hours of quality sleep per night.
- Include active recovery days with light activities like walking or yoga.

ENDOMORPH WORKOUT PLAN: MUSCLE GAIN AND INCREASED WEIGHT

Goal: Build Lean Muscle Mass and Increase Weight
Endomorphs, who may have a tendency to store fat and find it challenging to gain muscle, can follow this workout plan to build lean muscle mass effectively and support weight gain.

Weekly Workout Schedule:

Day 1: Full-Body Strength Training

- Squats: 4 sets of 8-10 reps
- Bench Press: 4 sets of 8-10 reps
- Bent-Over Rows: 4 sets of 8-10 reps
- Dumbbell Lunges: 4 sets of 10 reps per leg
- Planks: 4 sets of 30-60 seconds

Day 2: Rest or Low-Intensity Activity

Day 3: Upper Body Strength

- Pull-Ups or Lat Pulldowns: 4 sets of 8-10 reps
- Push-Ups or Chest Flyes: 4 sets of 8-10 reps
- Dumbbell Bicep Curls: 4 sets of 10-12 reps
- Tricep Dips: 4 sets of 10-12 reps

Day 4: Rest or Low-Intensity Activity

Day 5: Lower Body Strength

- Deadlifts: 4 sets of 8-10 reps
- Leg Press: 4 sets of 8-10 reps
- Leg Curls: 4 sets of 10 reps
- Standing Calf Raises: 4 sets of 12-15 reps

Day 6: Rest or Low-Intensity Activity

Day 7: Full-Body Strength Training (Different Exercises)

- Romanian Deadlifts: 4 sets of 8-10 reps
- Incline Bench Press: 4 sets of 8-10 reps
- Pull-Ups or Lat Pulldowns: 4 sets of 8-10 reps
- Leg Press: 4 sets of 8-10 reps
- Planks: 4 sets of 30-60 seconds

Workout Tips:

- Focus on compound exercises that engage multiple muscle groups.
- Lift with proper form and progressively increase weights as you progress.
- Execute each exercise with controlled movements and a full range of motion.
- Rest for 1-2 minutes between sets.

- Stay well-hydrated throughout the day.
- Ensure proper nutrition to support muscle growth and recovery.

Additional Tips:

- Consume a protein-rich diet to facilitate muscle recovery and growth.
- Maintain a slight calorie surplus to support weight gain.
- Get 7-9 hours of quality sleep each night for muscle repair and growth.
- Incorporate active recovery days with low-intensity activities like walking or yoga.
- Consider seeking guidance from a fitness professional for personalized assistance.

ENDOMORPH: BUILDING STRENGTH AND TONING

This plan is designed to help Endomorphs build strength and tone their physique effectively through a balanced approach to training, nutrition, and recovery. Customize it based on individual preferences and progress.

Strength Training Routine:

- **Frequency**: 3-5 days a week.
- **Duration**: 30-60 minutes per session.
- **Exercises:** Combine strength training with aerobic exercises like running or cycling. Include compound exercises for full-body workouts.
- **Sets and Repetitions:** 3-4 sets of 8-15 repetitions.
- **Rest:** Allow at least 48 hours of rest between intense strength workouts.

Dietary Guidance:

- Maintain a balanced diet with a slight calorie surplus or maintenance level.
- Include a variety of nutrients from lean proteins, whole grains, fruits, and vegetables.
- Macros Ratio:
    - Protein: 20-30% of total daily calories
    - Carbohydrates: 40-50% of total daily calories
    - Fats: 30-40% of total daily calories

Recovery and Rest:

- Stay well-hydrated throughout the day.
- Add stretching and flexibility exercises to your routine.
- Allow at least 48 hours of rest between intense strength workouts.

ENDOMORPH WORKOUT PLAN: BUILDING STRENGTH AND TONING

Goal: *Build Strength and Achieve Toning*
Endomorphs, you can build strength and achieve a toned physique effectively while maintaining a balanced approach to training, nutrition, and recovery by following this workout plan.

Weekly Workout Schedule:

Day 1: Full-Body Strength Training
- Squats: 4 sets of 8-10 reps
- Bench Press: 4 sets of 8-10 reps
- Bent-Over Rows: 4 sets of 8-10 reps
- Dumbbell Lunges: 4 sets of 10 reps per leg
- Planks: 4 sets of 30-60 seconds

Day 2: Rest or Low-Intensity Activity

Day 3: Upper Body Strength
- Pull-Ups or Lat Pulldowns: 4 sets of 8-10 reps
- Push-Ups or Chest Flyes: 4 sets of 8-10 reps
- Dumbbell Bicep Curls: 4 sets of 10-12 reps
- Tricep Dips: 4 sets of 10-12 reps

Day 4: Rest or Low-Intensity Activity

Day 5: Lower Body Strength
- Deadlifts: 4 sets of 8-10 reps
- Leg Press: 4 sets of 8-10 reps
- Leg Curls: 4 sets of 10 reps
- Standing Calf Raises: 4 sets of 12-15 reps

Day 6: Rest or Low-Intensity Activity

Day 7: Full-Body Strength Training (Different Exercises)
- Romanian Deadlifts: 4 sets of 8-10 reps
- Incline Bench Press: 4 sets of 8-10 reps
- Pull-Ups or Lat Pulldowns: 4 sets of 8-10 reps
- Leg Press: 4 sets of 8-10 reps
- Planks: 4 sets of 30-60 seconds

Workout Tips:
- Focus on compound exercises that work multiple muscle groups.
- Maintain proper form and gradually increase weights as you progress.
- Execute each exercise with controlled movements and a full range of motion.
- Rest for 1-2 minutes between sets.
- Stay well-hydrated throughout the day.
- Ensure a balanced diet with a focus on nutrient-dense foods.

Additional Tips:
- Include stretching and flexibility exercises in your routine.
- Allow at least 48 hours of rest between intense strength workouts.
- Aim to maintain a balanced diet with a slight calorie surplus or maintenance level.
- Get 7-9 hours of quality sleep each night for muscle recovery.
- Incorporate active recovery days with low-intensity activities like walking or yoga.

ENDOMORPH: WEIGHT MANAGEMENT AND FAT LOSS

This plan is designed to help Endomorphs effectively manage their weight and reduce body fat. It combines cardio and strength training to enhance calorie burn, along with dietary guidance for calorie control. Proper hydration and recovery are emphasized for successful weight management and fat loss. Customize the plan to align with individual preferences and goals.

Cardio and Strength Training Routine:

- **Frequency**: 4-6 days a week.
- **Duration**: Alternate between 30-45 minutes of cardiovascular exercise (e.g., running, cycling) and 30-45 minutes of strength training on different days.
- **Cardio Intensity**: Include both steady-state and high-intensity interval training (HIIT) sessions for fat burning.

Dietary Guidance:

- Consume a calorie deficit to support fat loss.
- Emphasize lean proteins, vegetables, and whole grains.
- Monitor portion sizes and avoid excessive calorie consumption.
- Macros Ratio:
    - Protein: 20-30% of total daily calories
    - Carbohydrates: 30-40% of total daily calories
    - Fats: 30-40% of total daily calories

Flexibility and Recovery:

- Stay well-hydrated throughout the day.
- Ensure 7-9 hours of quality sleep per night.
- Incorporate active recovery days with low-intensity activities like walking or yoga.

ENDOMORPH WORKOUT PLAN: WEIGHT MANAGEMENT AND FAT LOSS

Goal: Effective Weight Management and Fat Loss
Endomorphs, you can effectively manage your weight and reduce body fat with this structured workout plan.

Weekly Workout Schedule:

Day 1: Full-Body Strength and Cardio

- Squats: 3 sets of 8-10 reps
- Push-Ups: 3 sets of 8-10 reps
- Bent-Over Rows: 3 sets of 8-10 reps
- Planks: 3 sets of 30-60 seconds
- Cardio: 30-40 minutes of moderate-intensity (e.g., brisk walking or cycling)

Day 2: Rest or Low-Intensity Activity

Day 3: Upper Body Strength and Cardio

- Pull-Ups or Lat Pulldowns: 3 sets of 8-10 reps
- Bench Press: 3 sets of 8-10 reps
- Dumbbell Bicep Curls: 3 sets of 10-12 reps
- Tricep Dips: 3 sets of 10-12 reps
- Cardio: 30-40 minutes of moderate-intensity (e.g., brisk walking or cycling)

Day 4: Rest or Low-Intensity Activity

Day 5: Lower Body Strength and Cardio

- Deadlifts: 3 sets of 8-10 reps
- Leg Press: 3 sets of 8-10 reps
- Leg Curls: 3 sets of 10 reps
- Standing Calf Raises: 3 sets of 12-15 reps
- Cardio: 30-40 minutes of moderate-intensity (e.g., brisk walking or cycling)

Day 6: Rest or Low-Intensity Activity

Day 7: Full-Body Strength and Cardio (Different Exercises)

- Romanian Deadlifts: 3 sets of 8-10 reps
- Incline Bench Press: 3 sets of 8-10 reps
- Pull-Ups or Lat Pulldowns: 3 sets of 8-10 reps
- Leg Press: 3 sets of 8-10 reps
- Planks: 3 sets of 30-60 seconds
- Cardio: 30-40 minutes of moderate-intensity (e.g., brisk walking or cycling)

Workout Tips:

- Focus on compound exercises to engage multiple muscle groups.
- Use proper form and progressively increase the weights.
- Perform exercises with controlled movements and full range of motion.
- Rest for 1-2 minutes between sets.
- Stay hydrated and maintain a balanced diet.

Additional Tips:

- Create a calorie deficit through diet and exercise to support fat loss.
- Emphasize lean proteins, vegetables, and whole grains in your diet.
- Monitor portion sizes and avoid excessive calorie consumption.
- Ensure you stay well-hydrated throughout the day.
- Get 7-9 hours of quality sleep each night.
- Incorporate active recovery days with low-intensity activities like walking or yoga.

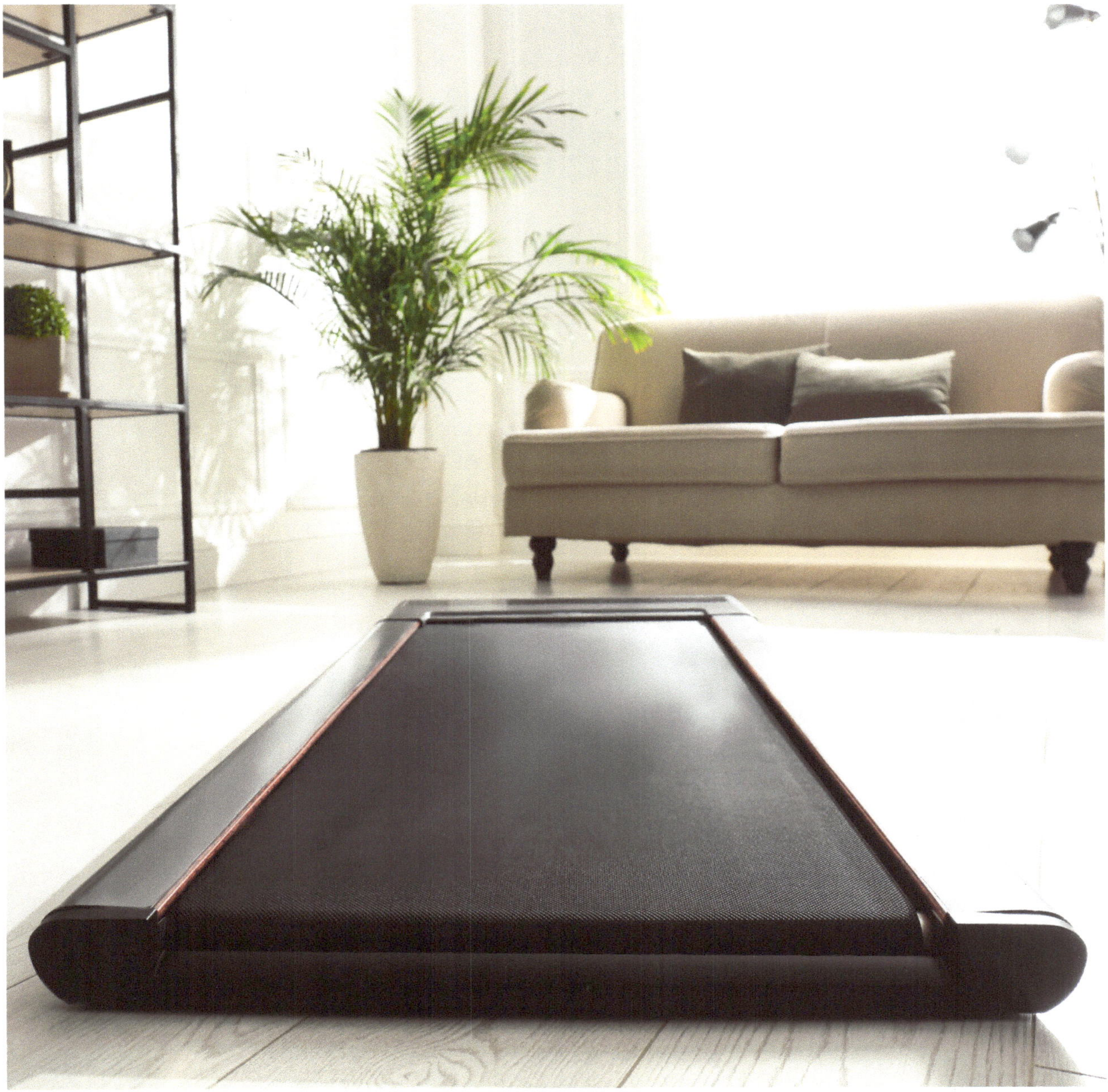

"Wellness Insights: *Did You Know?*"

- ***Did you know...*** that regular exercise not only strengthens your muscles but also improves your mood and boosts your energy levels?
- ***Did you know...*** that walking is a simple and accessible way to start your fitness journey? Incorporating walking into your daily routine can help with weight loss, improve cardiovascular health, and boost overall fitness. Start by walking for 10-15 minutes a day at a comfortable pace, and gradually increase the duration and intensity as you build endurance.

COMPREHENSIVE LIST OF Exercises and Mind-Body Practices

In addition to your tailored workout plans, here is a comprehensive list of exercises and mind-body practices. This list includes a wide variety of movements and techniques to support all aspects of fitness, from strength and cardio to flexibility, balance, and mental well-being. Use this as a resource to diversify your workouts and enhance your overall fitness journey.

LIST OF EXERCISES:

Lower Body Strength, Upper Body Strength, Cardio for Low-Intensity, Cardio for High-Intensity:

Lower Body Strength	Upper Body Strength	Cardio for Low-Intensity	Cardio for High-Intensity
Squats Deadlifts Leg Press Lunges (Forward, Reverse, Walking) Leg Curls (Machine or Dumbbell) Standing Calf Raises Romanian Deadlifts Box Jumps Step-Ups Glute Bridges	Bench Press (Barbell or Dumbbell) Pull-Ups Lat Pulldowns Rows (Bent-Over, Seated) Push-Ups Dumbbell Bicep Curls Tricep Dips Shoulder Press (Barbell or Dumbbell) Chest Flyes Lateral Raises	Brisk Walking Cycling (Leisurely) Swimming (Leisurely) Elliptical Machine (Low Resistance) Yoga Tai Chi Pilates Low-Intensity Aerobics Hiking (Easy Trails) Stretching Exercises	Running Sprinting High-Intensity Interval Training (HIIT) Jump Rope Cycling (High Intensity/ Spinning) Swimming (Vigorous) Burpees Mountain Climbers Tabata Workouts CrossFit Workouts

Compound Movements/Exercises, Isolation Exercises, Core and Abdominal Exercises:

Compound Movements/ Exercises	Isolation Exercises	Core and Abdominal Exercises
Squats Deadlifts Bench Press Pull-Ups Lat Pulldowns Rows (Various Types) Lunges Clean and Jerk Snatch Push Press	Bicep Curls (Dumbbell or Barbell) Tricep Extensions (Dumbbell or Barbell) Leg Curls Leg Extensions Dumbbell Flyes Lateral Raises Front Raises Calf Raises (Seated or Standing) Concentration Curls Tricep Kickbacks	Planks (Front and Side) Russian Twists Bicycle Crunches Leg Raises Sit-Ups V-Ups Medicine Ball Slams Hanging Leg Raises Woodchoppers Stability Ball Rollouts

"The journey of a thousand miles begins with a single step."

— *Lao Tzu*

Flexibility and Mobility Exercises, Balance and Stability, Core Strengthening Exercises, Functional Movement Patterns:

Flexibility and Mobility Exercises	Balance and Stability	Core Strengthening Exercises	Functional Movement Patterns
Yoga Poses (e.g., Downward Dog, Cobra) Pilates Movements (incorporates flexibility and core strength) Stretching Exercises (Dynamic and Static – e.g., leg swings, arm circles) Foam Rolling Resistance Band Mobility Drills Tai Chi Movements Active Isolated Stretching (AIS) Myofascial Release Techniques Mobility Circuits Feldenkrais Method Exercises	Single-Leg Balance Exercises (e.g., single-leg stands) Stability Ball Workouts (e.g., stability ball squats, planks) Balance Board Exercises Bosu Ball Exercises Yoga for Balance (e.g., Tree Pose, Warrior III) Standing Leg Swings Clock Lunges Balance Beam Walks Romanian Deadlifts with Dumbbells (for stability) Standing Medicine Ball Twists	Bicycle Crunches Russian Twists Leg Raises Plank Variations (e.g., side plank, forearm plank) Hanging Leg Raises (using a pull-up bar) Mountain Climbers V-Ups Swiss Ball Rollouts Windshield Wipers Captain's Chair Leg Raises	Squat to Press (simulates picking up an object) Lunge and Twist (simulates reaching for something) Farmer's Walk (carrying heavy objects) Pushing and Pulling Exercises (e.g., sled pushes, cable rows) Bodyweight Movements (e.g., climbing, crawling) Kettlebell Swings Medicine Ball Slams Tire Flips Box Jumps Sled Drags

> **"Strength does not come from physical capacity. It comes from an indomitable will."**
>
> — *Mahatma Gandhi*

MIND-BODY PRACTICES

1. **Yoga:** Yoga offers various styles, such as Hatha, Vinyasa, Ashtanga, Bikram, and more, to suit different preferences and fitness levels. It combines physical postures, breathing exercises, and meditation for holistic well-being. To get started with yoga, find a local class or use online resources to learn basic poses and sequences. Consider investing in a yoga mat for added comfort.

2. **Tai Chi:** This ancient Chinese martial art focuses on slow, flowing movements and deep breathing to enhance balance, flexibility, and relaxation. To begin Tai Chi, seek local classes or online tutorials. Wear loose, comfortable clothing and practice in a peaceful environment, like a park or quiet room.

3. **Qi Gong (Chi Kung)**: Qi Gong involves gentle movements, deep breathing, and meditation to cultivate and balance the body's vital energy (Qi or Chi). Explore Qi Gong through instructional videos or classes, ensuring a calm and focused setting for practice.

4. **Meditation:** Meditation techniques like mindfulness meditation, guided meditation, or others can help reduce stress, improve focus, and promote mental clarity. Start with short sessions and gradually increase meditation duration. Use meditation apps or guided recordings to assist you.

5. **Pilates:** While often considered a form of strength training, Pilates also emphasizes mindfulness, breathing, and body awareness. It can be an excellent choice for core strength and flexibility. Join a local Pilates class or follow online tutorials with a Pilates mat or equipment.

6. **Breathing Exercises**: Practice specific breathing techniques, such as diaphragmatic breathing or the 4-7-8 technique, to reduce stress and improve lung function. Learn these techniques through online resources and integrate them into your daily routine.

7. **Holistic Stretching:** Holistic stretching routines, like the Feldenkrais Method or Alexander Technique, focus on mindful movement, body awareness, and improving flexibility. Explore these practices with certified instructors or online tutorials.

8. **Mindful Walking:** This involves walking slowly and deliberately while paying attention to each step and your surroundings, promoting relaxation and mental clarity. Find a peaceful outdoor location, like a

park or nature trail, and practice mindful walking regularly.

9. **Body Scan:** Learn the body scan technique to systematically relax and release tension in different parts of the body. You can find guided body scan meditations online or consider enrolling in mindfulness programs that teach this technique.
10. **Visualization:** Visualization exercises involve creating mental images of peaceful and calming scenes to reduce stress and anxiety. Begin by finding a quiet space, close your eyes, and use guided visualization scripts or apps to help you practice.
11. **Progressive Muscle Relaxation:** This technique involves tensing and then relaxing different muscle groups to promote relaxation and reduce muscle tension. Find guided progressive muscle relaxation exercises online or consider therapy or counseling for more structured training.
12. **Holistic Mind-Body Classes:** Some fitness centers and studios offer holistic mind-body classes that combine various practices, allowing clients to explore different options. Check local listings for classes or explore online platforms that offer a variety of holistic classes.

TIPS FOR INCORPORATING Exercise into Daily Life

Incorporating exercise into your daily routine can seem challenging, but with a few practical strategies, it can become a seamless part of your lifestyle. Regardless of your body type, maintaining an active lifestyle is key for overall health and well-being. By finding activities you enjoy, setting realistic goals, and staying consistent, you can make exercise a regular and enjoyable part of your life.

- **Find Activities You Enjoy:** Choose exercises and activities that you find enjoyable. Whether it's dancing, hiking, or playing a sport, engaging in activities you love makes it easier to stay consistent.
- **Schedule Your Workouts:** Treat your workouts like important appointments. Schedule them into your calendar and commit to them as you would with any other meeting.
- **Set Realistic Goals:** Start with achievable goals and gradually increase the intensity and duration of your workouts. Setting realistic goals helps you stay motivated and track your progress.

- **Incorporate Movement Throughout the Day:** Look for opportunities to stay active throughout the day. Take the stairs instead of the elevator, walk or bike to nearby destinations, and take short activity breaks if you have a sedentary job.
- **Stay Consistent:** Consistency is key to achieving long-term fitness goals. Even on days when you feel less motivated, try to engage in some form of physical activity, even if it's just a short walk.
- **Find a Workout Buddy:** Exercising with a friend or joining a fitness community can provide accountability and make workouts more enjoyable.
- **Listen to Your Body:** Pay attention to how your body feels and adjust your workouts accordingly. Rest when needed and avoid overexertion to prevent injuries.

> **"It does not matter how slowly you go as long as you do not stop."**
>
> — *Confucius*

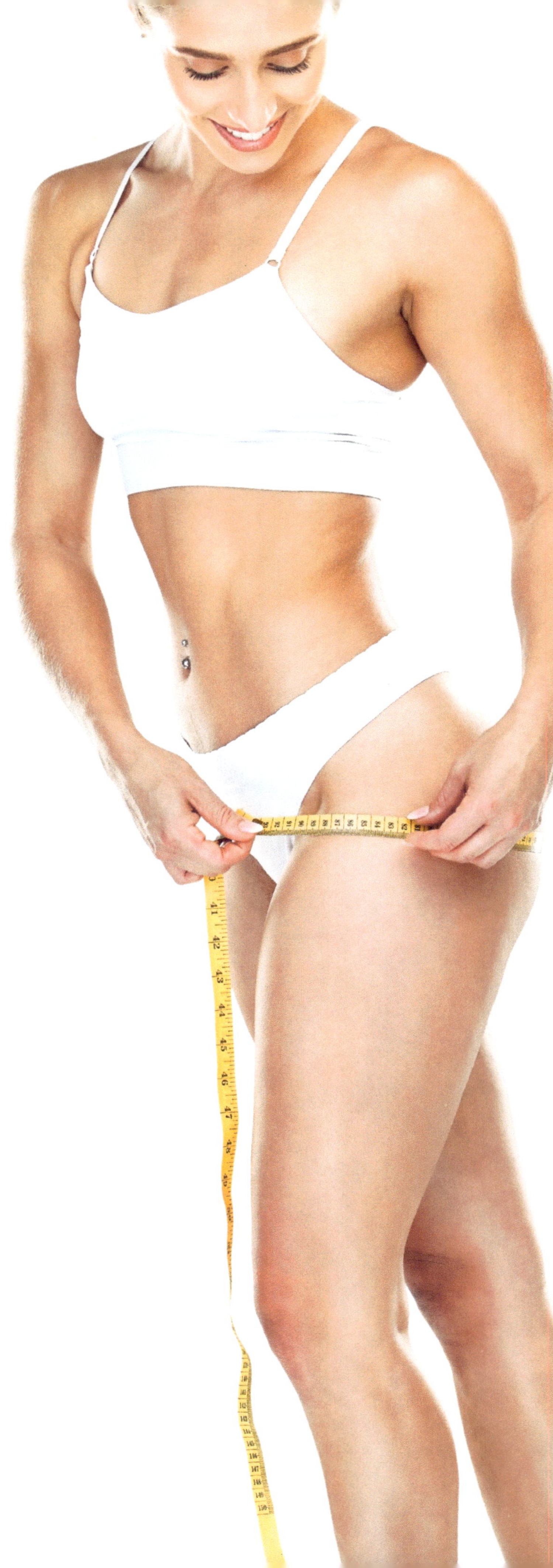

TRACKING AND Progress

WORKOUT TRACKER TEMPLATE

Keeping track of your progress is essential for staying motivated and reaching your wellness goals. This section provides tools and strategies to help you monitor your achievements and make adjustments as needed.

A workout tracker helps you log your exercise routines, monitor your performance, and identify areas for improvement. Here's an example of how to track and fill out the template for your weekly workout:

WEEKLY WORKOUT TRACKER EXAMPLE:

Day	Workout Type	Exercises Performed	Sets	Reps	Duration	Notes
Monday	Upper Body	Bench Press, Rows	4	10	45 mins	Felt strong, increased weight
Tuesday	Cardio	HIIT, Jump Rope	N/A	N/A	30 mins	High intensity, good sweat
Wednesday	Lower Body	Squats, Deadlifts	4	12	50 mins	Legs sore, need more stretching
Thursday	Rest		N/A	N/A	N/A	Rest day
Friday	Full Body	Kettlebell Swings, Push-Ups	3	15	40 mins	Increased reps, felt great
Saturday	Cardio	Cycling, Running	N/A	N/A	60 mins	Good endurance
Sunday	Rest		N/A	N/A	N/A	Rest day

Use the blank Weekly Workout Sheet template provided to log your workouts each week, noting the exercises performed, sets, reps, duration, and any relevant observations. This will help you stay organized and see your progress over time.

WORKOUT TRACKER

__/__/__

	Workout Type	Exercises Performed	Sets	Reps	Duration	Notes
Monday						
Tuesday						
Wednesday						
Thursday						
Friday						
Saturday						
Sunday						

DAILY MEAL LOG TEMPLATE

While you have a comprehensive meal plan provided in this book, this weekly meal tracker is offered for those who find it helpful to monitor their daily intake and make necessary adjustments. Some may choose to use this tracker to get started, while others may prefer to focus on learning how to listen to their body's cues without tracking. Use this tool if it supports your journey, but remember, the ultimate goal is to develop a healthy, balanced relationship with food and exercise.

Maintaining a meal and fitness log helps you keep track of your dietary habits and exercise routines, ensuring you stay on course towards your goals. Keeping your weekly workout sheets and daily meal trackers together provides a comprehensive overview of your progress. Here's an example of how to fill out your meal tracker:

DAILY MEAL LOG EXAMPLE:

Time	Meal/ Snack	Food and Drink Consumed	Portion Size	Calories	Notes
7:00 AM	Breakfast	Smoothie with Spinach and Banana	1 glass	250	Added extra spinach
10:00 AM	Snack	Greek Yogurt with Berries	1 cup	150	Felt full until lunch
12:30 PM	Lunch	Quinoa Salad with Chickpeas	1 bowl	400	Very satisfying
3:00 PM	Snack	Nuts and Dried Fruit	1 handful	200	Good energy boost
6:30 PM	Dinner	Baked Salmon with Asparagus	1 plate	500	Delicious and filling
8:30 PM	Snack	Dark Chocolate	2 squares	100	Indulgent treat

Use the blank Daily Meal Tracker template to log your meals and snacks each day. Note the portion sizes, calorie intake, and any observations about how you felt or adjustments you made.

DAILY MEAL TRACKER

___ / ___ / ___

Time	Meal	Food/Drink Consumed	Portion	Protein	Carbs	Fat	Calories
	Breakfast						
	Snack						
	Lunch						
	Snack						
	Dinner						
	Snack						

NOTES:

GOAL SETTING AND Progress Tracking

Achieving your fitness goals starts with setting clear, actionable objectives and consistently tracking your progress. Clear goals help you maintain motivation, measure your success, and make necessary adjustments along the way. By using the SMART criteria—Specific, Measurable, Achievable, Relevant, and Time-Bound—you can set effective goals and track your progress efficiently. Here's how:

SMART GOALS:

Specific: Clearly define your goal. Instead of saying "I want to get fit," specify "I want to run a 5K in 30 minutes."

Measurable: Ensure your goal can be measured. Track your progress with metrics such as weight, body measurements, or performance improvements.

Achievable: Set realistic goals that challenge you but are attainable. Consider your current fitness level and resources.

Relevant: Align your goals with your personal values and long-term objectives. Ensure they are meaningful to you.

Time-Bound: Set a deadline for achieving your goal. This creates a sense of urgency and helps you stay focused.

Example SMART Goal: "I will lose 10 pounds in 3 months by following a balanced diet and exercising 4 times a week."

SMART GOALS

When setting goals, ensure they follow the SMART structure. Use the questions below to create your goals. Start with five goals, but feel free to create as many as you like. Each goal should be detailed on a separate sheet, and you can track them on your Progress Tracking Sheet.

S	**SPECIFIC** WHAT SPECIFIC ASPECT OF MY HEALTH DO I WANT TO IMPROVE?	
M	**MEASURABLE** HOW WILL I MEASURE MY PROGRESS?	
A	**ACHIEVABLE** WHAT STEPS WILL I TAKE TO REACH THIS GOAL?	
R	**RELEVANT** WHY IS THIS GOAL IMPORTANT TO MY OVERALL HEALTH/WELLNESS?	
T	**TIME BOUND** WHAT IS MY DEADLINE FOR ACHIEVING THIS GOAL?	

TRACKING PROGRESS:

- Regular Check-Ins: Schedule regular check-ins (e.g., weekly or monthly) to assess your progress. Use measurements, photos, and performance metrics to evaluate your achievements.
- Adjust as Needed: If you're not seeing the desired progress, adjust your plan. This might involve changing your workout routine, modifying your diet, or setting new goals.
- Celebrate Milestones: Celebrate your achievements along the way. Recognizing your progress boosts motivation and reinforces positive behavior.

PROGRESS TRACKING SHEET

Here's an example of a progress tracking sheet to help you create your own:

Date	Goal	Current Status	Notes/Adjustments
January 1	Lose 10 pounds	150 pounds	Starting point
February 1	Lose 10 pounds	145 pounds	On track, keep it up
March 1	Lose 10 pounds	142 pounds	Adjust diet, increase cardio
April 1	Lose 10 pounds	140 pounds	Goal achieved, celebrate!

SECTION 13

ADDITIONAL
Resources

ONLINE SUPPORT AND Community Information

Building a support network and connecting with a community can significantly enhance your wellness journey. Here are some ways to find support and engage with like-minded individuals:

Join Online Communities:

- Evolutionary Body System Community: Join our online community to connect with others, share your progress, and find motivation. Participate in forums, join group challenges, and access exclusive content.
- Social Media Groups: Look for Facebook groups, Reddit communities, and other social media platforms focused on holistic wellness, nutrition, and fitness. Engaging with these groups can provide additional support and inspiration.

Attend Workshops and Webinars:

- Webinars: Participate in webinars hosted by wellness experts to gain deeper insights into various topics, such as nutrition, mindfulness, and fitness.
- Workshops: Attend local or virtual workshops that focus on holistic health practices. These events often provide practical tips and techniques to enhance your well-being.

Find a Mentor:

- Wellness Coaches and Practitioners: Consider working with a wellness coach or a Holistic Health Practitioner (HHP) who can provide personalized guidance and support. A coach or HHP can help you set goals, create action plans, and stay accountable. Many coaches and practitioners offer one-on-one or group support, providing valuable insights, shared experiences, and collective motivation to help you maintain a balanced lifestyle and overcome challenges.
- Mentorship Programs: Look for mentorship programs within wellness communities where experienced individuals offer guidance and support to newcomers.

FAQ'S

Frequently Asked Questions

Q: How can I start incorporating holistic wellness into my busy schedule?

- A: Start small by integrating one or two practices, such as mindful eating or a short daily meditation. Gradually add more as you become comfortable. Even simple changes, like drinking more water or taking a short walk during breaks, can make a big difference.

Q: Are the recipes in this guide suitable for people with dietary restrictions?

- A: Many recipes can be adapted for various dietary needs, such as gluten-free, dairy-free, or vegetarian. Always check the ingredients and make substitutions as necessary. Feel free to experiment and adjust recipes to suit your personal preferences and dietary requirements.

Q: How do I stay motivated to follow the meal and workout plans?

- A: Set clear, achievable goals and track your progress regularly. Celebrate small victories along the way and remind yourself of the benefits you're experiencing. Engaging with the community for support and accountability can also help you stay motivated.

Q: Can I still enjoy my favorite foods while following the holistic wellness guide?

- A: Absolutely! The 80/20 rule allows for flexibility and indulgence. Aim to make nutritious choices 80% of the time and enjoy your favorite treats in moderation. This approach helps maintain a balanced and sustainable lifestyle.

Q: How long will it take to see results from the holistic wellness practices?

- A: Everyone's journey is different, and results can vary based on individual factors. Consistency is key. Some people may start noticing changes within a few weeks, while others might take a bit longer. The important thing is to stay committed and patient with the process.

Q: What are the benefits of group coaching sessions?

- A: Group coaching sessions provide a supportive community environment where you can share experiences, gain insights from others, and stay motivated. These sessions offer collective accountability and the opportunity to learn from the diverse perspectives of group members.

Q: How do holistic health practices address mental well-being?

- A: Holistic health practices often include mindfulness, meditation, and stress management techniques that help improve mental clarity, reduce stress, and enhance emotional resilience. Integrating these practices can lead to a more balanced and fulfilling lifestyle.

Q: How do I handle setbacks in my wellness journey?

- A: Setbacks are a natural part of any journey. The key is to stay resilient and view them as learning opportunities. Adjust your goals if necessary, seek support from your community or coach, and remember to be patient with yourself as you progress.

SELF-CARE Practices

ESSENTIAL SELF-CARE PRACTICES

Taking time for self-care is essential for maintaining a balanced and healthy lifestyle. Incorporating these practices into your daily routine can help you manage stress, improve mental clarity, and enhance your overall well-being. Here are some essential self-care practices to support your holistic wellness journey:

Meditation:

Set aside 10-15 minutes each day for meditation. Find a quiet space, sit comfortably, and focus on your breath. Meditation helps reduce stress, improve focus, and enhance mental clarity.

Journaling:

Use journaling as a tool to process emotions, set goals, and reflect on your wellness journey. Spend a few minutes each day writing about your thoughts, experiences, and progress. This practice can provide valuable insights and promote emotional well-being.

Nature Walks:

Spend time in nature to rejuvenate your mind and body. Whether it's a walk in the park, a hike in the woods, or simply sitting in a garden, connecting with nature can reduce stress and improve your mood.

Deep Breathing Exercises:

Incorporate deep breathing exercises into your daily routine. Take slow, deep breaths in through your nose, hold for a few seconds, and exhale slowly through your mouth. This simple practice can help calm your mind and relax your body.

Digital Detox:

Take regular breaks from digital devices to reduce screen time and prevent burnout. Spend time engaging in activities that don't involve screens, such as reading a book, doing a puzzle, or enjoying a hobby.

Gratitude Practice:

Cultivate a gratitude practice by writing down three things you're grateful for each day. Focusing on the positive aspects of your life can improve your mood and overall outlook.

"Wellness Insights: *Did You Know?*"

» ***Did you know...*** that poor sleep can affect your hunger hormones and increase cravings for unhealthy foods?

4-WEEK WELLNESS TRANSFORMATION PLAN

To help you effectively implement the holistic health principles and self-care practices discussed, I've outlined a comprehensive 4-week plan. This plan will guide you week by week, focusing on nutrition, exercise, mindfulness, and self-care. By following this structured approach, you can ease into these practices, establishing a strong foundation for a healthier, more balanced lifestyle.

This plan serves as an accessible starting point to help you get started right away, building confidence and momentum. While you follow this 4-week plan, you can also spend time creating your SMART goals to further personalize your wellness journey. After completing the initial 4 weeks, you can move on to more customized meal and workout plans tailored to your body type and specific goals, ensuring continued progress and success.

Week 1: Establishing Healthy Foundations

Nutrition

- Eat Whole Foods: Focus on fresh, unprocessed foods. Incorporate plenty of fruits, vegetables, lean proteins, whole grains, and healthy fats.
- Stay Hydrated: Drink at least 8 glasses of water daily.
- Balanced Meals: Follow the Comprehensive 4-Week Meal Plan and stick to the 80/20 rule—eat nutritious foods 80% of the time and allow 20% for treats.

Exercise

- Daily Movement: Aim for at least 30 minutes of physical activity each day. This can include walking, yoga, or any activity you enjoy. If starting with 30 minutes feels too challenging, begin with 10 minutes and gradually increase your time.
- Strength Training: Include strength training exercises twice a week to build muscle and boost metabolism. These sessions can be part of your overall physical activity for the week.

Mindfulness

- Mindful Eating: Pay attention to what you eat. Chew slowly and savor each bite.
- Daily Meditation: Practice 5-10 minutes of meditation each morning to reduce stress and increase focus.

Self-Care

- Sleep: Aim for 7-9 hours of quality sleep each night.
- Journaling: Spend a few minutes each day writing about your thoughts and goals.

Week 2: Building Momentum

Continue the practices from Week 1, and layer in the following:

Nutrition

- Meal Prep: Prepare meals in advance to ensure you stick to your healthy eating plan.

- Try New Recipes: Experiment with new healthy recipes from the book to keep meals exciting.

Exercise
- Increase Intensity: Gradually increase the intensity of your workouts. Add an extra 10 minutes to your daily activity.
- Variety: Incorporate different types of exercises into your daily movement to keep your routine interesting and discover what you enjoy, such as cycling, swimming, or pilates.

Mindfulness
- Gratitude Practice: Write down three things you're grateful for each day.
- Mindful Breathing: Practice deep breathing exercises when you feel stressed.

Self-Care
- Digital Detox: Spend one hour each day away from screens.
- Nature Walks: Spend time outdoors to connect with nature.

Week 3: Enhancing Wellness

Continue the practices from Weeks 1 and 2, and layer in the following:

Nutrition
- Reduce Sugar: Cut down on sugary snacks and beverages.
- Healthy Snacks: Keep healthy snacks like nuts, fruits, and yogurt on hand.

Exercise
- Cardio Focus: Include at least three cardio sessions this week, such as running, brisk walking, or aerobics.
- Flexibility: Add stretching or a yoga session to improve flexibility.

Mindfulness
- Positive Affirmations: Start your day with positive affirmations.
- Mindful Moments: Take short breaks throughout the day to pause and reflect.

Self-Care
- Pamper Yourself: Treat yourself to a relaxing bath or a massage.
- Connect: Spend quality time with loved ones.

Week 4: Reflecting and Sustaining

Continue the practices from Weeks 1, 2, and 3, and layer in the following:

Nutrition
- Evaluate Progress: Reflect on your eating habits and make adjustments as needed. Use this time to consider what has worked well for you and where you can make improvements.

- Sustainability: You can move on to customized meal plans tailored to your body type and goals. Additionally, you may consider adding the 21-day smoothie challenge to focus on specific wellness objectives. Plan how you will continue your healthy eating habits beyond the 30 days.

Exercise

- Review Routine: Assess your fitness progress and set new goals to challenge yourself. Consider how you can build on the foundation you've established over the past month.
- Customized Workout Plans: Transition to workout plans tailored to your body type and fitness goals to continue your progress effectively.
- Celebrate Milestones: Reward yourself for sticking to your exercise plan. Recognize your achievements and use them as motivation to keep going.

Mindfulness

- Deepen Practice: Increase your meditation time to 15-20 minutes. Explore different mindfulness techniques to find what works best for you.
- Mindful Living: Integrate mindfulness into daily activities like eating, walking, and working. Make it a habit to be present in each moment.

Self-Care

- Regular Check-ins: Continue journaling and reflecting on your progress. Make it a regular practice to stay connected with your thoughts and feelings.
- Plan Ahead: Schedule regular self-care activities to maintain your well-being. Think about how you can continue to prioritize self-care in your daily routine.

By following this 4-week plan and building on the practices from each week, you can set the foundation for a healthier, more balanced lifestyle and experience a positive transformation. After completing the initial four weeks, consider moving on to more personalized plans to continue your wellness journey. Whether you choose customized meal and workout plans based on your body type and goals, or embark on the 21-day smoothie challenge, there are many paths to explore that will help you maintain and enhance your holistic wellness.

SEASONAL Wellness Tips

TIPS FOR MAINTAINING WELLNESS THROUGHOUT THE SEASONS

Spring:

- Hydration: As temperatures rise, it's important to stay hydrated. Drink plenty of water and include hydrating foods like cucumbers, melons, and leafy greens in your diet.
- Allergy Management: Spring can bring seasonal allergies. Incorporate local honey, herbal teas, and anti-inflammatory foods to help manage symptoms.
- Outdoor Activities: Take advantage of the warmer weather by engaging in outdoor activities like hiking, biking, or gardening.

Summer:

- Sun Protection: Protect your skin from the sun by using natural sunscreens, wearing hats, and seeking shade during peak sunlight hours.
- Light Meals: Opt for light, refreshing meals like salads, smoothies, and chilled soups to stay cool and nourished.
- Stay Active: Enjoy summer activities like swimming, paddleboarding, and outdoor sports to stay active and fit.

Fall:

- Immune Support: Boost your immune system with seasonal foods rich in vitamins and minerals, such as squash, apples, and root vegetables.
- Warm Comfort Foods: As the weather cools, enjoy warm, comforting meals like soups, stews, and roasted vegetables.
- Mindful Transitions: Use the change in seasons as an opportunity to reflect on your goals and make any necessary adjustments to your wellness routine.

Winter:

- Vitamin D: Ensure you're getting enough vitamin D, especially if you have limited sun exposure. Consider supplements or vitamin D-rich foods like fatty fish and fortified products.
- Cozy Self-Care: Embrace cozy self-care practices like reading, hot baths, and enjoying warm beverages to stay relaxed and content.
- Stay Active Indoors: Find ways to stay active indoors, such as yoga, home workouts, or indoor sports, to maintain your fitness during colder months.

HOLISTIC HEALTH Myths and Facts

COMMON MYTHS AND FACTS ABOUT HOLISTIC HEALTH

There are many misconceptions about holistic health that can prevent people from fully embracing its benefits. By debunking these myths, you can gain a clearer understanding of what holistic health truly entails and how it can enhance your overall well-being. Here are some common myths and the facts that dispel them:

Myth: Holistic health practices are not scientifically backed.

Fact: Many holistic health practices, such as mindfulness, yoga, and nutrition-based therapies, are supported by scientific research and have proven health benefits.

Myth: Holistic health is only about diet and exercise.

Fact: Holistic health encompasses physical, mental, emotional, and spiritual well-being, integrating various practices to achieve overall wellness.

Myth: Holistic health is expensive.

Fact: Many holistic health practices, such as meditation, walking in nature, and mindful eating, are low-cost or free. It's about making conscious lifestyle choices that support your well-being.

Myth: You have to follow a strict regimen to benefit from holistic health.

Fact: Holistic health is about balance and flexibility. It's more effective to adopt sustainable practices that fit into your lifestyle rather than following strict regimens.

Myth: Holistic health is only for people with health issues.

Fact: Holistic health is beneficial for everyone, regardless of their current health status. It promotes prevention, well-being, and a higher quality of life.

FURTHER READING AND Interactive Elements

Books:
The Omnivore's Dilemma: A Natural History of Four Meals by Michael Pollan
How Not to Die: Discover the Foods Scientifically Proven to Prevent and Reverse Disease by Michael Greger
You Are a Badass: How to Stop Doubting Your Greatness and Start Living an Awesome Life by Jen Sincero
The Body Keeps the Score: Brain, Mind, and Body in the Healing of Trauma by Bessel van der Kolk

Websites:
EvolutionaryBodySystem.com: www.evolutionarybodysystem.com
NutritionFacts.org: www.nutritionfacts.org
Mindful.org: www.mindful.org
Bodybuilding.com: www.bodybuilding.com

Apps:
MyFitnessPal: www.myfitnesspal.com
Fig: www.foodisgood.com
Headspace: www.headspace.com
Strava: www.strava.com

Video Links:
Guided Meditation: Follow along with a calming guided meditation to reduce stress and enhance mindfulness. https://youtu.be/MIr3RsUWrdo?si=SHrOp3CsEYohIm0K
Cooking Demonstrations: Learn how to prepare some of the delicious recipes from this guide with step-by-step video tutorials. https://tasty.co/

Quizzes:
Nutrition Knowledge Quiz: Test your knowledge about nutrition and learn more about how to make healthy choices. https://www.healthshots.com/quiz/nutrition-quiz/

Guided Meditations:
Mindfulness Meditation: A 10-minute mindfulness meditation to help you stay present and focused. https://youtu.be/ZToicYcHIOU?si=f_eQqCH1M8Wr5629
Sleep Meditation: A relaxing meditation to help you unwind and prepare for a restful night's sleep. https://youtu.be/BI8YfvXBL3E?si=iOWjVOEHxV08IRTs

CONCLUSION

CONCLUSION

As you reach the end of "The Evolutionary Plate: From Taste to Transformation," I hope you feel inspired, empowered, and equipped with the knowledge and tools to embark on your holistic wellness journey. This guide is more than a collection of recipes and fitness plans; it's a comprehensive approach to living a balanced, healthy, and fulfilling life.

This book is a reflection of my own journey and the principles that have transformed my life. The experiences, lessons, and insights shared within these pages come from my personal path to holistic wellness. I have poured my heart and soul into creating a resource that can guide you towards the same sense of balance and well-being that I have found.

Remember, the journey to holistic wellness is personal and unique to each individual. Embrace the changes at your own pace, and don't be afraid to adapt the practices to fit your lifestyle. The key is consistency, patience, and self-compassion.

I encourage you to revisit the various sections of this book as you progress on your journey. The recipes, fitness plans, self-care practices, and additional resources are here to support you every step of the way. Stay connected with your community, seek support when needed, and celebrate your progress, no matter how small it may seem.

Thank you for choosing to make this journey with "The Evolutionary Plate: From Taste to Transformation—4 Weeks to Balanced and Sustainable Nutrition." Your commitment to your health and well-being is commendable, be proud of yourself! I am honored to be a part of your path to transformation. Here's to a healthier, happier, and more balanced you.

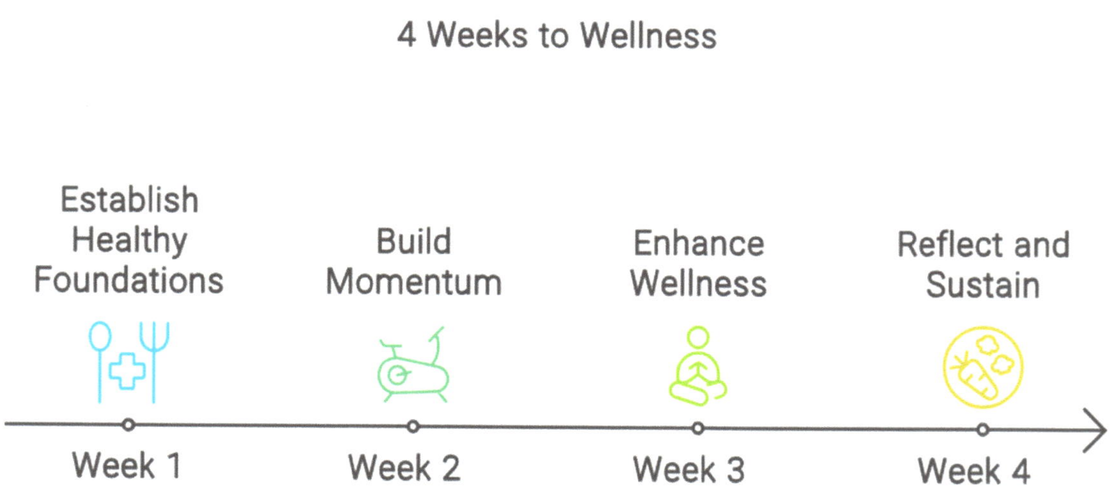
4 Weeks to Wellness
Establish Healthy Foundations
Build Momentum
Enhance Wellness
Reflect and Sustain
Week 1
Week 2
Week 3
Week 4

ENCOURAGEMENT and Final Thoughts

A Journey of Transformation:

Starting a journey of transformation is both brave and rewarding. By integrating the principles of holistic wellness, you can achieve not only physical health but also mental, emotional, and spiritual well-being. Celebrate every small step towards a healthier lifestyle, no matter how incremental it may seem.

Staying consistent is key to lasting change. Even when faced with challenges, remain committed to your wellness goals. There will be tough days, but focusing on the bigger picture will help you stay on track. Trust the process and believe in your ability to achieve your goals.

Your body is an incredible source of wisdom. Listen to its signals and needs. Whether it's taking a rest day, modifying your diet, or finding new ways to relax and rejuvenate, paying attention to your body will guide you towards making the best choices for your health.

Holistic wellness is an ongoing, ever-evolving journey. Embrace the changes and growth that come with it. As you continue to learn and adapt, you'll discover new aspects of yourself and your capabilities. This evolution is a testament to your strength and resilience.

Remember, you are not alone on this journey. Connect with the Evolutionary Body System community and other like-minded individuals who share your commitment to health and wellness. Support, motivate, and inspire each other to stay on track and reach your goals.

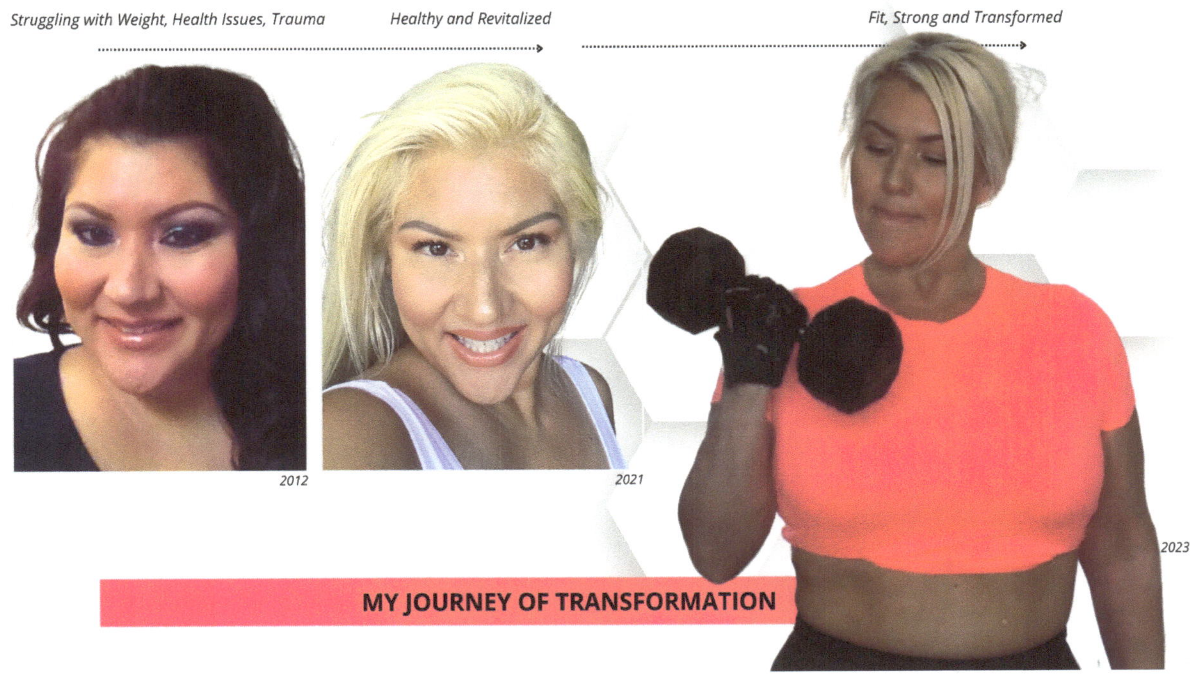

FINAL Words:

Thank you for allowing me to be a part of your wellness journey. It's been an honor to share my experiences, insights, and practices with you. I am confident that with dedication, mindfulness, and the tools provided in this guide, you will transform your health and life. Here's to a future filled with vitality, balance, and joy—one delicious bite at a time.

With heartfelt gratitude,
Yolanda Trevino

INVITATION TO JOIN YOLANDA ON Continued Wellness Journey

Stay Connected:

I invite you to stay connected and continue your wellness journey with Evolutionary Body System. Visit our website, participate in our programs and events, and join our online community. Together, we can achieve our health goals and support each other in living our best lives.

Explore Further Resources:

Explore the additional resources provided in this guide, including books, websites, and apps that can further support your journey. Continuous learning and staying informed are essential for maintaining holistic wellness.

Share Your Story:

Your story is powerful. Share your progress, challenges, and successes with the community. Your experiences can inspire and motivate others who are on a similar path. Together, we can create a supportive and uplifting environment for everyone striving for better health.

Commit to Ongoing Growth:

Commit to ongoing growth and self-improvement. The principles you've learned in this guide are just the beginning. Continue to seek new knowledge, embrace new practices, and evolve in your wellness journey.

EVOLUTIONARY BODY SYSTEM

SECTION 15

SOURCES

The Evolutionary Plate Philosophy

Liska, D., et al. (2019). "Nutrition and integrative medicine: a primer for clinicians." *Integrative Medicine* (4th Ed.). Elsevier.

Pollan, M. (2009). *"Food Rules: An Eater's Manual." Penguin.*

Willett, W.C., et al. (1995). "Mediterranean diet pyramid: a cultural model for healthy eating." *American Journal of Clinical Nutrition*, 61(6), 1402S-1406S.

Estruch, R., et al. (2018). "Primary prevention of cardiovascular disease with a Mediterranean diet supplemented with extra-virgin olive oil or nuts." *New England Journal of Medicine,* 378(25), e34.

Kuhnlein, H.V., & Receveur, O. (1996). "Dietary change and traditional food systems of indigenous peoples." *Annual Review of Nutrition,* 16(1), 417-442.

Pollan, Michael. *The Omnivore's Dilemma: A Natural History of Four Meals.* Penguin Press, 2006.

Meal Planning and Preparation

Lutz, C.A., & Przytulski, K.R. (2010). "Nutrition and diet therapy." *F.A. Davis Company.*

Heller, J., et al. (2020). *"Meal planning and time management for health professionals."* Routledge.

Bittman, M. (2014). *"How to Cook Everything Fast: A Better Way to Cook Great Food."* Houghton Mifflin Harcourt.

Patel, R., & Wardle, J. (2011). "Mindful eating and meal preparation." *International Journal of Behavioral Nutrition and Physical Activity,* 8, 22.

Trichopoulou, A., et al. (2003). "Adherence to a Mediterranean diet and survival in a Greek population." *New England Journal of Medicine,* 348(26), 2599-2608.

USDA National Nutrient Database. (2019). "FoodData Central." USDA.

Personalized Nutrition

Liska, D., et al. (2019). "Nutrition and integrative medicine: a primer for clinicians." *Integrative Medicine* (4th Ed.). Elsevier.

Walden, P., & Jones, M. (2011). *"Body Type and Fitness."* Human Kinetics.

Lee, J.D. (2001). *"The Body Type Diet."* HarperCollins.

Helms, E.R., et al. (2014). "Evidence-based recommendations for natural bodybuilding contest preparation: nutrition and supplementation." *Journal of the International Society of Sports Nutrition*, 11(1), 20.

Pollan, M. (2009). "*Food Rules*: An Eater's Manual." Penguin.

Stoppani, J. (2014). *"Encyclopedia of Muscle & Strength."* Human Kinetics.

Byrd-Bredbenner, C. (2000). *"Perspectives in Nutrition."* McGraw-Hill Education.

Mindful Eating Practices

Kabat-Zinn, J. (1994). "*Wherever You Go, There You Are: Mindfulness Meditation in Everyday Life.*" Hyperion.

Albers, S. (2012). "*Eating Mindfully: How to End Mindless Eating and Enjoy a Balanced Relationship with Food.*" New Harbinger Publications.

Kristeller, J.L., & Wolever, R.Q. (2011). "Mindfulness-based eating awareness training for treating binge eating disorder: the conceptual foundation." *Eating Disorders*, 19(1), 49-61.

Detoxification

Dunn, R.D. (2012). "*The Wild Life of Our Bodies: Predators, Parasites, and Partners That Shape Who We Are Today.*" HarperCollins.

Crook, W.G. (1984). "*The Yeast Connection: A Medical Breakthrough.*" Vintage.

Cabot, S., & Cabot, S. (2010). "*The Liver Cleansing Diet: Love Your Liver and Live Longer.*" SCB International.

Murray, M.T. (1997). "*The Complete Book of Juicing: Your Delicious Guide to Youthful Vitality.*" Three Rivers Press.

Rogers, S.A. (2002). "*Detoxify or Die.*" Prestige Publishing.

Everlywell: https://www.everlywell.com/

Genova Diagnostics: https://www.gdx.net/

Dr. Clark Store: https://www.drclarkstore.com/

Herbs and Supplements

Gladstar, R. (2012). "*Medicinal Herbs: A Beginner's Guide.*" Storey Publishing.

Murray, M.T., & Pizzorno, J. (2006). "*The Encyclopedia of Healing Foods.*" Atria Books.

Manson, J.E., et al. (2020). "The role of dietary supplements and botanicals in maintaining health and preventing disease." *JAMA*, 324(15), 1500-1509.

Starwest Botanicals: https://www.starwest-botanicals.com/

Supreme Nutrition Products: https://www.supremenutritionproducts.com/

Holistic Wellness Practices

Chopra, D. (2015). "*The Healing Self: A Revolutionary New Plan to Supercharge Your Immunity and Stay Well for Life.*" Harmony.

Micozzi, M.S. (2010). "*Fundamentals of Complementary and Alternative Medicine.*" Elsevier.

Workout Plans

Kravitz, L., & Green, D.J. (2002). "*Essentials of Strength Training and Conditioning.*" Human Kinetics.

Bompa, T.O., & Buzzichelli, C. (2015). "*Periodization Training for Sports.*" Human Kinetics.

Delavier, F. (2010). "*Strength Training Anatomy.*" Human Kinetics.

Feuerstein, G. (2008). "*The Yoga Tradition: Its History, Literature, Philosophy and Practice.*" Hohm Press.

Baechle, T.R., & Earle, R.W. (2008). "*Essentials of Strength Training and Conditioning.*" Human Kinetics.

Tracking and Progress

Locke, E.A., & Latham, G.P. (2002). "Building a practically useful theory of goal setting and task motivation." *American Psychologist*, 57(9), 705.

Self-Care Practices

Nhat Hanh, T. (2011). "*The Art of Power.*" HarperOne.

Seasonal Wellness Tips

Foster, S., & Duke, J.A. (2000). "*A Field Guide to Medicinal Plants and Herbs: Of Eastern and Central North America.*" Houghton Mifflin Harcourt.

Holistic Health Myths and Facts

Edzard, E. (2019). "*Alternative Medicine: A Critical Assessment of 150 Modalities.*" Springer.

SECTION 16

ABOUT THE author

About the Author

Yolanda Trevino, PLC, HHP, HWC

Founder of Evolutionary Body System | Author | Entrepreneur

Yolanda Trevino is a dedicated wellness expert, certified as a Professional Life Coach, Holistic Health Practitioner, and Holistic Wellness Coach. With a profound commitment to holistic health and a passion for helping others, Yolanda has dedicated her life to empowering individuals to achieve their wellness goals and transform their lives.

Yolanda's journey to holistic wellness began with personal health struggles. After years of facing various health challenges, she made a pivotal decision to reclaim her life through holistic practices. By integrating nutrition, mindfulness, and physical activity, she not only healed her body but also transformed her entire being, shedding 77 pounds as a result of her overall wellness journey.

Driven by her transformative experience, Yolanda founded the Evolutionary Body System, a hub for holistic wellness and transformative programs. Through this platform, she created the Holistic Growth Reset, a comprehensive 6-week program designed to help individuals overcome personal challenges, rebuild from trauma, and embrace a journey toward comprehensive well-being. This program offers a dynamic approach to personal transformation, blending established wellness techniques with innovative holistic practices.

In addition to her work with the Evolutionary Body System, Yolanda is a multi-published author and entrepreneur. Her ventures, such as Microhair Aesthetics, focus on hair and skin wellness, further demonstrating her commitment to holistic health. Yolanda's expertise has been featured in national and local magazines, showcasing her as a leading voice in the wellness industry.

Yolanda's mission is to empower others to take control of their health and well-being. Through her books, products and programs, she provides invaluable guidance and support to those seeking to transform their lives. Whether you're looking to heal, improve your health, or simply live a more balanced and fulfilling life, Yolanda's expertise and compassionate guidance can help you achieve your aspirations. Her holistic approach emphasizes the importance of integrating body, mind, and spirit, helping individuals achieve lasting wellness and fulfillment.

Stay connected with Yolanda and the Evolutionary Body System community through our website and social media channels. Share your progress, seek support, and join a network of like-minded individuals committed to holistic health.

Website: Evolutionary Body System
Facebook: Evolutionary Body System on Facebook
Instagram: @EvolutionaryBodySystem

www.ingramcontent.com/pod-product-compliance
Lightning Source LLC
LaVergne TN
LVHW071243210926
848486LV00007B/330

9781737159568